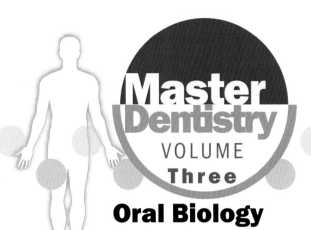

Master Dentistry

VOLUME

Three

Oral Biology

Commissioning Editor: Alison Taylor
Development Editor: Clive Hewat
Project Manager: Frances Affleck
Designer/Design Direction: Stewart Larking
Illustration Manager: Bruce Hogarth
Illustrator: Robert Britton

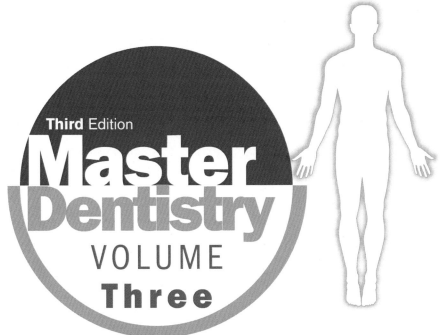

Third Edition

Master Dentistry

VOLUME Three

Oral Biology

B. K. B. Berkovitz
BDS MSc PhD FDS (Eng)
Emeritus Reader,
Anatomy and Human Sciences,
Biomedical and Health Sciences,
King's College, London, UK

B. J. Moxham
BSc BDS PhD
Professor of Anatomy,
Cardiff School of Biosciences,
Cardiff University, Cardiff, UK

R. W. A. Linden
BDS PhD MFDS RCS
Professor of Craniofacial Biology,
King's College, London, UK

A. J. Sloan
BSc PhD
Reader in Bone Biology &
Tissue Engineering,
School of Dentistry,
Cardiff University,
Cardiff, UK

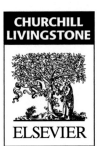

CHURCHILL LIVINGSTONE

ELSEVIER

Edinburgh   London   New York   Oxford   Philadelphia   St Louis   Sydney   Toronto   2011

CHURCHILL
LIVINGSTONE
ELSEVIER

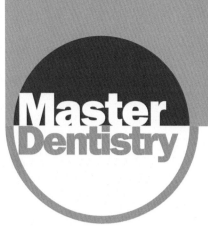

ISBN 978-0-702-03122-9

British Library Cataloguing in Publication Data
A catalogue record for this book is available from the British Library

Library of Congress Cataloging in Publication Data
A catalog record for this book is available from the Library of Congress

Notices
Knowledge and best practice in this field are constantly changing. As new research and experience broaden our understanding, changes in research methods, professional practices, or medical treatment may become necessary.

Practitioners and researchers must always rely on their own experience and knowledge in evaluating and using any information, methods, compounds, or experiments described herein. In using such information or methods they should be mindful of their own safety and the safety of others, including parties for whom they have a professional responsibility.

With respect to any drug or pharmaceutical products identified, readers are advised to check the most current information provided (i) on procedures featured or (ii) by the manufacturer of each product to be administered, to verify the recommended dose or formula, the method and duration of administration, and contraindications. It is the responsibility of practitioners, relying on their own experience and knowledge of their patients, to make diagnoses, to determine dosages and the best treatment for each individual patient, and to take all appropriate safety precautions.

To the fullest extent of the law, neither the Publisher nor the authors, contributors, or editors, assume any liability for any injury and/or damage to persons or property as a matter of products liability, negligence or otherwise, or from any use or operation of any methods, products, instructions, or ideas contained in the material herein.

ELSEVIER your source for books, journals and multimedia in the health sciences
www.elsevierhealth.com

Working together to grow libraries in developing countries

www.elsevier.com | www.bookaid.org | www.sabre.org

ELSEVIER   BOOK AID International   Sabre Foundation

The Publisher's policy is to use **paper manufactured from sustainable forests**

Transferred to Digital Printing in 2013

Printed in China

Contents

Preface vii

1. **Anatomy of the oral cavity and the jaws** 1

2. **Temporomandibular (craniomandibular) joint** 10

3. **Human dentition: tooth morphology and occlusion** 18

4. **Orofacial musculature, mastication and swallowing** 36

5. **Tongue, flavour, thermoreception and speech** 51

6. **Vasculature, lymphatics and innervation of the orodental tissues** 67

7. **Salivary glands, saliva and salivation** 79

8. **Investing organic layers on enamel surfaces** 94

9. **Development of the craniofacial complex** 101

10. **Early tooth development, root development (including cementogenesis) and tooth eruption** . . . 113

11. **Mechanisms of mineralization** 135

12. **Dental tissues. I.** Enamel: structure, composition and development 142

13. **Dental tissues. II.** Dentine/pulp complex: structure, composition, development and oral pain 161

14. **Dental tissues. III.** Cementum: structure and composition 194

15. **Periodontal ligament (including oral and periodontal mechanoreception and the tooth support mechanism)** 203

16. **Alveolar bone: structure and composition** 221

17. **Oral mucosa and gingival crevicular fluid: structure and composition** 235

18. **Revision summary charts** 250

Further reading 289

Index 291

Preface

Long gone are the days when all that was necessary to receive a university education in dentistry was to enrol, attend the lectures and practicals, read the recommended textbooks, occasionally use library resources and present oneself for examinations – the ending of such practices has come not a day too soon, say most students and academic staff! Nowadays, students expect feedback concerning their academic progress and performance, and there is as much emphasis on learning as on teaching. Furthermore, the courses must be integrated and clinically relevant. The learning objectives must be clearly stated and promulgated, core material must be properly identified, and students must be made explicitly aware of the examination process and the way in which their studies strategically relate to assessment.

This book aims to address many of these issues with respect to the teaching and learning of oral biology. Accordingly, most of the chapters integrate anatomical, biochemical and physiological core, clinically important material. In addition, to guide students in their studies, each chapter has a brief overview of the topic and lists the essential learning objectives. This is followed by a concise exposition of core material and by an extensive section providing self-assessment questions (consisting of true/false questions, extended matching questions, picture questions and essay questions). Answers are provided and give detailed feedback information; outline/model answers are included for the essay questions. The book ends with a series of summary sheets – a unique feature. These sheets provide, in 'mind-map' format, the crucial information in a pictorial form that should aid the learning of the topics by the reader. Overall, it is the authors' intention that our approach will prove beneficial to today's dental students who are at the early stages of their professional development. However, we do not intend for the present text to be a substitute for more extensive textbooks in oral biology. Indeed, it remains our conviction that a good dentist is one who, throughout his/her training and professional life, not only understands the requirement to take strategic approaches but also values a deeper approach that aids competency and leads to mastery. Accordingly, this book should be regarded as providing the first, important stage in learning oral biology that will stimulate students to seek a more in-depth appreciation of the subject and its contribution to the scientific foundation of dentistry.

BKB Berkovitz and RWA Linden (London)
BJ Moxham and AJ Sloan (Cardiff)

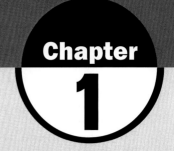

Anatomy of the oral cavity and the jaws

Chapter 1

Lips   1
Cheeks   1
Oral vestibule   1
Palate   1
Floor of the mouth   2
Maxillary bones   2
Maxillary sinus   2
Bones contributing to the hard palate   2
Mandible   2
    Self-assessment: questions   4
    Self-assessment: answers   7

Overview

The mouth (oral cavity) is concerned with the ingestion (and selection) of food, with its subsequent mastication and swallowing, and with speech and breathing. It extends from the lips and cheeks externally to the pillars of the fauces at the oropharyngeal isthmus internally. The palate forms the roof of the mouth and the tongue occupies the floor of the mouth. The lateral walls of the oral cavity are defined by the cheeks and retromolar regions. The jaws are the tooth-bearing bones, comprising two maxillary bones forming the upper jaw and a single bone, the mandible, forming the lower jaw.

Learning objectives

Using correct and appropriate anatomical and dental terminologies, you must:
* be able to describe, accurately and in detail, all the visible features present in the mouth
* be able to describe the anatomical features of the bones (mandible and maxilla) that comprise the jaws.

Lips

The lips (labia) are covered externally by skin and internally by mucous membrane. The red portion of the lip (the vermilion) is a human characteristic. Laterally, the upper lip is separated from the cheeks by nasolabial grooves. The labiomarginal sulci delineate the lower lip from the cheeks. A labiomental groove separates the lower lip from the chin. In the midline of the upper lip runs the philtrum.

The corners of the lips are termed the labial commissures. Lips that are lightly closed at rest are described as being 'competent'; 'incompetent' lips describe a situation where, with the facial muscles relaxed, a lip seal is not produced. The position of the lips is important in controlling protrusion of the incisors. With 'competent' lips, the tips of the maxillary incisors lie below the upper border of the lower lip and thus maintain the 'normal' inclination of the incisors. With 'incompetent' lips, the maxillary incisors may not be so controlled and the lower lip may even lie behind them, thus producing an exaggerated proclination.

Cheeks

The cheeks (buccae) extend intra-orally from the labial commissures to the ridge of mucosa overlying the ascending ramus of the mandible. Its mucosa is non-keratinized and is tightly adherent to the buccinator muscle. The parotid duct drains into the cheek opposite the maxillary second molar. A hyperkeratinized line called the linea alba may be seen at a position related to the occlusal plane. In the retromolar region, in front of the pillars of the fauces, a fold of mucosa containing the pterygomandibular raphe extends from the upper to the lower alveolus.

Oral vestibule

The oral vestibule is the space between the lips and cheeks and the teeth and alveolus. The mucosa covering the alveolus is reflected onto the lips and cheeks to form a trough or sulcus called the vestibular fornix. Here, the mucosa may show sickle-shaped folds called frena that contain loose connective tissue. The gums (gingivae) are described on pages 238–239.

Palate

The palate forms the roof of the mouth and separates the oral and nasal cavities. The immovable hard palate lies anteriorly and the movable soft palate posteriorly. The skeleton of the hard palate is bony while that of the soft palate is fibrous. The hard palate is covered by a keratinized mucosa, which is firmly bound to underlying bone. The incisive papilla immediately behind the maxillary central incisors covers the nasopalatine nerves as they emerge from the incisive fossa. In the midline, and extending posteriorly from the incisive papilla, is the palatine raphe. Here, the oral mucosa is attached directly to bone without a submucous layer. Palatine rugae are elevated ridges that radiate from the incisive papilla and the anterior part of the palatine raphe. At the junction of the palate and the alveolus lies a submucosa in which run the greater palatine nerves and vessels. The shape and size of the dome of the palate vary considerably. The boundary between the soft palate and the hard palate may be distinguished by a change in colour, the soft palate being a darker red with a yellowish tint. Extending laterally from the free border of the soft palate are the palatoglossal and palatopharyngeal folds (the palatoglossal fold being anterior). These folds cover the palatoglossus and palatopharyngeus muscles and between them lies the palatine tonsil. This tonsil is a collection of lymphoid material. At the free edge of the soft palate, in the midline, is the palatal uvula. The oropharyngeal isthmus is where the oral cavity and the oropharynx meet (at the pillars of the fauces).

Floor of the mouth

The floor of the mouth proper is a horseshoe-shaped region above the mylohyoid muscles and beneath the movable part of the tongue. It is covered by a lining of non-keratinized mucosa. In the midline, near the base of the tongue, the lingual frenum extends on to the inferior surface of the tongue. The sublingual papilla, onto which the submandibular salivary ducts open, is centrally positioned at the base of the tongue. On either side of this papilla are the sublingual folds, beneath which lie the submandibular ducts and sublingual salivary glands. The floor of the mouth is occupied by the tongue and this is described on pages 51–53.

Maxillary bones

The maxillary bone consists of a body, frontal, zygomatic, alveolar and palatine processes, and an orbital plate. The body of the maxilla forms the skeleton of the anterior part of the cheek. The posterior convexity of the body is the maxillary tuberosity and it has several small foramina for the passage of the posterior superior alveolar nerves. In the midline, the alveolar processes of the two maxillae meet at the intermaxillary suture, whence they diverge to form the opening into the nasal fossae. At the lower border of this nasal aperture, in the midline, lies the anterior nasal spine. The frontal process extends above the nasal aperture towards the bridge of the nose. The orbital plate forms the floor of the orbit and below the orbital rim lies the infra-orbital foramen (through which the infra-orbital branch of the maxillary nerve emerges). The zygomatic process extends upwards to articulate with the zygoma. From the entire lower surface of the body arises the alveolar process supporting the maxillary teeth. The structure of the alveolus is described on pages 221–225. The medial aspect of the

maxilla forms the lateral wall of the nose. The maxillary palatine process extends horizontally from the medial surface of the maxilla where the body meets the alveolar process.

Maxillary sinus

The maxillary sinus (antrum) is situated in the body of the maxilla. It is pyramidal in shape. The base (medial wall) forms part of the lateral wall of the nose. The apex extends into the zygomatic process of the maxilla. The roof of the sinus is part of the floor of the orbit, and the floor of the sinus is formed by the alveolar process and part of the palatine process of the maxilla. The anterior wall of the sinus is the facial surface of the maxilla and the posterior wall is the infratemporal surface of the maxilla. Running in the roof of the sinus are the infra-orbital nerve and vessels. The anterior superior alveolar nerve and vessels run in the anterior wall of the sinus. The posterior superior alveolar nerve and vessels pass through canals in the posterior surface of the sinus. The medial wall of the maxillary sinus contains the opening (ostium) of the sinus that leads into the middle meatus of the nose. As this opening lies well above the floor of the sinus, its position is unfavourable for drainage. The roots of the cheek teeth are related to the floor of the maxillary sinus. The maxillary air sinus is lined by respiratory epithelium (a ciliated columnar epithelium), with numerous goblet cells. The sinus is innervated by the infra-orbital nerve and the superior alveolar branches of the maxillary nerve.

Bones contributing to the hard palate

The four major bones contributing to the hard palate are the palatine processes of the maxillae and the horizontal plates of the palatine bones. The junction between the palatine processes is the median palatine suture. Anteriorly, behind the central incisors, is the incisive fossa through which pass the nasopalatine nerves. The posterior edges of the palatine processes articulate with the horizontal plates of the two palatine bones to form the transverse palatine suture. Laterally, this junction is incomplete, forming the greater palatine foramina, through which pass the greater palatine nerves and vessels. Behind the greater palatine foramina lie the lesser palatine foramina, through which pass the lesser palatine nerves and vessels. The junction of the two palatine bones in the midline completes the median palatine suture. At the posterior border of the horizontal palatine plates is the posterior nasal spine.

Mandible

The mandible consists of a horizontal body and two vertical rami. The body of the mandible carries the mandibular teeth and their associated alveolar processes. The mental protuberance constitutes the chin. Above the mental protuberance lies a shallow depression termed the incisive fossa. Midway in the height of the body of the mandible, related to the premolar teeth, is the mental foramen, through which pass the mental branches of the inferior alveolar nerve. The inferior margin of the body meets the posterior margin of the ramus at the angle of the mandible. This is the site of insertion of the masseter muscle and stylomandibular ligament. The alveolus forms the superior margin of the mandibular body. The junction of the alveolus and ramus is demarcated by an external oblique ridge, which runs across the body of the mandible towards the mental foramen. The coronoid and condylar processes are at the superior border of the ramus. The coronoid process provides attachment for the temporalis muscle. The condylar process has a neck supporting an articular surface, which fits into the mandibular fossa of the temporal bone to form the temporomandibular joint. Close to the midline, on the inferior surface of the mandibular body, lie the digastric fossae, into which are inserted the anterior bellies of the digastric muscles. Above the fossae are the genial spines that serve as attachments for the geniohyoid muscles and the genioglossus muscles. Passing upwards and backwards across the medial surface of the body of the mandible is the internal oblique ridge. From this ridge, the mylohyoid muscle takes origin. Around the angle of the mandible, the bone is roughened for the attachment of the medial pterygoid muscle. In the centre of the medial surface of the ramus lies the mandibular foramen, through which the inferior alveolar nerve and artery pass into the mandibular canal. A bony process, the lingula, extends from the anterosuperior surface of the foramen. The mylohyoid groove may be seen running down from the postero-inferior surface of the foramen. The mandibular canal begins at the mandibular foramen and extends to the region of the premolar teeth, where it bifurcates into the mental and incisive canals.

One

Self-assessment: questions

True/false statements

Which of the following statements are true and which are false?

a. The oral cavity is demarcated from the oropharynx by the palatoglossal folds.
b. When the teeth are in occlusion, the vestibule of the mouth communicates with the oral cavity proper in the retromolar region.
c. The linea alba in the cheek is a hyperkeratinized line representing the site of the occlusal plane.
d. The parotid gland usually drains opposite the maxillary second molar tooth.
e. The soft palate during swallowing is depressed to meet Passavant's ridge on the posterior wall of the pharynx.
f. 'Incompetent' lips describes a situation where, at rest, the lips are closed without muscle strain and there is an 'anterior oral seal'.
g. Waldeyer's ring consists solely of the lymphatic tissue of the palatine tonsils and the lingual tonsils.
h. The jaws are part of the viscerocranium that houses and protects the cranial parts of the respiratory and digestive tracts.
i. The infra-orbital foramen in the maxilla transmits the infra-orbital branch of the ophthalmic division of the trigeminal nerve.
j. The genial (mental) tubercles (spines) provide attachments for the digastric muscles.
k. The muscle forming the floor of the mouth is the geniohyoid.
l. A submucosa exists beneath the palatine raphe.
m. The mental foramen lies beneath the mesial root of the first permanent molar tooth.
n. The opening of the maxillary sinus lies low down near its floor.
o. The lingula of the mandible gives attachment to the pterygomandibular raphe.

Extended matching questions

Theme: Floor of mouth

Lead-in

Select the most appropriate option to answer items 1–5. Each option can be used once, more than once or not at all.

Item list

1. Location of the opening of the submandibular salivary duct
2. Location of the sublingual salivary glands
3. Name of muscle underlying the mucosa and forming a diaphragm for the floor of the mouth
4. Name given to bony exostoses that extend from the mandibular alveolus into the floor of the mouth
5. The location of the attachment of the frenum from the ventral surface of the tongue

Option list

A. Buccinator
B. Deep lingual folds
C. Digastric
D. Epulides
E. Fimbriated folds
F. Genial tubercles
G. Geniohyoid
H. Incisive papilla
I. Lingual frenum
J. Mylohyoid
K. Stylohyoid
L. Sublingual folds
M. Sublingual papilla
N. Tori mandibulares

Picture questions

Figure 1.1

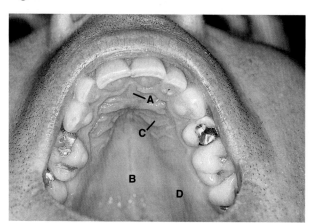

This is a picture of the hard palate in the roof of the mouth.

a. Identify the features labelled A–D.
b. What type of mucosa covers this region?
c. Where precisely would you locate the major nerves supplying the hard palate?
d. Why is it difficult for infections (pus) arising from a maxillary tooth to spread along the hard palate?

Self-assessment: questions

Figure 1.2

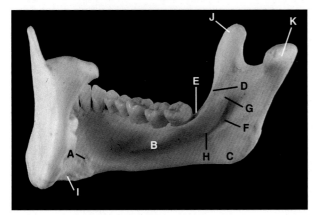

This is a picture of the inner (medial) surface of the mandible.
a. Identify the features labelled A–K.
b. What is attached to G and what is its embryological origin?
c. Which muscles gain attachment to A, B, C, D and I?
d. What structure running close to E is endangered when the mandibular third molar tooth is surgically removed?

Figure 1.3 (Courtesy of Professor C. Franklyn)

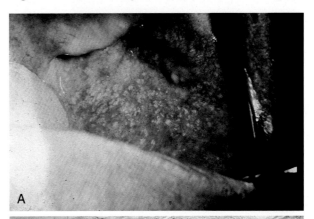

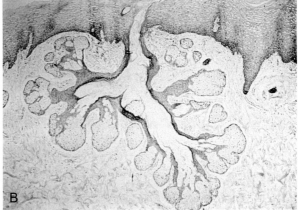

An 18-year-old woman, on cleaning her teeth, noticed for the first time that there were numerous small, light yellow spots in the mucosa of the cheeks (Figure 1.3A). Close inspection by her dentist revealed occasional ducts from which a greasy substance was exuding. A biopsy was taken and the histology of the region is shown in Figure 1.3B.
a. What are these structures?
b. Why are they present in the cheek region?
c. Why did they appear at this age?

Self-assessment: questions

Figure 1.4

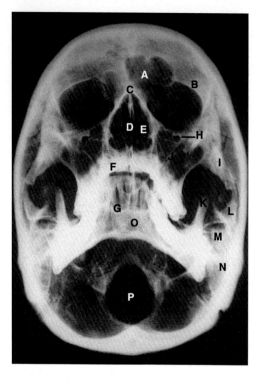

This is a skull radiograph.

a. What is the projection used for radiographing this skull?
b. Identify the structures labelled A–P.
c. What is the clinical significance of taking this type of radiograph?
d. What features indicate that this is a radiograph of an anatomical specimen and not of a living patient?

Figure 1.5

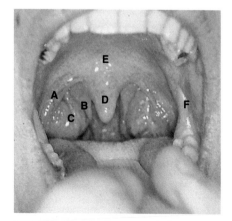

a. Identify the structures A–E.
b. What is the name of the underlying structure that produces the ridge-like elevation F and what is its clinical significance?
c. Describe the sensory and motor innervation of the soft palate.

Figure 1.6

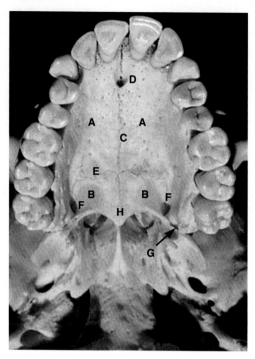

a. Identify the structures A–H.
b. What is the origin of the structures entering and leaving the foramina labelled D, F and G?

Essay questions

1. Compare and contrast the hard and soft palates.
2. Describe the muscle attachments for the mandible and indicate how knowledge of these attachments may aid our understanding of the displacement of bony fragments following fractures of the body of the mandible.

Self-assessment: answers

True/false answers

a. **True**. The palatoglossal folds and the palatopharyngeal folds are respectively the anterior and posterior pillars of the fauces at the oropharyngeal isthmus.

b. **True**. Clinically, this communication permits the passage of liquid foods when the teeth are 'wired' together as treatment following fractures of the jaws.

c. **True**. Hyperkeratinization is a common reaction of the oral mucosa to trauma.

d. **True**. The opening of the parotid duct may present as a papilla or as a simple opening into the cheek.

e. **False**. The soft palate is raised during swallowing by the combined actions of the levator and tensor veli palatini muscles.

f. **False**. Competent lips produce an anterior oral seal and ensure the correct inclination of the incisors since the competent lower lip pushes against both the lower and the upper incisors.

g. **False**. Waldeyer's tonsillar ring 'guarding' the openings of the pharynx also includes the tubal and pharyngeal tonsils in the nasopharynx.

h. **True**. The neurocranium houses and protects the brain and the organs of special sense.

i. **False**. The infra-orbital foramen does transmit the infra-orbital nerve (and associated blood vessels) but this nerve is a branch of the maxillary division of the trigeminal.

j. **False**. The superior genial tubercles give rise to the genioglossus muscles and the inferior tubercles give rise to the geniohyoid muscles. The anterior bellies of the digastric muscles are attached to the digastric fossae below the genial tubercles and at the inferior border of the mandible.

k. **False**. The mylohyoid muscles (attached together at the midline by a raphe) form the diaphragm for the floor of the mouth.

l. **False**. The palatine raphe in the centre of the hard palate is firmly bound to the underlying bone (forming a mucoperiosteum).

m. **False**. It is said that the mental foramen usually lies beneath the roots of a premolar tooth.

n. **False**. The opening of the maxillary air sinus (ostium) lies high up towards the roof of the sinus (an unfavourable location for drainage of the mucus into the lateral wall of the nose, hiatus semilunaris of the middle meatus).

o. **False**. The lingula gives a site for attachment of the sphenomandibular ligament. Both the lingula and the sphenomandibular ligament are remains of the fetal Meckel's cartilage (1st pharyngeal arch cartilage). The pterygomandibular raphe extends from the pterygoid hamulus to the retromolar fossa behind the mandibular third molar tooth.

Extended matching answers

Item 1 = Option M. The sublingual papilla is the site of opening of the submandibular ducts (it is also the site of opening of one of the major ducts of the sublingual gland (Bartholin's duct), although most of the ducts of the sublingual gland do not form a main duct but drain directly into the floor of the mouth at the location of the sublingual fold).

Item 2 = Option L. The sublingual glands lie below the sublingual folds (see also Item 1 above).

Item 3 = Option J. The two mylohyoid muscles together form the diaphragm for the mouth and delineate the floor of the mouth from the suprahyoid region of the neck (although both regions communicate at the posterior edges of the diaphragm).

Item 4 = Option N. Tori mandibulares are bony exostoses extending from the mandibular alveolus into the region of the floor of the mouth. They are not pathological. Torus palatinus is a bony exostosis in the hard palate.

Item 5 = Option M. As well as being the sites of opening of the submandibular duct and of Bartholin's duct (see Item 1 above), the sublingual papilla is the normal site of termination of the sublingual frenum from the ventral surface of the tongue.

Picture answers

Figure 1.1

a. A = incisive papilla. B = palatine raphe. C = palatine rugae. D = soft tissue masses where greater palatine nerves and vessels run.

b. The mucosa over the hard palate has a keratinized (masticatory) stratified squamous epithelium. For most parts, there is no submucosa and the tissue presents as a mucoperiosteum.

c. The nasopalatine nerves exit at the incisive fossa and are thus located below the incisive papilla and behind the maxillary central incisor teeth. The greater palatine nerves run in a submucosa, each along a lateral channel between the maxillary alveolar and the maxillary palatine processes.

d. The mucoperiosteum is an effective barrier to the spread of infection from the maxillary teeth into the hard palate. Therefore, palatal abscesses tend to be discrete and well defined.

Figure 1.2

a. A = genial (mental) spines (tubercles). B = internal oblique (mylohyoid) ridge. C = angle of mandible. D = temporal crest. E = retromolar triangle. F = mandibular foramen. G = lingula. H = mylohyoid groove. I = digastric fossa. J = coronoid process. K = condylar process.

Self-assessment: answers

b. At G, the lingula, is attached the sphenomandibular ligament (an accessory ligament of the temporomandibular joint). This ligament is the remains of the perichondrium of Meckel's cartilage (the cartilage of the 1st pharyngeal arch).

c. At A, the genial spines, are attached the genioglossus muscles (superior spines) and geniohyoid muscles (inferior spines). At B, the mylohyoid ridge, is attached the mylohyoid muscle which contributes to the diaphragm for the floor of the mouth. At C, the inner aspect of the angle of the mandible, is attached the medial pterygoid muscle. At D, the temporal crest, is attached (in part) the temporalis muscle. At I, the digastric fossa, is attached the anterior belly of the digastric muscle.

d. The lingual branch of the mandibular nerve runs on the lingual alveolar plate of the permanent mandibular third molar tooth and must therefore be protected during surgical extraction of this tooth. If the nerve is damaged, there will be: (i) loss of general sensation to the tongue (ventral and dorsal surfaces), floor of mouth and lingual gingivae; (ii) loss of special sensation (taste) to the anterior two-thirds of the tongue; and (iii) loss of secretomotor supply to the submandibular and sublingual salivary glands. The losses associated with (ii) and (iii) result from damage to the fibres from the chorda tympani branch of the facial nerve (nervus intermedius) which passes with the lingual nerve.

Figure 1.3

a. The patches are termed 'Fordyce spots' and are ectopic sebaceous glands (structures normally restricted to the skin).

b. Developmentally, the mouth is a region where both ectoderm and endoderm make contributions.

c. Hormonal changes at puberty stimulate the formation and secretion of sebaceous glands.

Figure 1.4

a. Occipitomental radiograph of the skull.

b. A = frontal air sinus. B = margin of orbit. C = nasal bones. D = nasal septum. E = nasal fossa with superimposed shadows of ethmoidal air cells. F = maxilla and teeth. G = body of mandible and teeth. H = infra-orbital foramen and canal. I = zygoma. J = maxillary air sinus. K = coronoid process of mandible. L = zygomatic process of temporal bone. M = condyle of mandible. N = mastoid air cells. O = occipital condyle. P = foramen magnum.

c. This radiograph is useful for obtaining clear views of the paranasal air sinuses; postero-anterior (PA) views of the skull show too much superimposition of structures over the sinuses.

d. We know the radiograph is of an anatomical specimen because of the absence of the vertebral column.

Figure 1.5

a. A = palatoglossal arch (anterior pillar of fauces). B = palatopharyngeal arch (posterior pillar of fauces). C = palatine tonsil. D = uvula. E = soft palate.

b. F is the ridge produced by the pterygomandibular raphe, which passes from the pterygoid hamulus to the posterior end of the mylohyoid line. Its clinical significance is as a landmark for an inferior alveolar nerve block (see page 69).

c. Four of the muscles of the palate (palatoglossus, palatopharyngeus, musculus uvulae and levator veli palatini) derive their nerve supply from the pharyngeal plexus, while the remaining muscle (tensor veli palatini) is supplied by a branch of the mandibular nerve. The sensory supply to the soft palate is via the greater and lesser palatine nerves. Additional sensory branches arise from the glossopharyngeal nerve. Minor salivary glands in the soft palate derive their secretomotor supply from the greater petrosal nerve via the pterygopalatine ganglion.

Figure 1.6

a. A = palatine process of maxilla. B = horizontal plate of palatine bone. C = median palatine suture. D = incisive fossa. E = transverse palatine suture. F = greater palatine foramen. G = lesser palatine foramen. H = posterior nasal spine.

b. At D, the incisive fossa, emerge the nasopalatine nerves via the pterygopalatine ganglion; these are branches of the maxillary nerve. At F, the greater palatine foramen, emerge the greater palatine nerve, also from the maxillary nerve via the pterygopalatine ganglion, and the greater palatine artery, a branch from the third part of the maxillary artery. At G, the lesser palatine foramen, emerge the lesser palatine nerves, again from the maxillary nerve via the pterygopalatine ganglion, accompanied by the lesser palatine artery, a branch from the third part of the maxillary artery.

Outline essay answers
Question 1

Writing essays requires a logical ordering of information and, wherever possible, some evidence of analysis and critical thinking. Consequently, there should be an introductory paragraph that provides the very basic information, an outline of how the essay is to be structured and, where appropriate, indication of any recent evidence/discoveries, controversies or other aspects that require analysis and

Self-assessment: answers

Table 1.1 Features of the hard and soft palates

Feature	Hard palate	Soft palate
Location	Anterior two-thirds of palate	Posterior third of palate
Appearance	Red	Red with yellowish tint
Skeleton	Bony	Fibrous (palatine aponeurosis)
Functions	Immovable; bounds oral and nasal cavities	Movable; protects nasopharynx during swallowing
Features	Incisive papilla; palatine raphe; rugae	Uvula; pillars of fauces
Musculature	None	Musculus uvulae; tensor and levator veli palatini; palatoglossus; palatopharyngeus
Innervation and vasculature	Nasopalatine; greater palatine	Lesser palatine

Table 1.2 Muscle classification according to attachment to body or rami

Muscles attached to body of mandible	Muscles attached to ramus
Platysma and other muscles of facial expression	Masseter
Digastric	Temporalis
Geniohyoid and genioglossus muscles	Medial and lateral pterygoids
Mylohyoid	
Buccinator	

synthesis of information and concepts. Where the question asks for comparisons, it is important that you do not just describe one element and then another without juxtaposing information. Thus, for the palate, information relating to the hard palate must be immediately juxtaposed with information relating to the soft palate.

The introductory paragraph to this question should be brief and general; it should emphasize that the palate is the roof of mouth (subdividing oral cavity and nasal cavity) and that there are important functional as well as structural differences. Subsequent paragraphs should directly compare and contrast the hard and soft palates with respect to the following 'features':

- Location
- Appearance in vivo
- Skeleton and musculature
- Innervation and vasculature
- Functional aspects: swallowing and speech
- Material beyond core (e.g. clinical considerations, such as torus palatinus, clefts).

For a summary, see Table 1.1.

Note that for scientific essays it is acceptable (indeed, desirable) to provide diagrams and also to provide headings.

A concluding paragraph should be provided that summarizes the essential/important differences.

Question 2

The introduction to this essay should be general and brief, highlighting essential information about the mandible, the temporomandibular joint and the process of mastication (a characteristic of mammals). The essay should be structured so that the muscles are classified according to the general subdivision of mandible into a body and the rami (see Table 1.2).

For all the muscles listed in the table, the attachments should be clearly described and the use of diagrams is encouraged.

After describing the muscles and their attachments, the clinical significance of these in relation to understanding the effects of fractures of the mandible should be discussed. The account should highlight some general comments regarding mandibular fractures and the 'principles of displacement' according to the line/direction of the fracture and the location of muscle attachments in relation to the line of the fracture.

Chapter 2

Temporomandibular (craniomandibular) joint

Gross anatomy	**10**
Mandibular fossa	10
Mandibular condyle	10
Joint capsule	10
Synovial membrane	11
Temporomandibular ligament	11
Accessory ligaments	11
Intra-articular disc	11
Nerves	11
Blood supply	11
Histology	**11**
Articular surfaces	12
Intra-articular disc	12
Synovial membrane	12
Mandibular condyle of the child	12
Self-assessment: questions	13
Self-assessment: answers	15

Overview

The temporomandibular joint (TMJ) is the synovial joint whereby the condyle of the mandible attaches to the mandibular fossa at the base of the skull. The joint cavity is subdivided into upper and lower compartments by an intra-articular disc. Movement at this joint is essential for mastication and speech. Movement at one TMJ will have a reaction in the TMJ of the other side.

Learning objectives

You should:
* know the structure of the TMJ at both the gross and the microscopic levels
* appreciate the differences between the joint of a child and that of an adult
* be able to compare and contrast the TMJ with more typical synovial joints
* appreciate the clinical importance of the joint, which can give rise to pain and restriction of jaw movements.

Gross anatomy

The temporomandibular joint (TMJ) is the synovial articulation between the condylar process of the mandible and the mandibular (glenoid) fossa of the temporal bone. The joint space is divided into two joint cavities (upper and lower) by an intra-articular disc. The upper joint space allows for gliding movements down a bony prominence (the articular eminence) immediately anterior to the mandibular fossa, while the lower joint space allows for hinge movements. With opening and closing of the jaws, a combination of rotation and translation occurs. During wide opening, about 75% of the movement can be explained by rotation in the lower compartment. Movement of the joint is influenced by the teeth. Movements of the joint can be considered as symmetrical (opening, closing, protrusion, retrusion) or asymmetrical (lateral).

Mandibular fossa

The mandibular fossa is an oval depression in the temporal bone, lying immediately anterior to the external acoustic meatus. Its mediolateral dimension is greater than its anteroposterior one in order to accommodate the mandibular condyle, and it is wider laterally than medially. The bone of the central part of the mandibular fossa is thin. The fossa is bounded anteriorly by the articular eminence, laterally by the zygomatic process, and posteriorly by the tympanic plate.

Mandibular condyle

When viewed from above, the mandibular condyle is roughly ovoid in outline, the anteroposterior dimension (approximately 1 cm) being about half the mediolateral dimension. The medial aspect is wider than the lateral. The long axis of the condyle is not, however, at right angles to the ramus, but angled so that the lateral pole of the condyle lies slightly anterior to the medial pole. The convex anterior and superior surfaces of the head of the condyle are the articular surfaces. The broad articular head of the condyle joins the ramus through a thin bony projection termed the neck of the condyle. A small depression, the pterygoid fovea, marks part of the attachment of the inferior head of the lateral pterygoid muscle.

Joint capsule

The capsule of the TMJ is thin and is attached to the margins of the mandibular fossa above and to the neck of the condyle of the mandible below. Posteriorly, the capsule is associated with the thick, vascular but loosely arranged connective tissue of the bilaminar zone of the intra-articular disc (the retrodiscal pad). Internally, the capsule is attached to the intra-articular disc and is lined by synovial membrane. The collagen fibres of the capsule run predominantly in a vertical direction. The capsule is richly innervated.

Synovial membrane

The synovial membrane lines the inner surface of the fibrous capsule and the margins of the intra-articular disc, but does not cover the articular surfaces of the joint. The synovial membrane secretes the synovial fluid that occupies the joint cavities. Important components of the synovial fluid are the proteoglycans, which aid lubrication of the joint. At rest, the hydrostatic pressure of the synovial fluid has been reported as being subatmospheric, but this is greatly elevated during mastication.

Temporomandibular ligament

The main ligament strengthening the joint capsule is the temporomandibular (lateral) ligament. It takes origin from the lateral surface of the articular eminence of the temporal bone (at the site of a small bony protrusion, the articular tubercle). The temporomandibular ligament inserts on to the posterior surface of the condyle. This ligament provides the main means of support for the joint, restricting backward and inferior movements of the mandible and resisting dislocation during forward movements. The temporomandibular ligament is reinforced by a horizontal band of fibres running from the articular tubercle to the lateral surface of the condyle. These horizontal fibres restrict posterior movement of the condyle. There is little evidence of any comparable ligament on the medial aspect of the joint capsule, so medial displacement is prevented by the temporomandibular ligament of the opposite side.

Accessory ligaments

The accessory ligaments of the TMJ traditionally described are the stylomandibular ligament, the sphenomandibular ligament and the pterygomandibular raphe. However, only the sphenomandibular ligament is likely to have any significant influence upon mandibular movements.

- The sphenomandibular ligament (a remnant of the perichondrium of Meckel's cartilage) extends from the spine of the sphenoid bone to the lingula near the mandibular foramen.
- The stylomandibular ligament is a reinforced lamina of the deep cervical fascia as it passes medially to the parotid salivary gland. It extends from the tip of the styloid process and the stylohyoid ligament to the angle of the mandible.
- The pterygomandibular raphe extends from the pterygoid hamulus to the posterior end of the mylohyoid line in the retromolar region of the mandible.

Intra-articular disc

The intra-articular disc (meniscus) is a dense, fibrous structure moulded to the bony joint surfaces above and below. Blood vessels are evident only at the periphery of the intra-articular disc, the bulk of it being avascular. Above, the disc covers the slope of the articular eminence in front while below it covers the condyle. When viewed in sagittal section, the upper surface of the disc is concavo-convex from front to back and the lower surface is concave. The disc is of variable thickness, being thinnest in its central part. In centric occlusal position, the articular surface of the condyle lies against the thinner, intermediate part of the intra-articular disc and faces the posterior slope of the articular eminence.

The margin of the intra-articular disc merges peripherally with the joint capsule. Posteriorly, it is attached to the capsule by a bilaminar zone (retrodiscal tissue/pad). The superior lamina is loose and possesses numerous vascular elements and elastin fibres. The inferior lamina is relatively avascular and less extensible, and is attached to the posterior margin of the condyle.

Nerves

The nerves providing the rich innervation for the joint are the auriculotemporal, masseteric and deep temporal nerves of the mandibular division of the trigeminal nerve. The largest is the auriculotemporal nerve, supplying the medial, lateral and posterior parts of the joint. The remaining two nerves supply the anterior parts of the joint. Although free nerve endings associated with nociception are found everywhere in the joint capsule, of particular functional importance are more complex endings (i.e. Ruffini-like endings) associated with proprioception and important in the control of mastication. Joint receptors, along with Golgi tendon organs in the tendons and muscle spindles in the muscles, are called proprioceptors because of their role in position sense. When the joint capsule is compressed or stretched during movement of the joint, Ruffini-like (slowly adapting) mechanoreceptor endings will signal not only the position of the joint, but also the direction and velocity of the movement; they will not, however, be able to signal the force developed between the teeth.

Blood supply

The blood supply to the joint is supplied mainly from the superficial temporal and maxillary arteries.

Histology

Two unusual histological features of the TMJ are that:

- the articular surfaces are not lined by hyaline cartilage like the majority of synovial joints, but by fibrous

tissue (reflecting the intramembranous development of the bones of the joint)
- a secondary cartilage is present in the head of the mandibular condyle until adolescence.

Articular surfaces

Four distinct layers have been described covering the bony head of the adult condyle:

- The most superficial layer forms the articular surface and is composed of fibrous tissue (mainly collagen, but with some elastin fibres). Fibroblasts/fibrocytes within the surface layer are sparsely distributed.
- Beneath the articular surface layer is a more cellular zone (cell-rich zone).
- Beneath the cell-rich zone is another fibrous layer in which a number of the cells are rounded, and have an appearance reminiscent of cartilage-like cells; this layer is generally referred to as the fibrocartilaginous layer.
- Immediately covering the bone is a thin zone of calcified cartilage, distinguished from the underlying bone of the mandibular condyle by its different staining properties. This calcified cartilage is a remnant of the secondary condylar cartilage.

The articular surface covering the mandibular fossa of the temporal bone is similar to that of the condyle. Although generally thinner, it thickens as it passes over the articular eminence.

Intra-articular disc

The intra-articular disc contains cells embedded in a matrix composed of fibres and ground substance. The majority of fibres consist of type I collagen, although traces of other types of collagen have been recorded. There is also a small quantity of elastin fibres present in the disc.

Collagen fibres in the thinner, central region of the intra-articular disc (also known as the intermediate zone) run mainly in an anteroposterior direction. In the thicker, anterior and posterior portions (also known as the anterior and posterior bands respectively), prominent fibre bundles also run transversely (mediolateral orientation) and superoinferiorly, giving the fibres a much more convoluted appearance. Around the periphery of the disc, the collagen fibre bundles are arranged circumferentially. When viewed in polarized light, the collagen fibres show alternating dark and light bands, indicating that they are wavy or crimped.

Ground substance

The ground substance of the disc comprises about 5% of its dry weight. The major glycosaminoglycans are chondroitin sulphate and dermatan sulphate that, by their anionic charge, can absorb water and help resist compressive loading.

Cells

The cells of the intra-articular disc are numerous at the time of birth and become more sparsely distributed in the adult. They display a varied outline, varying between flattened (fibroblast-like) and rounded (chondrocyte-like). The cells show moderate amounts of the intracellular organelles associated with the synthesis and secretion of components of the extracellular matrix (such as endoplasmic reticulum, mitochondria, Golgi material and vesicles).

The cells possess numerous fine processes, many extending for considerable distances; these processes are rich in the gap junction protein, connexin 43. This might allow for the passage of nutrients and fluid from the peripheral blood vessels to the central avascular regions of the disc. Occasionally, cells may have a rounded, cartilage-like appearance that is age-related.

Blood vessels

Although blood vessels are present in the articular disc at the time of birth, the majority are soon lost and the bulk of the intra-articular disc, especially the central region, soon becomes avascular.

Synovial membrane

The synovial membrane consists of a layer of flattened endothelial-like cells resting on a vascular layer. The cells comprising the superficial layer are of two types:

- A macrophage-like cell type that is phagocytic
- A fibroblast-like cell.

Histological appearance varies according to age. This is due to the presence of the secondary condylar cartilage during childhood. This cartilage appears initially at about the tenth week of intrauterine life and remains as a zone of proliferating cartilage until adolescence.

Mandibular condyle of the child

Like that of the adult, the mandibular condyle of a child is lined by a layer of fibrous tissue, beneath which is a proliferative layer of undifferentiated cells that shows more activity. Cells from this proliferative layer divide to give rise to fibroblast-like cells that subsequently differentiate into chondrocytes, which form the secondary condylar cartilage. Like cartilage elsewhere, the collagen is chiefly type II. Chondrocytes in the deep part of the condylar cartilage hypertrophy and synthesize type X collagen, following which the matrix undergoes endochondral ossification. The possible role of the condylar cartilage in growth of the mandible is controversial. Unlike that of the adult, the condyle of the young child is not lined by a distinct layer of compact bone.

Self-assessment: questions

True/false statements

Which of the following statements are true and which are false?

a. The upper joint cavity of the temporomandibular joint is primarily associated with hinge movements of the mandible.
b. The articular disc of the temporomandibular joint gains an attachment anteriorly to the medial pterygoid muscle.
c. Like other synovial joints, the articular surfaces of the temporomandibular joint are covered by hyaline cartilage.
d. The bone of the mandibular (glenoid) fossa is thick in order to withstand loading during mastication.
e. The sensory supply to the temporomandibular joint is derived primarily from the great auricular nerve.
f. The attachments of the articular capsule of the temporomandibular joint do not enclose the petrotympanic fissure.
g. Lateral excursions of the mandible are the only bilaterally asymmetrical movements of this bone.
h. The capsule of the temporomandibular joint is strengthened medially by the temporomandibular ligament.
i. The condylar cartilage is a primary cartilage.
j. The central region of the intra-articular disc is avascular.
k. Like fibroblasts elsewhere, those in the intra-articular disc possess a few short cell processes.
l. Ruffini-like mechanoreceptors in the temporomandibular joint signal the position of the joint, and the direction and velocity of the movement of the joint, as well as the force developed between the teeth.

Extended matching questions

Theme: Temporomandibular joint

Lead-in

Select the most appropriate option to answer items 1–6. Each option can be used once, more than once or not at all.

Item list
1. Synovial membrane
2. Temporomandibular (lateral) ligament
3. Intra-articular disc
4. Articular surface of condyle
5. Cells of the secondary condylar cartilage
6. Upper joint cavity

Option list
A. It is composed of hyaline cartilage
B. Hinge movements primarily occur here
C. It lines the articular surfaces of the joint
D. It lines the inner surface of the joint capsule
E. They are aligned in columns to allow for growth
F. They have mainly disappeared by the late teens
G. It has high amounts of type III collagen
H. Translational (forward) movements primarily occur here
I. Its type I collagen fibres are not crimped
J. The processes of its cells are long and show rich branching
K. It is attached to the articular tubercle
L. Unlike most other synovial joints, it is composed of fibrous tissue

Picture questions

Figure 2.1

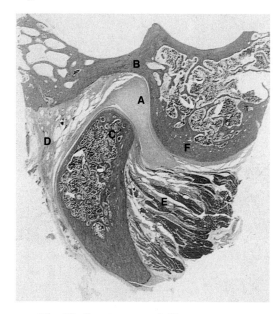

a. Identify the structures A–F.
b. What is the innervation of E?

Figure 2.2

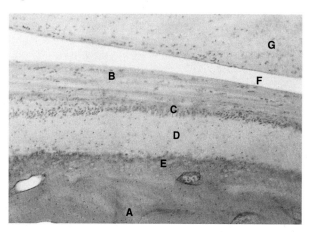

Self-assessment: questions

This is a micrograph of part of the mandibular condyle.
a. Identify A–G.
b. Is this from a young or old patient?

Figure 2.3

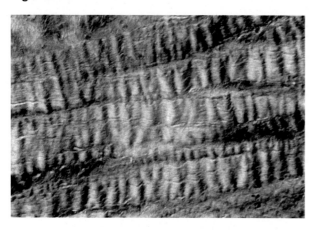

a. What feature of the collagen of the intra-articular disc is evident from this micrograph viewed with interference microscopy? (Magnification × 150)

Figure 2.4 (Courtesy of Professor D. A. Luke)

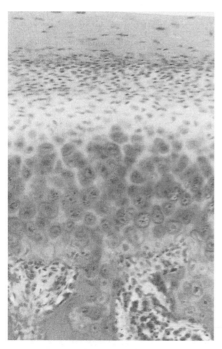

This is a micrograph of part of the mandibular condyle.
a. Is this from a young or an old person? Give the reason for your choice.

Figure 2.5 (Courtesy of Professor J. D. Langdon)

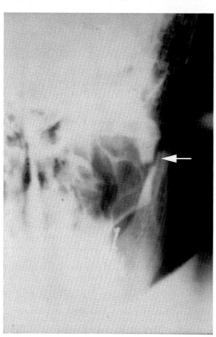

a. A footballer was taken to hospital after being involved in a clash of heads during a match. On examination, the attending doctor observed that the region around the left ear was painful and swollen, and exhibited some bleeding. On looking into the mouth, the doctor discovered that the teeth on the left side were seen to come into premature contact before those on the right side. Movement of the jaw was painful and, on opening, the jaw deviated to the left. A postero-anterior radiograph of the left ramus is shown here. Explain the symptoms.

Essay questions

1. What are the possible functions of the temporomandibular joint?
2. How does the temporomandibular joint compare with other synovial joints?
3. How does the condylar cartilage differ from a primary cartilage, such as the spheno-occipital synchondrosis?
4. Give some examples of the clinical relevance of a knowledge of the temporomandibular joint.

Self-assessment: answers

True/false answers

a. **False.** The upper joint cavity is associated with forward translocatory movements of the mandible. It is the lower joint cavity in which hinge movements occur.

b. **False.** The attachment is to the lateral pterygoid muscle.

c. **False.** As the forming articular bones develop intra-membranously, the articular surfaces are lined by fibrous tissue.

d. **False.** The loads directly impinging on the condyle are small and so the bone of the mandibular fossa is thin. The loads are buttressed by adjacent struts of bone and may be taken up by the occlusion of the teeth.

e. **False.** The auriculotemporal (and masseteric) nerve supplies the main sensory component. The great auricular nerve is sensory to skin at the angle of the mandible (and the parotid capsule).

f. **True.** Otherwise, the chorda tympani nerve would lie within the capsule of the joint.

g. **True.** The other movements (i.e. opening, closing, protraction, retraction) are symmetrical.

h. **False.** This ligament is found laterally and prevents lateral displacement of the joint. Medial displacement of the joint is limited by the action of the lateral ligament of the opposite side.

i. **False.** It is a secondary cartilage, as it appears after the mandibular condyle has been formed intramembranously.

j. **True.** This may help explain the apparently poor healing properties of the disc following surgery.

k. **False.** The cell processes are numerous and may be of considerable length. This may be related to the lack of blood vessels and may provide a mechanism for transporting nutritional elements.

l. **False.** Ruffini-like mechanoreceptors in the joint can signal the position of the joint, and the direction and velocity of the movement, but are unable to signal the force developed between the teeth.

Extended matching answers

Item 1 = Option D. Synovial membrane is limited to the inner surface of the joint capsule as, if it was reflected on to the articular surfaces, it would be worn away during movement of the joint.

Item 2 = Option K. The temporomandibular ligament is attached to the articular tubercle on the zygomatic process of the temporal bone. The ligament limits lateral movement of the mandibular condyle on its own side. Medial movement at the joint is limited by the temporomandibular ligament on the opposite side.

Item 3 = Option J. This unusual cell morphology may be related to the fact that the bulk of the intra-articular disc is avascular, and may provide a mechanism that allows for the distribution of nutritional requirements between cells.

Item 4 = Option L. The fibrous tissue lining the articular surfaces of the temporomandibular joint reflects the fact that the bones are developed intramembranously (and not endochondrally).

Item 5 = Option F. The cartilage cells associated with secondary condylar cartilage have disappeared by late teens. Evidence of the original existence of a condylar cartilage in the adult condyle may be inferred from the presence of a layer of calcified cartilage.

Item 6 = Option H. Translational (forward) movements occur in the upper joint cavity, while a hinge move-ment occurs in the lower joint cavity. In normal jaw opening, movement occurs in both joint cavities.

Picture answers

Figure 2.1

a. A = articular disc. B = mandibular fossa. C = condyle of mandible. D = capsule of joint. E = lateral ptery-goid muscle. F = articular eminence.

b. The lateral pterygoid muscle is supplied by a branch from the anterior division of the mandibular nerve.

Figure 2.2

a. A = bone of condylar cartilage. B = fibrous layer cov-ering articular surface. C = cell-rich layer of prolif-erative zone. D = layer of fibrocartilage. E = layer of calcified cartilage. F = lower joint space. G = articular disc.

b. As there is no evidence of an active secondary condy-lar cartilage, it is from an older patient.

Figure 2.3

a. The micrograph demonstrates crimping along the length of the collagen fibres. This would indicate that the fibres are subjected to tensional loading. Similar crimping is seen in the fibrous articular layer.

Figure 2.4

a. This is a section taken through the condylar region of a child, as an active secondary condylar cartilage is still evident. This cartilage disappears at the age of approximately 15 years.

Figure 2.5

a. The signs are compatible with a unilateral fracture of the left mandibular condyle (arrowed in the radio-graph). The bleeding may be the result of damage to the external acoustic meatus. The premature contact of the teeth on the left side is due to displacement of the left mandibular condyle and the resulting loss

Self-assessment: answers

in height of the left ramus. The jaw deviates to the left on opening because of the unopposed activity of the unaffected right lateral pterygoid muscle. The diagnosis can be confirmed by radiography. About 30% of all mandibular fractures involve the condyles and occur in the region of the narrow neck.

Outline essay answers

Question 1

Although the precise function(s) of the temporomandibular joint is not known, the following are among the roles attributed to the intra-articular disc:

- It improves the fit between the bony articulating surfaces.
- It provides stability during mandibular movements.
- It acts as a shock absorber and distributes loads over a large area.
- It protects the articular surfaces, especially from shear forces generated during condylar movements.
- It spreads the synovial fluid.
- Instead of stabilizing the condyle (see second bullet point above), it acts primarily as a destabilizing agent for the condyle and permits it to move more freely.

Question 2

Although having a number of features typical of synovial joints in other regions (e.g. a joint capsule, a synovial membrane secreting synovial fluid, ligaments to limit movement), the temporomandibular joint also has some unusual features:

- The joint space is divided into two joint cavities (upper and lower) by an intra-articular disc; the upper joint space allows for gliding movements, the lower joint space for hinge movements.
- The articular surfaces are not composed of hyaline cartilage but of fibrous tissue. This reflects the joint's intramembranous ossification as compared with the endochondral ossification of most other synovial joints.
- A secondary condylar cartilage is present in the head of the condyle until adolescence.
- Movement of the joint is influenced by the teeth.
- There are two temporomandibular joints associated with the single mandible; this has considerable functional significance, as movement at one joint is accompanied by movement at the other.

Question 3

Developmentally, a primary cartilage appears first and maps out the shape of the future bone, which develops by endochondral ossification. In the case of the condylar cartilage, the ramus has already formed in membrane before this secondary cartilage appears.

Primary cartilages have inherent growth potential, as is evidenced when they are transferred to tissue culture. The condylar cartilage has little intrinsic growth potential when placed in tissue culture.

In the spheno-occipital synchondrosis, proliferative zones lie on either side of the central region of the cartilage, and proliferation involves cartilage cells. This contrasts with the condylar cartilage, where it is undifferentiated fibroblast-like cells that undergo proliferation.

In the synchondrosis, the chondrocytes are aligned in columns in the direction of growth on both sides of the cartilage, and there is considerable production of extracellular matrix which, together with the original cell proliferation and the absorption of water by the proteoglycans, is responsible for providing the growth force. In the secondary condylar cartilage, however, there is far less production of extracellular matrix and there is no alignment of the hypertrophic chondrocytes into columns. In the case of an epiphyseal growth plate (as opposed to a synchondrosis), columns of cartilage cells are produced only on one side of the cartilage.

Question 4

During dental procedures, such as tooth extraction (or even yawning), excessive force may result in the head of the condyle being drawn anteriorly and over the articular eminence. This will result in a dislocation of the jaw and prevent the jaw from being closed. If unilateral, the jaw will deviate towards the unaffected side.

The intra-articular disc may gradually become displaced from its normal position between the articular surfaces. Most commonly it is displaced anteromedially. The posterior part of the disc may end up between the bony articular surfaces and be subjected to abnormal loading. The synovial fluid in temporomandibular joint disorders may show an increased content in molecules such as pro-inflammatory cytokines (e.g. interleukin, tumour necrosis factor), matrix metalloproteinases and vascular endothelial growth factor.

Like other synovial joints, the temporomandibular joint is prone to inflammatory and degenerative conditions, such as rheumatoid arthritis and osteoarthritis. In these situations, damage to the articular surfaces will subject the articular disc to increased friction that may lead to degenerative changes within the disc.

Common symptoms associated with temporomandibular joint syndrome include pain in the jaw joint, clicking sounds in the joint and limited mouth opening. These disorders are not easily treated, perhaps because of the lack of blood vessels in the disc.

Fractures of the mandible are common and often involve the condyle. If unilateral, the bite will be abnormal, with premature contact of the teeth on the affected side. When the patient is asked to close, the jaw will deviate to the

Self-assessment: answers

affected side. The condyle is usually displaced anteromedially, as a result of the pull of the lateral pterygoid muscle. If a fracture in a child is left untreated, abnormal healing may result in fusion of the mandible to the articular fossa. This ankylosis may result in limitation of movement and facial disharmony.

During examination of children in their early teens, it may be evident that the mandible is developing at a greater or lesser rate than the maxillae and that this imbalance is likely to lead to a malocclusion and/or facial disharmony. Unlike aspects of sutural growth in the upper jaw that are amenable to intervention and improvement, growth is less easy to modulate in the mandible.

Nevertheless, orthodontic appliances have been designed to try to modify any growth contributed by the condylar cartilage (although there is little evidence that the cartilage plays any significant role in the growth process). Thus, appliances that push the mandible back and compress the condylar cartilage against the mandibular fossa are used to try to retard mandibular growth. Conversely, in situations where the mandible is underdeveloped, appliances that reposition the condyle in a forward position have been used to enhance development of the condyle in an attempt to produce a more forward-positioned lower dental arch. However, the success of such procedures is not always predictable.

Human dentition: tooth morphology and occlusion

Tooth morphology	18
Dental notation	18
Differences between teeth of the deciduous and permanent dentitions	19
Incisors	19
Canines	21
Premolars	21
Molars	22
Pulp morphology	24
The occlusion of the permanent teeth	24
Centric occlusal position	24
Malocclusions	25
Self-assessment: questions	27
Self-assessment: answers	33

Overview

The human dentition, structurally and functionally, is characteristic of an omnivorous mammal. Indeed, the heterodonty includes all basic tooth forms in the dentition (i.e. incisors, canines and molars). The dentition is diphyodontic (having two generations or series of teeth – there being a primary or deciduous dentition that is succeeded by a secondary or permanent dentition). Occlusion of the dentition refers to the way in which the teeth bite together. Its main feature relates to the fact that, in normal (or anatomical) centric occlusion, a maxillary (upper) tooth occludes with its opposite tooth in the mandible plus the tooth located distally. Thus, the maxillary first (central) incisor occludes with the mandibular first (central) and second (lateral) incisors.

Learning objectives

You must:
- be able to identify precisely a tooth from either the permanent or the deciduous dentition (excepting the variable permanent third molar teeth)
- be able to describe the typical pulp morphologies for such teeth
- be able to describe the relationships of permanent teeth within the dental arches
- be able to describe the characteristics of normal (anatomical) centric occlusal position
- be able to categorize malocclusions in terms of Angle's classification and the incisor relationship classification.

Tooth morphology

Humans have two generations of teeth: the deciduous (or primary) dentition and the permanent (or secondary) dentition. This is termed diphyodonty. In both dentitions, there are three basic tooth forms: incisiform, caniniform and molariform.

- Incisiform teeth (incisors, I in dental notation) are cutting teeth, with thin, blade-like crowns.
- Caniniform teeth (canines, C) are piercing/tearing teeth, having a single cone-shaped cusp on their crowns.
- Molariform teeth (molars, M, and premolars, PM) are grinding teeth, possessing more than onecusp on an otherwise flattened biting surface. Premolars are bicuspid teeth; they are unique to the permanent dentition and replace the deciduous molars.

Table 3.1 gives definitions of terms used for the descriptions of tooth form.

Dental notation

The types and numbers of teeth in any mammalian dentition can be expressed using dental formulae. The formula for the deciduous human dentition is DI 2/2 DC 1/1 DM 2/2 = 20, and for the permanent dentition I 2/2 C 1/1 PM 2/2 M 3/3 = 32, where the numbers following each letter refer to the number of teeth of each type in the upper and lower jaws on one side only. In both the permanent and deciduous dentitions, the incisors may be distinguished according to their relationship to the midline. Thus, the incisor nearest the midline is the first (or central) incisor and the more laterally positioned incisor the second (or lateral) incisor. The permanent premolars and the permanent and deciduous molars can also be distinguished according to their mesiodistal relationships. The molar most mesially positioned is designated the first molar, the one behind it being the second molar. In the permanent dentition, the tooth most distally positioned is the third molar. The mesial premolar is the first premolar, the premolar behind it being the second premolar.

Table 3.1 Terms used for the description of tooth form

Term	Definition
Crown	Clinical crown – that portion of a tooth visible in the oral cavity
	Anatomical crown – that portion of a tooth covered with enamel
Root	Clinical root – that portion of a tooth lying within the alveolus
	Anatomical root – that portion of a tooth covered by cementum
Cervical margin	The junction of the anatomical crown and the anatomical root
Occlusal surface	The biting surface of a posterior tooth (molar or premolar)
Cusp	A pronounced elevation on the occlusal surface of a tooth
Incisal margin	The cutting edge of anterior teeth, analogous to the occlusal surface of the posterior teeth
Tubercle	A small elevation on the crown
Cingulum	A bulbous convexity near the cervical region of a tooth
Ridge	A linear elevation on the surface of a tooth
Marginal ridge	A ridge at the mesial or distal edge of the occlusal surface of posterior teeth. Some anterior teeth have equivalent ridges
Fissure	A long cleft between cusps or ridges
Fossa	A rounded depression in a surface of a tooth
Buccal	Towards or adjacent to the cheek. The term buccal surface is reserved for that surface of a premolar or molar which is positioned immediately adjacent to the cheek
Labial	Towards or adjacent to the lips. The term labial surface is reserved for that surface of an incisor or canine which is positioned immediately adjacent to the lips
Palatal	Towards or adjacent to the palate. The term palatal surface is reserved for that surface of a maxillary tooth which is positioned immediately adjacent to the palate
Lingual	Towards or adjacent to the tongue. The term lingual surface is reserved for that surface of a mandibular tooth which lies immediately adjacent to the tongue
Mesial	Towards the median. The mesial surface is that surface which faces towards the median line following the curve of the dental arch
Distal	Away from the median. The distal surface is that surface which faces away from the median line following the curve of the dental arch

Differences between teeth of the deciduous and permanent dentitions

The crowns of deciduous and permanent teeth are distinguished essentially by:

- size
- the greater constancy of shape of the deciduous teeth
- the crowns of deciduous teeth appearing bulbous and often with pronounced labial or buccal cingula

- the cervical margins of deciduous teeth being more sharply demarcated and pronounced
- the cusps of newly erupted deciduous teeth being more pointed
- the opacity, whiteness and thinner covering of the enamel of deciduous teeth
- the enamel of deciduous teeth being more permeable, softer and more easily worn
- the lack of neonatal lines in deciduous teeth.

The roots of deciduous and permanent teeth are distinguished essentially by:

- being shorter and less robust in deciduous teeth
- the fact that the roots of the deciduous incisors and canines are longer in proportion to the crown than those of their permanent counterparts
- the roots of the deciduous molars being more widely divergent.

The pulps of deciduous and permanent teeth are distinguished essentially by:

- the fact that the pulp chambers of deciduous teeth are proportionally larger in relation to the crown
- the pulp horns in deciduous teeth being more prominent
- the root canals of deciduous teeth being extremely fine.

Incisors

Maxillary first (central) permanent incisor

The maxillary first (central) permanent incisor is the widest mesiodistally of all the permanent incisors and canines, the crown being almost as wide as it is long. Like all incisors, it is basically wedge- or chisel-shaped and has a single conical root. From the incisal view, the crown and incisal margin are centrally positioned over the root of the tooth. The incisal margin may be grooved by two troughs, the labial lobe grooves, which correspond to the divisions between three developmental lobes (or mammelons) seen on newly erupted incisors. The mammelons are lost by attrition soon after eruption. From the labial view, the crown length can be seen to be almost as great as the root length. The convex labial surface may be marked by two faint grooves that run vertically towards the cervical margin and which are extensions of the labial lobe grooves. The mesial surface is straight and approximately at right angles to the incisal margin. The disto-incisal angle, however, is more rounded and the distal outline more convex. Viewed palatally, the crown has a slightly shovel-shaped appearance and is bordered by mesial and distal marginal ridges. Near the cervical margin lies a prominent cingulum. The sinuous cervical margin is concave towards the crown on the palatal and labial surfaces, and convex towards the crown on the mesial and distal surfaces, the curvature on the mesial surface being the most pronounced of any tooth in the dentition. The single root of the first incisor tapers towards the apex and is conical in cross-section.

Maxillary second (lateral) permanent incisor

The maxillary second (lateral) permanent incisor is one of the most variable teeth in the dentition, although generally it is morphologically a diminutive form of the maxillary first incisor. The crown is much narrower and shorter than that of the first incisor, though the crown:root length ratio is considerably decreased. From the incisal aspect, the crown has a more rounded outline than the adjacent first incisor. Viewed labially, the mesio-incisal and disto-incisal angles, and the mesial and distal crown margins are more rounded than those of the first incisor. From the palatal aspect, lying in front of the cingulum is a pit (foramen caecum) that may extend some way into the root. A common morphological variation is the so-called 'peg-shaped' lateral incisor. The course of the cervical margin and the shape of the root are similar to those of the first incisor.

Mandibular first (central) permanent incisor

The mandibular incisors have the smallest mesiodistal dimensions of any teeth in the permanent dentition. They can be distinguished from the maxillary incisors by:

- the marked lingual inclination of the crowns over the roots
- the mesiodistal compression of their roots
- the poor development of the marginal ridges and cingula.

The mandibular first (central) permanent incisor has a bilaterally symmetrical triangular shape. In the newly erupted tooth, three mammelons are usually present. The incisal margin is at right angles to a line bisecting the tooth labiolingually. The mesio-incisal and disto-incisal angles are sharp and the mesial and distal surfaces are approximately at right angles to the incisal margin. The profiles of the mesial and distal surfaces appear very similar, being convex in their incisal thirds and relatively flattened in the middle and cervical thirds. The lingual cingulum and mesial and distal marginal ridges appear less distinct than those of the maxillary incisors. The cervical margins on the labial and lingual surfaces show their maximum convexities midway between the mesial and distal borders of the root. The cervical margin on the distal surface is less curved than that on the mesial surface. The root is narrow and conical, though flattened mesiodistally, and is frequently grooved on the mesial and distal surfaces (the distal groove being more marked).

Mandibular second (lateral) permanent incisor

The mandibular second (lateral) permanent incisor closely resembles the mandibular first incisor. However, it is slightly wider mesiodistally and is more asymmetric in shape. The distal surface diverges at a greater angle from the long axis of the tooth, giving it a fan-shaped appearance, and the disto-incisal angle is more acute and rounded. Another distinguishing characteristic is the angulation of the incisal margin relative to the labiolingual axis of the tooth; in the first incisor, the incisal margin forms a right angle with the labiolingual axis, whereas that of the second incisor is 'twisted' distally in a lingual direction.

Maxillary first (central) deciduous incisor

The maxillary first (central) deciduous incisor is similar morphologically to the corresponding permanent tooth. However, because the width of the crown of the deciduous incisor nearly equals the length it appears plumper than its permanent successor. Unlike the permanent teeth, no mammelons are seen on the incisal margin. The labial surface is unmarked by grooves, lobes or depressions. The mesio-incisal angle is sharp and acute, while the disto-incisal angle is more rounded and obtuse. On the palatal surface, the cingulum is a very prominent bulge. Unlike those of its permanent successor, the marginal ridges are poorly defined and the concavity of the palatal surface is shallow. As with all deciduous teeth, the cervical margins are more pronounced, but less sinuous, than those of their permanent successors. The fully formed root is conical in shape, tapering apically to a rather blunt apex. Compared with the corresponding permanent tooth, the root is longer in proportion to the crown.

Maxillary second (lateral) deciduous incisor

The maxillary second (lateral) deciduous incisor is similar in shape to the maxillary first deciduous incisor, though smaller. One obvious difference is the more acute mesio-incisal angle and the more rounded disto-incisal angle. The palatal surface is more concave and the marginal ridges more pronounced. Viewed incisally, the crown appears almost circular (in contrast to the first incisor, which appears diamond shaped). The palatal cingulum is generally lower than that of the first deciduous incisor.

Mandibular first (central) deciduous incisor

The mandibular first (central) deciduous incisor is morphologically similar to its permanent successor. However, it is much shorter, has a low labial cingulum, and the marginal ridges are poorly defined. The mesio-incisal and disto-incisal angles are sharp right angles and the incisal margin is straight in the horizontal plane. The single root is more rounded than that of the corresponding permanent tooth and, when complete, tapers and tends to incline distally.

Mandibular second (lateral) deciduous incisor

The mandibular second (lateral) deciduous incisor is a bulbous tooth that resembles its permanent successor. It is wider than the mandibular first deciduous incisor and is asymmetric. The mesio-incisal angle is more obtuse and rounder than that of the mandibular first deciduous incisor, and the incisal margin slopes downwards distally. Unlike the permanent tooth, the root is rounded.

Canines

Canines are the only teeth in the dentition with a single cusp. Morphologically, they can be considered transitional between incisors and premolars.

Maxillary permanent canine

The maxillary permanent canine is a stout tooth with a well-developed cingulum and the longest root of any tooth. Viewed from its incisal aspect, it appears asymmetric such that the distal portion of the crown is much wider than the mesial portion. Prominent longitudinal ridges pass from the cusp tip down both the labial and palatal surfaces. The incisal part of the crown occupies at least one-third of the crown height. From this view, the mesial arm of the incisal margin is shorter than the distal arm, and the disto-incisal angle is more rounded than the mesio-incisal angle. The profiles of the mesial and distal surfaces converge markedly towards the cervix of the tooth. The mesial profile is slightly convex; the distal profile is markedly convex. The mesial surface of the crown forms a straight line with the root; the distal surface meets the root at an obtuse angle. The palatal surface shows distinct mesial and distal marginal ridges and a well-defined cingulum. The longitudinal ridge from the tip of the cusp meets the cingulum and is separated from the marginal ridges on either side by distinct grooves or fossae. Viewed mesially or distally, the distinctive feature is the stout character of the crown and the great width of the cervical third of both the crown and root. The cervical margin of this tooth follows a course similar to that of the incisors but the curves are less pronounced. The root is the largest, and stoutest, in the dentition and is triangular in cross-section. The mesial and distal surfaces of the root are often grooved longitudinally.

Mandibular permanent canine

The mandibular permanent canine is similar to the maxillary canine, but smaller, more slender and more symmetrical. The cusp is generally less well developed. From the incisal aspect, there are no distinct longitudinal ridges from the tip of the cusp on to the labial and lingual surfaces. Viewed labially, the incisal margin occupies only one-fifth of the crown height and the cusp is less pointed. The crown is narrower mesiodistally than that of the maxillary canine so it appears longer, narrower and more slender. The mesial and distal profiles tend to be parallel or only slightly convergent towards the cervix. The labial and mesial surfaces are clearly defined, being inclined acutely to each other, whereas the labial surface merges gradually into the distal surface. The lingual surface is flatter than the corresponding palatal surface of the maxillary permanent canine, and the cingulum, marginal ridges and fossae are indistinct. The mesial and distal surfaces are longer than those of the maxillary canine. The cervical margin of this tooth follows a course similar to that of the incisors. The root is normally single, though occasionally it may bifurcate. In cross-section, the root is oval, being flattened

mesially and distally. The root is grooved longitudinally on both its mesial and distal surfaces.

Maxillary deciduous canine

The maxillary deciduous canine has a fang-like appearance and is similar morphologically to its permanent successor, though more bulbous. It is generally symmetrical. Bulging of the tooth gives the crown a diamond-shaped appearance when viewed labially or palatally, with the crown margins overhanging the root profiles. The width of the crown is greater than its length. On the labial surface, there is a low cingulum cervically, from which runs a longitudinal ridge up to the tip of the cusp. A similar longitudinal ridge also runs on the palatal surface. This ridge extends from the cusp apex to the palatal cingulum and divides the palatal surface into two shallow pits. The marginal ridges on the palatal surface are low and indistinct. The root is long compared with the crown height and is triangular in cross-section.

Mandibular deciduous canine

The mandibular deciduous canine is more slender than the maxillary deciduous canine. The crown is asymmetrical and the cusp tip displaced mesially. Consequently, the mesial arm is shorter and more vertical than the distal arm. On the labial surface, there is a low cingulum. On the lingual surface, the cingulum and marginal ridges are less pronounced than the corresponding structures on the palatal surface of the maxillary deciduous canine. The longitudinal ridges on both the labial and lingual surfaces are poorly developed. The width of the crown is less than the length. The root is single and tends to be triangular in cross-section.

Premolars

Premolars are sometimes referred to as 'bicuspids', having a buccal and a palatal (or lingual) cusp.

Maxillary first premolar

The maxillary first premolar has an ovoid crown with distinct marginal ridges. The buccal and palatal cusps are separated by a central occlusal fissure running mesiodistally. The occlusal fissure crosses the mesial marginal ridge on to the mesial surface (the canine groove). Viewed buccally, the mesial slope of the buccal cusp is generally longer than the distal slope. Viewed palatally, the palatal cusp is lower than the buccal cusp and its tip lies more mesially. From the mesial aspect, the mesial surface is marked by a distinct concavity, the canine fossa. The cervical margin follows essentially a level course around the crown. There are usually two roots, a buccal and a palatal root.

Maxillary second premolar

The maxillary second premolar is similar in shape to the maxillary first premolar. However, the occlusal surface appears more compressed and the mesiodistal dimension of the crown is smaller. The central fissure does not cross the mesial marginal ridge. From the buccal aspect, the mesio- and disto-occlusal angles are less prominent and the two cusps are smaller and more equal in size than those of the first premolar. Like the first premolar, the tip of the palatal cusp lies more mesially. Viewed palatally, less of the buccal profile is visible. There is no canine fossa or canine groove on the mesial surface. The root is single.

Mandibular first premolar

The mandibular premolars differ from the maxillary premolars in that occlusally the crowns appear rounder and the cusps are of unequal size, the buccal cusp being the most prominent.

The mandibular first premolar has a dominant buccal cusp and a very small lingual cusp that appears not unlike a cingulum. The buccal and lingual cusps are connected by a ridge that divides the poorly developed mesiodistal occlusal fissure into mesial and distal fossae. The mesial fossa is generally smaller than the distal fossa. A canine groove often extends from the mesial fossa over the mesial marginal ridge on to the mesiolingual surface of the crown. The mandibular first premolar differs from other premolars in that the occlusal plane does not lie perpendicular to the long axis of the tooth but is included lingually. The cervical line follows an almost level course around the tooth. The root is single and is grooved longitudinally both mesially and distally, the mesial groove being more prominent.

Mandibular second premolar

The lingual cusp of the mandibular second premolar is better developed than that of the first premolar, although it is not as large as the buccal cusp. The occlusal outline is round or square. The mesiodistal occlusal fissure between the cusps is well defined. However, like the first premolar, the fissure ends in mesial and distal fossae, the distal fossa being the larger. Unlike the first premolar, a ridge does not usually join the apices of the cusps. The lingual cusp is usually subdivided into mesiolingual and distolingual cusps, the mesiolingual cusp being wider and higher than the distolingual. From the mesial and distal aspects, the occlusal surface appears horizontal to the long axis of the tooth, unlike the mandibular first premolar. The crown is wider buccolingually than that of the first premolar and the buccal cusp does not incline as far over the root. The mesial marginal ridge is higher than the distal marginal ridge. The cervical margin follows a level course around the tooth. The root is single and its apex may be curved distally.

Molars

Molars present the largest occlusal surfaces of all teeth. They have 3–5 major cusps (although the maxillary first deciduous molar has only two). Molars are the only teeth that have more than one buccal cusp. Generally, the lower molars have two roots while the upper have three. The permanent molars do not have deciduous predecessors.

Maxillary first permanent molar

The maxillary first permanent molar is usually the largest molar and the crown is rhombic in outline, the mesiopalatal and distobuccal angles being obtuse. It has four major cusps (mesiobuccal, mesiopalatal, distobuccal and distopalatal) separated by an irregular H-shaped occlusal fissure. The mesiopalatal cusp is the largest, the buccal cusps being smaller and of approximately equal size. An accessory cusplet of variable size is seen in 60% of first molars on the palatal surface of the mesiopalatal cusp (the tubercle of Carabelli). The distopalatal cusp is generally the smallest cusp of the tooth. A buccal groove extends from the occlusal table, passing between the cusps to end about halfway up the buccal surface. Viewed palatally, the disproportion in size between the mesiopalatal and distopalatal cusps is evident. A palatal groove extends from the occlusal surface, between the palatal cusps, to terminate approximately halfway up the palatal surface. The mesial marginal ridge is more prominent than the distal ridge and may have distinct tubercles. The cervical margin follows an even contour around the tooth. There are three roots, two buccal and one palatal, arising from a common root stalk. The palatal root is the longest and stoutest. The buccal roots are more slender and are flattened mesiodistally; the mesiobuccal root is usually the larger and wider of the two.

Maxillary second permanent molar

The maxillary second permanent molar closely resembles the maxillary first permanent molar but is reduced in size and has different cusp relationships. Viewed occlusally, the rhomboid form is more pronounced and the oblique ridge is smaller. The distopalatal cusp is considerably reduced. The occlusal fissure pattern is more variable and supplemental grooves are more numerous. A tubercle of Carabelli is not usually found on the mesiopalatal cusp and the tubercles on the mesial marginal ridge are less numerous or less pronounced. Like the first molar, the second molar has two buccal roots and one palatal. They are shorter and less divergent than those of the first molar and may be partly fused.

Maxillary third permanent molar

The maxillary third permanent molar is the most variable in the dentition. Most commonly, the crown is triangular in shape, having the three cusps of the trigon but no talon. The roots are often fused and irregular. Third permanent molars are the teeth most often absent congenitally.

Differences between maxillary and mandibular molars

The mandibular molars differ from the maxillary molars in many respects:

- Mandibular molars have two roots (mesial and distal).
- They are derived from a five-cusped form.

- The crowns of the lower molars are oblong, being broader mesiodistally than buccolingually.
- The fissure pattern is cross-shaped.
- The lingual cusps are of more equal size.
- The tips of the buccal cusps are shifted lingually so that, from the occlusal view, the whole of the buccal surface is visible.

Mandibular first permanent molar

The mandibular first permanent molar is pentagonal in outline. It is broader mesiodistally than buccolingually. The occlusal surface is divided into buccal and lingual parts by a mesiodistal occlusal fissure. The buccal side of the occlusal table has three distinct cusps: mesiobuccal, distobuccal and distal. Each cusp is separated by a groove, which joins the mesiodistal fissure. On the lingual side are two cusps: mesiolingual and distolingual. The fissure separating the lingual cusps joins the mesiodistal fissure in the region of the central fossa. The lingual cusps tend to be larger and more pointed. The tips of the buccal cusps are displaced lingually, are rounded and are lower than the lingual cusps. The smallest cusp is the distal cusp. In 90% of cases, the mesiolingual cusp is joined to the distobuccal cusp across the floor of the central fossa. This feature, together with the five-cusped pattern, is termed the *Dryopithecus* pattern. The buccal surface appears markedly convex. The fissure separating the mesiobuccal and distobuccal cusps terminates halfway up the buccal surface in a buccal pit. From the lingual aspect, the mesiolingual cusp appears slightly larger. Both the mesial and distal marginal ridges are V-shaped, being notched at their midpoint. The cervical margin follows a uniform contour around the tooth. The two roots, one mesial and one distal, arise from a common root stalk. They are markedly flattened mesiodistally and the mesial root is usually deeply grooved.

Mandibular second permanent molar

The mandibular second permanent molar has a rectangular shape viewed occlusally; the buccal profile is thus nearly equal in length to the lingual profile, unlike the mandibular first permanent molar. There are four cusps, the mesiobuccal and mesiolingual cusps being slightly larger than the distobuccal and distolingual cusps. The cusps are separated by a cross-shaped occlusal fissure pattern. From the buccal aspect, a fissure extends between the buccal cusps and terminates approximately halfway up the buccal surface. Because there is no distal cusp, the mesial and distal surfaces are more equal in terms of their convexity. The mesial and distal marginal ridges are not as markedly notched at their midpoint. The mesial and distal roots are flattened mesiodistally and are smaller, and less divergent, than those of the first molar. They may be partly fused.

Mandibular third permanent molar

The mandibular third permanent molar has a variable morphology, though not as variable as that of the maxillary third permanent molar. It is the smallest of the mandibular

molars. The crown usually has four or five cusps. In shape, it is normally a rounded rectangle or is circular. Its occlusal fissure pattern is very irregular. The roots are greatly reduced in size and are often fused.

Maxillary first deciduous molar

The maxillary first deciduous molar is the most atypical of all molars, deciduous or permanent, appearing intermediate between a premolar and a molar. Viewed occlusally, the crown is an irregular quadrilateral with the mesiobuccal corner producing a prominent bulge, the molar tubercle. The mesiopalatal angle is markedly obtuse. The tooth is generally bicuspid; the buccal (more pronounced) and palatal cusps are separated by an occlusal fissure that runs mesiodistally. The lingual cusp may be subdivided into two. On the mesial side lies the buccal cingulum, which extends to the molar tubercle. Marginal ridges link the buccal and palatal cusps. The tooth has three roots (two buccal and one palatal), which arise from a common root stalk. The mesiobuccal root is flattened mesiodistally; the distobuccal root is smaller and more circular; the palatal root is the largest and is round in cross-section. The distobuccal and palatal roots may be partly fused.

Maxillary second deciduous molar

The maxillary second deciduous molar closely resembles the maxillary first permanent molar. A tubercle of Carabelli on the mesiopalatal cusp is often well developed.

Mandibular first deciduous molar

The mandibular first deciduous molar has several unique features. From the occlusal aspect, the crown appears elongated mesiodistally and is an irregular quadrilateral with parallel buccal and lingual surfaces. The mesiobuccal corner is extended, forming a molar tubercle, and the mesiolingual angle is markedly obtuse. The occlusal table can be divided into buccal and lingual parts by a mesiodistal fissure. The buccal part consists of two cusps, the mesiobuccal cusp being larger than the distobuccal cusp. The lingual part of the tooth is narrower than the buccal part and has two cusps separated by a lingual fissure, the mesiolingual cusp being larger than the distolingual cusp. The buccal cusps are larger than the lingual cusps. A transverse ridge may connect the mesial cusps, dividing the mesiodistal fissure into a distal fissure and a mesial pit. From the buccal aspect, the mesiobuccal cusp occupies at least two-thirds of the crown area and projects higher occlusally than the distobuccal cusp. The molar tubercle on the mesial corner of the buccal surface can be seen in this view. From the lingual aspect the cusps are conical in shape. The distolingual cusp appears only as a bulging protuberance on the distal margin. The mesial marginal ridge is more prominent than the distal marginal ridge. The mandibular first deciduous molar has two divergent roots, mesial and distal, which are flattened mesiodistally. The mesial root is often grooved.

Mandibular second deciduous molar

The mandibular second deciduous molar is a smaller version of the mandibular first permanent molar. Unlike the permanent tooth, there is a cingulum on the mesiobuccal corner of the crown. The mesiolingual and distobuccal cusps are not usually joined to give the *Dryopithecus* pattern.

Pulp morphology

Concerning pulp morphology, the dental pulp occupies the pulp chamber in the crown of the tooth and the root canal(s) in the root(s). The pulp chamber conforms, in basic shape, to the external form of the crown. Root canal anatomy varies with tooth type and root morphology. At the apex of the root, the root canal becomes continuous with the periapical periodontal tissues through an apical foramen. In anterior teeth, the pulp chambers merge almost imperceptibly into the root canals. In the premolar and molar teeth, the pulp chambers and root canals are distinct. Pulp horns (or cornua) extend from the pulp chambers to the mesial and distal angles of the incisor tooth crowns and towards the cusps of posterior teeth.

Each root most often contains one root canal, but two are not unusual (mandibular incisors can have two root canals and mandibular molars commonly have two root canals in their mesial roots). For the maxillary first permanent molar, there may be four root canals (the fourth canal being located in the mesiobuccal root), while the mesial root of the mandibular first molar invariably has two root canals. When roots are fused, the tooth still maintains the usual number of root canals. The size of the pulp chamber and the diameter of the root canals decrease significantly with age and in response to caries, attrition or other external stimuli due to the deposition of secondary (and sometimes tertiary) dentine (see pages 164–165).

When the tooth first erupts into the oral cavity, root development is incomplete and the apical foramen is wide. The apical foramen narrows with subsequent development of the root and a constriction formed from cementum develops. This constriction marks the boundary between pulpal and periapical tissue. For deciduous teeth, the pulp chamber is relatively large and the pulp horns are longer and closer to the surface of the tooth compared with permanent teeth. The pulp chambers of deciduous mandibular molars are proportionately larger than those of the deciduous maxillary molars. The mesiobuccal pulp horn in deciduous molars is particularly near to the occlusal surface and thus highly vulnerable to exposure by dental caries, trauma or cavity preparation.

Small canals running from the pulp chamber to the furcation region are common in deciduous molars. In the slender roots of deciduous molars, the root canals are narrower and more ribbon-shaped than those in permanent teeth. Note that the maxillary first deciduous molar has 2–4 root canals, with two canals in the mesiobuccal root in 75% of cases. The palatal and distobuccal roots are often fused (one-third of cases), but contain distinct canals.

Furthermore, the maxillary second deciduous molar has 2–5 root canals (the mesiobuccal root usually bifurcates or contains two canals). Palatal and distobuccal roots sometimes fuse and contain a single, common canal. The mandibular first deciduous molar may have 2–4 canals (most mesial roots have two); the mandibular second deciduous molar usually has three canals, but can vary from two to five (two are often seen in mesial roots).

The occlusion of the permanent teeth

Occlusion refers to the relationship of the dental arches when tooth contact is made. Both the maxillary and mandibular dental arches take the form of catenary curves. The positions of the teeth within the dental arch are determined by numerous factors and forces. Indeed, the spatial configuration of the arches is dependent upon an interaction between the eruptive movements carrying the teeth into their functional positions and, once the teeth have erupted, the forces brought to bear upon each tooth; the size of the dental arches varies considerably between individuals.

Viewed labially, the maxillary incisors have slight distal inclinations whereas the canine has a distinct mesial angulation. When these teeth are viewed distally, all show pronounced proclinations into the lip (although the canine is slightly more vertical). For the mandibular incisors and canine, when viewed labially, the incisors are more or less vertical and the canine has a slight mesial inclination. When viewed distally, these anterior mandibular teeth, like the anterior maxillary teeth, are proclined. When viewed buccally, the maxillary premolars and molars change from a slight mesial angulation (premolars) to a distal inclination (the third molar). This contrasts with the mandibular posterior teeth, which show increasing mesial inclination moving back through the arch. When the maxillary premolars and molars are viewed distally, the teeth change from being essentially vertical in the premolar region to being distinctly buccally inclined in the molars. This again contrasts with the mandibular premolars and molars, where the teeth become more lingually inclined moving through the arch.

The teeth align themselves such that the occlusal plane is not flat but describes a relatively linear curve in the anteroposterior direction, the curves of Spee. The occlusal curves of Wilson are aligned in the transverse plane. The curves of Wilson are such that the occlusal surfaces of the mandibular molars are directed lingually, while those of the maxillary molars are directed buccally. With age, and as a result of wear, the cusps of the teeth are worn away so that the curvatures of the occlusal plane are lost and the planes become flat.

Centric occlusal position

The centric occlusal position is the terminal position of physiological jaw movements and is the relationship between the two arches when the teeth are brought into contact with the mandibular condyles centrally positioned, at rest, in the mandibular fossae. The key to the intercuspal relationships between the teeth in the centric occlusal position is to be found in the relative positions of the maxillary and mandibular first permanent molars. In the normal centric occlusion, each arch is bilaterally symmetrical but, because the anterior maxillary segment is slightly larger than the corresponding mandibular segment (due to the unequal sizes of the maxillary and mandibular first incisors), each maxillary tooth will contact its corresponding mandibular antagonist and its distal neighbour. Thus, the maxillary first permanent molar will contact the distal part of the mandibular first permanent molar and the mesial part of the mandibular second permanent molar. The only exceptions are the mandibular first incisor and the maxillary third molar.

As the maxillary arch is a little larger and broader than the mandibular arch, there is a slight overlap of the mandibular arch by the maxillary arch such that the buccal cusps of the maxillary teeth extend a few millimetres beyond the buccal occlusal edge of the mandibular teeth. This overlap is termed overjet. When the buccolingual incisor relationships in anatomical centric occlusion are considered, two types of 'overlap' of the mandibular incisors by the maxillary incisors can be discerned. The overlap in the horizontal plane (overjet) is approximately 2–3 mm. The vertical overlap, specific to the incisors and canines, is termed overbite. The overbite in anatomical centric occlusion is such that the palatal surfaces of the maxillary incisors on average overlap the incisal third of the labial surfaces of the mandibular incisors.

'Centric stops' (sometimes referred to as 'holding contacts') represent the intercuspal contact positions. When the 32 teeth within the permanent dentition occlude, there are 138 centric stops, although this is seldom achieved during the normal bite. The major markings register on the occlusal surfaces of the posterior teeth. The slopes of the maxillary palatal cusps make stops coincident with the stops within the central fossae of the mandibular posterior teeth. The stops in the central fossae of the maxillary teeth coincide with the stops on the slopes of the buccal cusps of the mandibular posterior teeth. The cusps seated in the central fossae are sometimes referred to as 'supporting cusps'. As befits the anatomical overjet relationships, the tips of the maxillary buccal cusps and the mandibular lingual cusps remain relatively unmarked. For the anterior teeth, the mandibular incisors have the 'centric stops' on the incisal edges, whereas the stops on the maxillary incisors are positioned down the palatal surfaces.

Malocclusions

Malocclusions result from:

- malposition of individual teeth
- malrelationship of the dental arches
- variation in skeletal morphology of the jaws.

Two classifications describing malposition of teeth and malrelationship of the arches are in general use: Angle's classification and a classification based upon the relationships of the incisors. A classification of malocclusion based upon canine relationships is also available for clinical use. However, this is much less employed than Angle's classification and the incisor relationship classification.

Angle's classification of malocclusion

Angle's classification of malocclusion relies upon the relationship of the arches in the anteroposterior plane using the maxillary and mandibular first permanent molars as key teeth:

- For Angle's class I malocclusion, although one or more of the teeth are malpositioned, this does not affect the 'normal' relationship of the first permanent molars (i.e. the maxillary first molar occludes with the mandibular first and second molars).
- Angle's class II malocclusion is characterized by a 'prenormal' maxillary arch relationship, the maxillary first permanent molars occluding at least half a cusp more mesial to the mandibular first permanent molars than the 'normal' position:
  - Angle's class II (division 1) indicates that the maxillary incisors are proclined.
  - For Angle's class II malocclusion (division 2), the molar relationship is 'prenormal' but the maxillary incisors are retroclined. Frequently, only the first incisors are retroclined, the second incisors being proclined.
- Angle's class III malocclusion is characterized by a 'postnormal' maxillary arch relationship, the maxillary first permanent molars occluding at least half a cusp more distal to the mandibular first permanent molars than the 'standard' anatomical position. The incisor relationship varies from 'normal' overjet to an 'edge-to-edge' bite to reverse overjet (where the mandibular incisors lie labially to the maxillary incisors).

Classification based on incisor relationships

As the permanent molars do not have a fixed relationship in the arch and may migrate following early loss of deciduous teeth, the classification of malocclusion based upon incisor relationships is often preferred to Angle's classification. Furthermore, a classification of malocclusion related to the incisors is seen by many clinicians as being more appropriate because a major objective of orthodontic treatment is to establish an anatomical incisor relationship (patients being more concerned and aware of the aesthetics of the incisor relationship than they are of the molar relationship). As for Angle's classification, the classification of malocclusions based upon incisor relationships uses the categories class I, class II (division 1), class II (division 2) and class III. However, care must be taken not to confuse these classifications — for example, an Angle's class I molar relationship might exist alongside an incisor class III relationship in the same person! The classification relies upon the relationship of incisors relative to a specific landmark: the cingulum plateau on the maxillary first incisor.

- Class I incisor relationship represents a situation in which the incisors do not show any malposition. The incisal margins of the mandibular incisors occlude with, or lie directly below, the middle of the palatal surfaces of the maxillary incisors (i.e. on the cingulum plateau).
- For Class II incisor relationship, the incisal margins of the mandibular incisors lie behind the cingulum plateau on the palatal surfaces of the maxillary incisors:

- Division 1 indicates that the maxillary first incisors are proclined.
- Division 2 indicates that the maxillary first incisors are retroclined.
- For Class III incisor relationship, the incisal margins of the mandibular incisors lie in front of the cingulum plateau on the palatal surfaces of the maxillary incisors, providing reduced overjet, edge-to-edge bite or a reverse overjet.

Self-assessment: questions

True/false statements

Which of the following statements are true and which are false?

a. The maxillary first permanent incisor frequently exhibits a pit in front of the palatal cingulum.

b. The maxillary permanent canine presents a marked convexity at the junction of the mesial surface and incisal edge.

c. The maxillary first premolar has two pulp horns, one for each cusp, extending from the roof of the pulp chamber.

d. The tip of the palatal cusp of the maxillary second premolar is generally displaced towards the distal surface of the crown.

e. The outline of the maxillary first permanent molar is rhombic, the mesiopalatal and distobuccal angles being obtuse.

f. The distal root of the mandibular first permanent molar invariably contains two root canals.

g. The maxillary third permanent molar is the tooth most likely to become impacted.

h. Like their permanent successors, the roots of the mandibular deciduous incisors are compressed mesiodistally.

i. The buccal surface of the crown of the mandibular first deciduous molar shows a conspicuous bulge above the distal root.

j. A cusp of Carabelli is frequently found on the maxillary second deciduous molar.

k. Viewed occlusally, the dental arches are generally rectangular in form.

l. Normal (anatomical) occlusion represents the occlusion most prevalent in the community.

m. When the teeth are in centric occlusion, the mandibular condyles are centrally positioned in the mandibular (glenoid) fossae of the temporal bones.

n. All mandibular molars bear a distal relationship to the maxillary molars.

o. Excluding the permanent third molars, the most commonly malaligned tooth is the permanent maxillary canine.

Extended matching questions

Theme: The permanent dentition

Lead-in

Select the most appropriate option to answer items 1–5. Each option can be used once, more than once or not at all.

Item list

1. A tooth that consistently displays a tubercle of Carabelli
2. A tooth possessing a canine fossa on its mesial surface
3. A tooth possessing a foramen caecum
4. A tooth usually with two roots — buccal and palatal
5. A tooth that commonly has a cross-shaped fissure pattern

Option list

A. Deciduous mandibular molar (first)
B. Deciduous mandibular molar (second)
C. Deciduous maxillary molar (first)
D. Deciduous maxillary molar (second)
E. Permanent mandibular canine
F. Permanent mandibular incisor (first)
G. Permanent mandibular incisor (second)
H. Permanent mandibular premolar (first)
I. Permanent mandibular premolar (second)
J. Permanent mandibular molar (first)
K. Permanent mandibular molar (second)
L. Permanent maxillary canine
M. Permanent maxillary incisor (first)
N. Permanent maxillary incisor (second)
O. Permanent maxillary premolar (first)
P. Permanent maxillary premolar (second)
Q. Permanent maxillary molar (first)
R. Permanent maxillary molar (second)

Theme: Occlusion of the permanent dentition

Lead-in

Select the most appropriate option to answer items 1–5. Each option can be used once, more than once or not at all.

Item list

1. Term used to describe a position of equilibrium of forces tending to stabilize tooth position
2. Term used to describe the gap between the two dental arches at rest
3. Term used to describe the shape of a dental arch in the sagittal plane
4. Term used to describe the overlapping of the mandibular dental arch by the maxillary arch
5. Term used to describe an occlusion where one side of the maxilla lies inside the bite while the other side lies outside the bite

Option list

A. Centric stops
B. Competent overlap
C. Crossbite
D. Curve of Monson
E. Curve of Spee
F. Curve of Wilson
G. Freeway space
H. Neutral zone
I. Open bite
J. Overbite
K. Overclosure
L. Overjet
M. Proclination
N. Retroclination

Self-assessment: questions

Picture questions

Figure 3.1

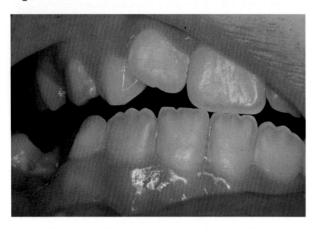

a. Is there anything unusual about the incisal margins of the mandibular permanent incisors?

Figure 3.2

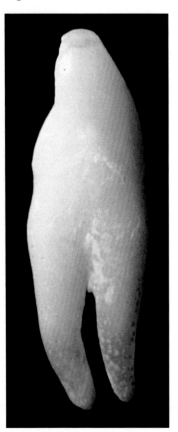

a. Is there anything unusual about this mandibular permanent canine?

Figure 3.3

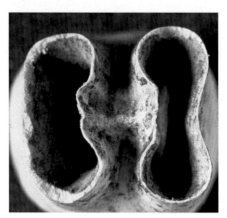

a. How do you account for the appearance of the roots of this tooth?

For each illustration (Figures 3.4–3.12)
a. Identify the tooth, indicating the surface viewed.
b. Give the age at which the crown of each tooth commences calcification.
c. Give the age at which each tooth erupts into the oral cavity.
d. For Figures 3.4, 3.7, 3.8 and 3.9, list the nerves which must be anaesthetized in order to extract the tooth.

Self-assessment: questions

Figure 3.4

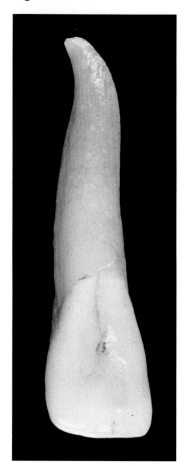

Figure 3.5

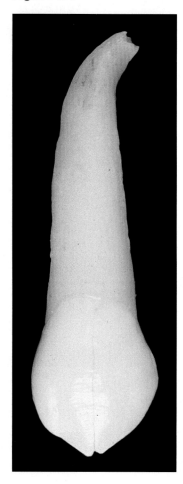

Figure 3.7

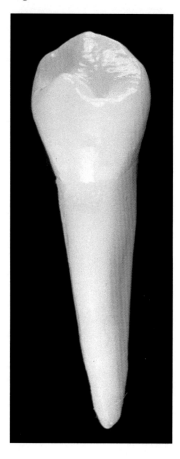

Figure 3.6

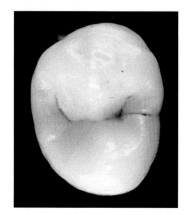

Self-assessment: questions

Figure 3.8

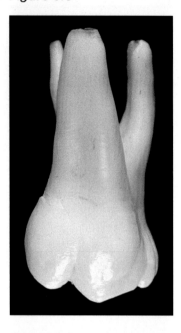

Figure 3.9

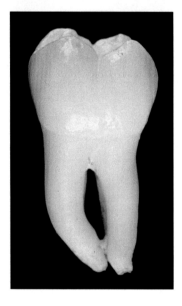

Figure 3.10

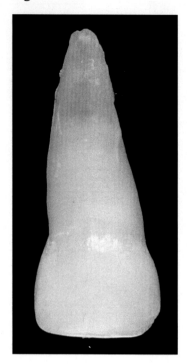

Figure 3.11

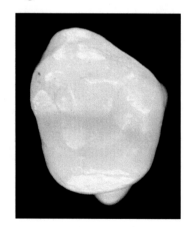

Self-assessment: questions

Figure 3.12

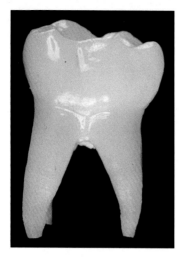

Figure 3.14 (Courtesy of Dr P. Smith)

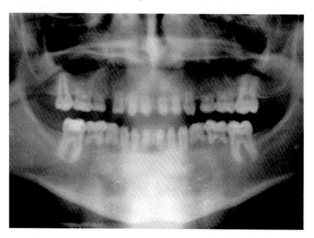

a. Is anything abnormal in this radiograph of the dentition?

Figure 3.13 (Courtesy of Dr P. Smith)

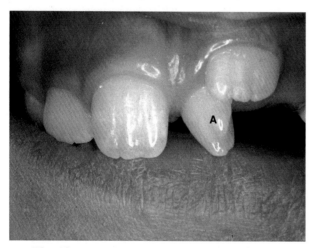

a. Identify structure A.
b. How else may it present clinically?

Figure 3.15

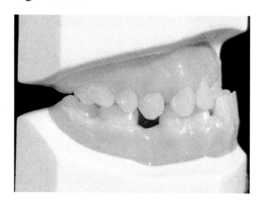

a. Using Angle's classification of occlusion, identify the occlusion illustrated here.

Self-assessment: questions

Figure 3.16

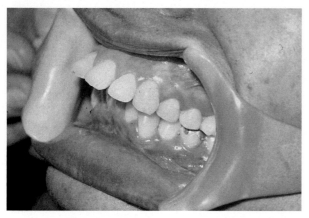

a. Using the incisor classification of occlusion, identify the malocclusion shown here.
b. Why is the incisor classification now preferred in the clinic to Angle's classification?

Figure 3.17

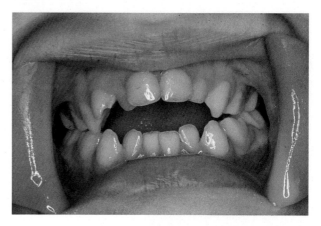

a. What malocclusion is evident in this patient and with what underlying condition may it be associated?

Essay questions

1. Compare and contrast permanent molars with deciduous molars.
2. Describe root morphology in the permanent dentition highlighting, wherever possible, the clinical relevance.
3. Describe the various classifications used to categorize malocclusions and discuss whether these are clinically and functionally adequate as classifications.

Self-assessment: answers

True/false answers

a. **False**. It is the maxillary second permanent incisor that presents the pit (foramen caecum).

b. **False**. The convexity lies at the junction of the incisal edge with the distal surface.

c. **True**. This is the normal pattern for cusps; however, a pulp horn is not found beneath the small lingual cusp of the mandibular first premolar.

d. **False**. The tip of the palatal cusp is generally displaced towards the mesial surface of the crown.

e. **True**. The acute angles of this tooth are the mesiobuccal and the distopalatal angles.

f. **False**. It is the mesial root that possesses two root canals.

g. **False**. The maxillary third permanent molar is rarely impacted, as it tends to be angled distally. It is the mandibular third molar that is most commonly impacted, being angled mesially.

h. **False**. The roots of the mandibular deciduous incisors have a rounded outline.

i. **False**. The bulge (molar tubercle) lies near the cervical margin above the mesial root.

j. **True**. A cusp of Carabelli is found frequently on this tooth, just as in the maxillary first permanent molar.

k. **False**. The dental arches are shaped as a catenary curve; rectangular forms are associated more with apes.

l. **False**. Malocclusion is most prevalent in the community. 'Normal' occlusion is found in only about 10% of the population (USA data).

m. **True**. Centric occlusal position is the standard occlusal position to assess the 'bite' of a patient. However, it is all too frequently difficult to achieve; palpation of the condyles in the mandibular (glenoid) fossae might aid the attainment of centric occlusal position.

n. **False**. In the 'normal' (or anatomical) occlusal position, a maxillary tooth will occlude with the distal portion of the corresponding mandibular tooth plus the mesial portion of the mandibular tooth distally.

o. **False**. Although the permanent maxillary canines are indeed frequently malaligned, the maxillary incisors are most often in malocclusion.

Extended matching answers

Theme: The permanent dentition

Item 1 = Option Q. A Carabelli trait (tubercle or even an extra cusp) is most commonly found on the permanent maxillary first molar tooth (60% of teeth). It can also be found, but rarely, on the second molar tooth. In the deciduous dentition, it can also be seen on the maxillary second molar.

Item 2 = Option O. A canine fossa is found on the mesial surface of the permanent maxillary first premolar tooth. Also on this surface is a canine groove (a continuation of the occlusal fissure across the mesial marginal ridge).

Item 3 = Option N. The foramen caecum is a pit characteristic of the permanent maxillary second (lateral) incisor tooth. It is located on the palatal surface close to the cingulum. The pit may extend some way from the crown and down into the root, and may be at risk from caries.

Item 4 = Option O. The permanent maxillary first premolar is the only premolar with more than one root.

Item 5 = Option K. The permanent mandibular second molar tooth has four cusps and a cross-shaped fissure pattern on the occlusal surface between the cusps.

Theme: Occlusion of the permanent dentition

Item 1 = Option H. Teeth are acted upon by many forces in the mouth – masticatory loads and forces from the tongue, lips and cheeks — and potentially the teeth move according to the direction and magnitude of these loads. 'Neutral zone' is a rather abstract term used to suggest that teeth will have their positions in the dental arches stabilized when there is an equilibrium of forces.

Item 2 = Option G. At rest, the teeth in the opposing dental arches do not bite together but show a slight gap (usually 2 mm) called 'freeway space'. This space is characteristic of the individual and is probably maintained by resting muscle length that controls mandibular posture. Dental procedures that unnecessarily affect 'freeway space' will result in unwanted strain on the facial musculature and can also badly affect facial profiles.

Item 3 = Option E. The curve of Spee describes the curvatures of the dental arches in the sagittal (anteroposterior) plane. The curves of Wilson describe the curvatures of the posterior teeth in the coronal (transverse) plane. The curves of Monson (often erroneously used to describe the curves of Wilson) combine both curves as if the teeth rested on a segment of a sphere of about 10 cm. This 'sphere', however, has not been successfully demonstrated.

Item 4 = Option L. The maxillary arch is slightly larger and broader than the mandibular arch and therefore usually overlaps the mandibular arch by a couple of millimetres. This overlap is termed overjet. Overbite refers to the way the maxillary incisors and canine vertically overlap the labial surfaces of the mandibular incisors and canine.

Item 5 = Option C. Crossbite is a transverse abnormality of the dental arches where there is an asymmetrical bite. It may be unilateral (as in this question) or bilateral. Crossbites are frequently related to discrepancies in the widths of the dental bases and may involve the displacement of the mandible to one side to obtain maximal intercuspation.

Self-assessment: answers

Picture answers

Figure 3.1

a. The notched incisal margin, containing three mammelons, is normal in the recently erupted tooth but is lost with attrition.

Figure 3.2

a. Yes, the tooth has two roots instead of its usual single root. This may be clinically significant during endodontic treatment or tooth extraction.

Figure 3.3

a. The wide-open pulp and the smooth, thin lining of dentine indicate that the root is incomplete and still forming.

Figure 3.4

a. Maxillary left second (lateral) permanent incisor. Palatal view.
b. 10–12 months.
c. 8–9 years.
d. Anterior superior alveolar nerve, infra-orbital nerve, nasopalatine nerve.

Figure 3.5

a. Maxillary left permanent canine. Labial view.
b. 4–5 months.
c. 11–12 years.

Figure 3.6

a. Maxillary right first premolar. Occlusal view.
b. 1½–2 years.
c. 10–11 years.

Figure 3.7

a. Mandibular right first premolar. Lingual view.
b. 1½–2 years.
c. 10–12 years.
d. Inferior alveolar nerve, mental nerve (possibly the buccal nerve), lingual nerve.

Figure 3.8

a. Maxillary left first permanent molar. Palatal view.
b. Birth.
c. 6–7 years.
d. Posterior and middle superior alveolar nerves, buccal nerve, greater palatine nerve.

Figure 3.9

a. Mandibular right second permanent molar. Buccal view.
b. 2½–3 years.
c. 12–13 years.
d. Inferior alveolar nerve, buccal nerve, lingual nerve.

Figure 3.10

a. Maxillary left first (central) deciduous incisor. Labial view.
b. 4 months in utero.
c. 7 months.

Figure 3.11

a. Maxillary left first deciduous molar. Occlusal view.
b. 5 months in utero.
c. 1–1½ years.

Figure 3.12

a. Mandibular left second deciduous molar. Buccal view.
b. 6 months in utero.
c. 1½–2½ years.

Figure 3.13

a. Structure A is a supernumerary tooth which has erupted into the palate behind the permanent incisors. The supernumerary tooth usually has a simplified cone-shaped form. It most commonly occurs in this region, when it is called a mesiodens. It may remain unerupted and be discovered on a radiograph when the patient presents with delayed eruption of the permanent maxillary incisor(s).

Figure 3.14

a. Yes. As evident from the fully erupted first permanent molars, the patient is about 9 years of age. However, all the remaining permanent teeth have failed to develop and the deciduous dentition has been completely retained.

Figure 3.15

a. Angle's class III malocclusion — the first permanent molars almost have a cusp-to-cusp relationship (the mandibular molars being 'prenormal' relative to the maxillary molars). Note that the reverse overjet for the incisors is not necessarily indicative of an Angle's class III malocclusion (there may be a normal overjet or edge-to-edge bite).

Self-assessment: answers

Figure 3.16

a. In terms of the incisor classification of occlusion, the malocclusion is designated class II division 1 — the tip of the mandibular incisors lying behind the cingulum of the maxillary incisors, which themselves show marked proclination.

b. Angle's classification, using the position of the permanent first molar teeth, may be affected by movement of these teeth in response to loss of other teeth in the arches or, being the first of the permanent teeth to erupt into the mouth, they may themselves be lost because of dental caries. Furthermore, patients are more likely to come to the orthodontist complaining of 'unsightly' malposition of their anterior teeth than about malposition of their molars.

Figure 3.17

a. This patient has an anterior open bite, the mandibular incisors not being overlapped (overbite) by the maxillary incisors. The condition may be associated with an anterior tongue thrust on swallowing, or the patient may be a habitual thumb sucker. It may also be associated with an abnormal and premature occlusal contact on the posterior teeth. It may also be related to underdevelopment of the anterior segment of the maxillae.

Outline essay answers

Question 1

The introductory paragraph should provide some general information concerning the human dentition, e.g. relating to diphyodonty, heterodonty and omnivorous diet. There should also be a definition of molars and a brief description of their functions.

A description of the general differences between deciduous and permanent teeth should follow, then descriptions of specific differences between deciduous and permanent molars (including numbers and location, chronology of development, and crown and root morphologies). Mention should be made of the fact that deciduous molars are replaced by permanent premolars and not molars.

For comparisons of the morphology of the teeth, diagrams are most useful (even if 'non-artistic'!).

The concluding paragraph should summarize the essential differences.

Question 2

The introductory paragraph should define roots (anatomical and clinical definitions) and mention the tissues comprising the roots (together with a diagram). Brief mention should also be made of root development (with a diagram) and of pulp morphology with respect to roots (again with a diagram).

There should follow a description of root morphology for each of the permanent incisors and canines (maxillary and mandibular), with appropriate diagrams.

The root morphology of the permanent premolars and molars (maxillary and mandibular) should be described, with appropriate diagrams.

Comparisons of deciduous versus permanent root morphologies can be briefly outlined.

General descriptions of the cervical margins (where anatomical crown meets anatomical root) can be provided, again with appropriate diagrams.

The final paragraph(s) should highlight some clinical considerations, for example:

- ageing
- pulp inflammation
- dental abscesses
- root canal therapy
- need to avoid pulps during conservation treatment
- pulpectomies
- others (e.g. pulp stones).

Question 3

The introductory paragraph should provide a definition of occlusion and include a discussion of the meaning of the word 'normal' as in 'normal centric occlusion'. Centric occlusion should be described, along with an explanation of how it is achieved in the patient (indeed, the difficulties of achieving centric occlusion should be alluded to).

A description of Angle's classification of malocclusion (with diagrams) should follow and then a description of the incisor and canine classifications of malocclusion (with diagrams). Comparisons of these classifications should highlight the relative merits (and demerits) of Angle's and incisor classifications. It should be emphasized that the classifications of occlusion and malocclusions are not functional and 'dynamic', but are 'static' morphological constructs.

The final paragraph should emphasize the controversies and difficulties outlined in the body of the essay and should end by discussing whether malocclusions are pathological or normal variations.

Chapter 4

Orofacial musculature, mastication and swallowing

Orofacial musculature	**36**
Muscles of mastication	36
Floor of the mouth	38
Muscles of the tongue	38
Muscles of facial expression	38
Muscles of the soft palate	39
Mastication	**39**
Chewing cycle	40
Control of mastication	41
Swallowing	**42**
Stages of swallowing	42
Swallowing centre	43
Swallowing reflexes	43
Self-assessment: questions	44
Self-assessment: answers	**47**

Overview

Extra-orally, the muscles of mastication move the mandible at the temporomandibular joint while the circumoral muscles of facial expression change the shapes and positions of the lips. In the suprahyoid region, the digastric, mylohyoid and geniohyoid muscles are located in the floor of the mouth. Intra-orally, the soft palate (the movable part of the palate) is raised and elevated by muscles during and after swallowing and the shape and position of the tongue is affected by intrinsic and extrinsic musculature (see pages 52–53). Chewing (mastication) and swallowing (deglutition) are important functions involving the orofacial musculature.

Learning objectives

You should:
- be able to describe the locations, attachments, functions and innervations of the muscles influencing mandibular movements and movements of the lips, cheeks and floor of the mouth, and the soft palate (for the musculature of the tongue, see pages 52–53)
- understand the physiological mechanisms underlying the processes (and control) of mastication and swallowing.

Orofacial musculature

Muscles of mastication

Although many muscles, both in the head and the neck, are involved in mastication, the 'muscles of mastication' is a collective term reserved for the masseter, temporalis, and medial and lateral pterygoid muscles. All the muscles of mastication receive their innervation from the mandibular division of the trigeminal nerve. Closely associated functionally with the muscles of mastication is the digastric muscle. The masseter and temporalis muscles lie on the superficial face, while the lateral and medial pterygoid muscles lie deeper within the infratemporal fossa.

Masseter

The masseter muscle consists of two overlapping heads:

- The superficial head arises from the zygomatic process of the maxilla and from the anterior two-thirds of the lower border of the zygomatic arch.
- The deep head arises from the deep surface of the zygomatic arch.

Internally, the muscle has many tendinous septa that greatly increase the area for muscle attachment and which provide a multipennate arrangement, thereby increasing its power. The superficial head passes downwards and backwards to insert into the lower half of the lateral surface of the ramus. The deep head, whose posterior fibres are more vertically oriented, inserts into the upper half of the lateral surface of the ramus, particularly over the coronoid process. The muscle elevates the mandible and is primarily active when grinding tough food. Indeed, the muscle exerts considerable power when the mandible is close to the centric occlusal position. On the basis of its fibre orientation, the posterior fibres of the deep head may have some retrusive capability for the mandible.

Temporalis

The temporalis muscle is the largest muscle of mastication. It takes origin from the floor of the temporal fossa of the lateral surface of the skull and from the overlying temporal fascia, and should thus be regarded as a bipennate muscle.

The attachment is limited above by the inferior temporal line. From this wide origin, the fibres converge towards their insertion on the apex, the anterior and posterior borders, and the medial surface of the coronoid process. Indeed, the insertion extends down the anterior border of the ramus almost as far as the third molar tooth. The posterior fibres of the muscle pass horizontally forwards while the anterior fibres pass vertically downwards on to the coronoid process. To reach the coronoid process, the muscle runs beneath the zygomatic arch. The anterior (vertical) part elevates the mandible, while the posterior (horizontal) part retracts the protruded mandible. In certain sites, the masseter and temporalis muscles are joined. This is particularly so for the deep fibres of the deep head of the masseter and the overlying temporalis muscle. The functional significance of this 'zygomatico-mandibular mass' is unclear.

Both the masseter and the temporalis muscles are innervated by branches of the anterior division of the mandibular nerve. Both receive their blood supply from the maxillary artery (masseteric and deep temporal branches), the superficial temporal artery (transverse facial and middle temporal branches) and, for the masseter muscle, the facial artery.

Pterygoids

Lateral pterygoid

The lateral pterygoid muscle lies in the roof of the infratemporal fossa and has essentially a horizontal alignment. It has two heads, superior and inferior:

- The superior (upper) head is the smaller and arises from the infratemporal surface of the greater wing of the sphenoid bone.
- The inferior (lower) head forms the bulk of the muscle and takes origin from the lateral surface of the lateral pterygoid plate of the sphenoid bone.

Both heads pass backwards and outwards and appear to merge before their areas of insertion. The fibres of the superior head insert into the capsule and possibly the medial aspect of the anterior border of the intra-articular disc of the TMJ. The fibres of the inferior head of the lateral pterygoid muscle insert into the pterygoid fovea of the mandibular condyle. However, the precise insertions of the muscle are still controversial and have clinical relevance with regard to TMJ disorders, particularly internal derangement, where the disc is displaced, usually in an anteromedial position, and the jaw may become locked. Such conditions may be associated with clicking joints, limited jaw movements and pain, and some have attributed variations in the attachment, and therefore function, of the superior head as an aetiological factor in the disease. Functionally, the superior and inferior heads should be considered as two separate muscles. The inferior head is concerned with mandibular protrusion, depression and lateral excursions. The superior head is activated during mandibular retrusion (providing controlled movements) and during clenching of the mandible.

Medial pterygoid

The medial pterygoid muscle consists of two heads:

- The bulk of the muscle arises as a deep head from the medial surface of the lateral pterygoid plate of the sphenoid bone.
- The smaller superficial head arises from the maxillary tuberosity and the neighbouring part of the palatine bone (pyramidal process).

From these sites of origin, the fibres of the medial pterygoid pass downwards, backwards and laterally to insert into the roughened surface of the medial aspect of the angle of the mandible. Tendinous septa within the muscle increase the surface area for muscle attachment, providing a multipennate arrangement and therefore increasing the power the muscle can exert. The main action of the muscle is to elevate the mandible, but it also assists in lateral and protrusive movements. An accessory medial pterygoid muscle has been described as a separate slip of muscle close to the deep surface of the medial pterygoid. This takes origin from the base of the skull close to the foramen ovale and merges with the deep head of the medial pterygoid. Its function is unknown. The masseter and medial pterygoid muscles together form a muscular sling that supports the mandible on the cranium.

The medial pterygoid muscle is innervated by a branch of the mandibular nerve that arises proximal to the division of the mandibular nerve into anterior and posterior trunks. The lateral pterygoid receives its nerve supply from the anterior trunk. Both muscles receive their blood supply as muscular branches from the maxillary artery.

Digastric

Because of its functional associations, the digastric muscle is described here, although it usually is not strictly classified as a 'muscle of mastication'. This muscle is located below the inferior border of the mandible and consists of an anterior and a posterior belly connected by an intermediate tendon:

- The posterior belly arises from the mastoid notch immediately behind the mastoid process of the temporal bone; it passes downwards and forwards towards the hyoid bone, where it becomes the digastric tendon. The digastric muscle passes through the insertion of the stylohyoid muscle and is attached to the greater horn of the hyoid bone by a fibrous loop.
- The anterior belly of the digastric muscle is attached to the digastric fossa on the inferior border of the mandible and runs downwards and backwards to the digastric tendon.

The digastric muscle depresses and retrudes the mandible, and is involved in stabilizing the position of the hyoid bone and in elevation of the hyoid during swallowing.

The anterior belly of the digastric muscle is innervated by the mylohyoid branch of the mandibular division of the trigeminal nerve, the posterior belly by the digastric branch of the facial nerve. This reflects different embryological origins, from first and second pharyngeal (branchial) arch mesenchyme respectively. The anterior belly receives its blood supply from the facial artery, the posterior belly from the posterior auricular and occipital arteries.

Floor of the mouth

The floor of the mouth is the region located between the medial surface of the mandible, the inferior surface of the tongue and the mylohyoid muscles. The mylohyoid muscles are attached to the mylohyoid lines of the mandible and consequently structures above these lines are related to the floor of the mouth, whereas structures below the lines are related to the upper part of the neck. This concept is of considerable clinical importance with respect to the spread of inflammation from infected teeth within the mandible. The two mylohyoid muscles form a muscular diaphragm for the floor of the mouth. Above this diaphragm are found the genioglossus and geniohyoid muscles medially and the hyoglossus laterally. Below the diaphragm lie the digastric and stylohyoid muscles.

Mylohyoid

The mylohyoid muscle arises from the mylohyoid line on the medial surface of the body of the mandible. Its fibres slope downwards, forwards and inwards. The anterior fibres of the mylohyoid muscle interdigitate with the corresponding fibres on the opposite side to form a median raphe. This raphe is attached above to the chin and below to the hyoid bone. The posterior fibres are inserted on to the anterior surface of the body of the hyoid bone. The muscle raises the floor of the mouth during the early stages of swallowing. It also helps to depress the mandible when the hyoid bone is fixed. The mylohyoid muscle is supplied by the mylohyoid branch of the inferior alveolar branch of the mandibular division of the trigeminal nerve. Its blood supply is derived from the lingual artery (sublingual branch), the maxillary artery (mylohyoid branch of the inferior alveolar artery) and the facial artery (submental branch).

Geniohyoid

The geniohyoid muscle originates from the inferior genial tubercle (mental spine). It passes backwards and slightly downwards to insert onto the anterior surface of the body of the hyoid bone. The geniohyoid muscle elevates the hyoid bone and is a weak depressor of the mandible. Its innervation is from the first cervical spinal nerve travelling with the hypoglossal nerve. Its blood supply is derived from the lingual artery (sublingual branch).

Muscles of the tongue

The intrinsic and extrinsic muscles of the tongue are described on pages 52–53.

Muscles of facial expression

The muscles of facial expression are characterized by:

• their superficial arrangement in the face
• their activities on the skin (brought about directly by their attachment to the facial integument)
• by their common motor innervation, the facial nerve.

Functionally, the muscles of facial expression are grouped around the orifices of the face (the orbit, nose, ear and mouth) and should be considered primarily as muscles controlling the degree of opening and closing of these apertures; the expressive functions of the muscles have developed secondarily. The muscles of facial expression vary considerably between individuals in terms of size, shape and strength. The superficial muscles around the lips and cheeks may be subdivided into two groups:

• The various parts of the orbicularis oris muscle
• Muscles that are radially arranged from the orbicularis oris muscle.

The fibres of orbicularis oris pass around the lips. The muscle is divided into four parts, each part corresponding to a quadrant of the lips. Its muscle fibres do not gain attachment directly to bone but occupy a central part of the lip. Muscle fibres in the philtrum insert onto the nasal septum. The range of movement produced by orbicularis oris includes lip closure, protrusion and pursing. The radial muscles can be divided into superficial and deep muscles of the upper and lower lips:

• The levator labii superioris, levator labii superioris alaeque nasi and zygomaticus major and minor are superficial muscles of the upper lip.
• The levator anguli oris is a deep muscle of the upper lip.
• The depressor anguli oris is a superficial muscle of the lower lip.
• The depressor labii inferioris and mentalis muscle are deep muscles of the lower lip.

As their names suggest, the levator labii superioris elevates the upper lip, the depressor labii inferioris depresses the lower lip, and the corners of the mouth are raised and lowered by the levator and depressor anguli oris muscles.

Two muscles extend to the corner of the mouth: the risorius and buccinator muscles, risorius lying superficial to the buccinator:

• The risorius muscle stretches the angles of the mouth laterally.
• The buccinator muscle arises from the pterygomandibular raphe and from the buccal side of the maxillary and mandibular alveoli above the molar teeth. Most of its fibres insert into mucous membrane covering the cheek; other fibres intercalate with orbicularis oris in the lips. As the fibres of the buccinator converge towards the angle of the mouth, the central fibres decussate. The main function of the buccinator muscle is to maintain the tension of the cheek against the teeth during mastication.

Muscles of the soft palate

The soft palate is supported by the fibrous palatine aponeurosis whose shape and position is altered by the activity of four pairs of muscles: the tensor veli palatini, the levator veli palatini, the palatoglossus and the palatopharyngeus muscles. In addition, there is the musculus uvulae intrinsic muscle of the soft palate.

Tensor veli palatini

The tensor veli palatini muscle arises from the scaphoid fossa of the sphenoid bone at the root of the pterygoid plates and from the lateral side of the cartilaginous part of the auditory (pharyngotympanic) tube. From its origin, the fibres converge towards the pterygoid hamulus, whence the muscle becomes tendinous, the tendon bending at right angles around the hamulus to become the palatine aponeurosis. The anterior border of the aponeurosis is attached to the posterior border of the hard palate. Medially, it merges with the aponeurosis of the other side. Posteriorly, it becomes indistinct, merging with submucosa at the posterior edge of the soft palate. When the tensor veli palatini muscle contracts, the aponeurosis becomes a taut, horizontal plate of tissue upon which other palatine muscles may act to change its position.

The motor innervation of the tensor veli palatini is derived from the mandibular branch of the trigeminal nerve (via the nerve to the medial pterygoid muscle and the otic ganglion).

Levator veli palatini

The levator veli palatini muscle originates from the base of the skull at the apex of the petrous part of the temporal bone, anterior to the opening of the carotid canal, and from the medial side of the cartilaginous part of the auditory tube. The muscle curves downwards, medially and forwards to enter the palate immediately below the opening of the auditory tube. The levator muscles of the palate form a U-shaped muscular sling. When the palatine aponeurosis is stiffened by the tensor muscles, contraction of the levator muscles produces an upwards and backwards movement of the soft palate. In this way, the nasopharynx is shut off from the oropharynx by the apposition of the soft palate on to the posterior wall of the pharynx.

Palatopharyngeus

The palatopharyngeus muscle arises from two heads: one from the posterior border of the hard palate, the other from the upper surface of the palatine aponeurosis. The two heads unite after arching over the lateral edge of the palatine aponeurosis, where the muscle passes downwards beneath the mucous membrane of the lateral wall of the oropharynx as the posterior pillar of the fauces (palatopharyngeal arch). The muscle is inserted into the posterior border of the thyroid cartilage of the larynx. The main action of the palatopharyngeus muscle is to elevate the larynx and pharynx, but it may also arch the relaxed palate and depress the tensed palate.

Palatoglossus

The palatoglossus muscle arises from the aponeurosis of the soft palate and descends to the tongue in the anterior pillar of the fauces, whence its fibres intercalate with the transverse fibres of the tongue. The action of the palatoglossus is to raise the tongue in order to narrow the transverse diameter of the oropharyngeal isthmus.

Musculus uvulae

The musculus uvulae muscle arises from the posterior nasal spine at the back of the hard palate and from the palatine aponeurosis. It passes backwards and downwards to insert into the mucosa of the uvula. It moves the uvula upwards and laterally, and helps to complete the seal between the soft palate and pharynx in the midline region when the palate is elevated.

With the exception of the tensor veli palatini muscle, the nerve supply to the muscles of the palate is derived from the cranial part of the accessory nerve via the pharyngeal plexus. The arterial supply to the muscles of the soft palate is derived from the facial artery (ascending palatine branch), the ascending pharyngeal artery and the maxillary artery (palatine branches).

Passavant's muscle

Passavant's muscle is a sphincter-like muscle that encircles the pharynx at the level of the palate, inside the fibres of the superior constrictor muscles. It is formed by fibres arising from the anterior and lateral part of the upper surface of the palatine aponeurosis. Contraction of this muscle forms a ridge (Passavant's ridge), against which the soft palate is elevated.

Mastication

The principal role of mastication in human beings is the mechanical breakdown of food placed in the mouth. In doing so it stimulates the secretion of saliva, which in turn assists in the digestive process due to the enzymes present in the saliva, and lubricates and binds the food particles, preparing them for swallowing. Mastication also releases substances from food that dissolve in the saliva and any other fluids taken into the mouth, which in turn contribute to the senses of taste and smell and also play a role in the cephalic phase of gastrointestinal secretions. The amount of mastication that food requires depends on the nature of the substance ingested. Solid substances are subjected to vigorous chewing before they are swallowed, whereas softer substances require less chewing and liquids require no chewing at all and are simply transported to the back of the mouth for swallowing. It has been shown that mastication is necessary for some foods, such as red meats, chicken and vegetables, to be fully absorbed by the

Four

rest of the gastrointestinal tract, whereas fish, eggs, rice, bread and cheese do not require to be chewed for complete absorption in the rest of the tract.

Mastication involves the coordinated activities of a number of structures in and around the mouth, primarily the teeth, jaw elevator (closing) and depressor (opening) muscles, temporomandibular joint, tongue, lips, palate and salivary glands. These are collectively called the masticatory apparatus.

Feeding (eating and drinking) is basically a process in which food is ingested and transported along the alimentary tract. For the more solid foods, the process of transportation is interrupted early by the need for mechanical breakdown and mixing by chewing. In the past, all the events that occur from the ingestion of the food to the beginning of the swallow were termed mastication. However, it is now thought that the term should be confined to the process of mechanical reduction of food particles by the act of chewing.

The teeth are the main organ of mastication and are adapted for the functional requirements of the diet. Man is omnivorous (meat and vegetable eater) and consequently the teeth are heterodont in character, in that they have different anatomical forms and functions in different parts of the dental arch. The anterior teeth have sharp edges for grasping, incising and tearing foods, while the posterior teeth are specialized for cutting flesh and grinding fibrous plant material. The teeth in humans are relatively unspecialized in contrast with the specialized dentitions of carnivorous mammals, such as cats and dogs, or herbivorous mammals, such as horses and cattle.

The upper and lower teeth of humans occlude, in that both the maxillary and mandibular teeth meet. Studies of the cusps of posterior teeth in hominids and early man have shown that they are worn down early in life and that the occlusal surfaces are flat and lack any distinctive cuspal features. This suggests that the role of the cusps of human posterior teeth in establishing tooth position and relationships during growth and eruption may be more important than their dietary role.

Mastication in humans involves both vertical and lateral movements of the jaws, like most herbivores (cattle, horses, rabbits and so on) but unlike pure carnivores (cats and dogs) that have only vertical movement of the jaw. Essentially, following breaking of the food using the incisors, the posterior teeth on the side breaking down the food, the so-called working side, are brought into vertical alignment, whilst the posterior teeth on the non-working side may, or may not, be in contact. The food is then crushed and ground by the opposing teeth on the working side, first by a vertical force and movement and then by a bucco–lingual horizontal force and movement. The process by which this occurs is described as the chewing cycle.

Chewing cycle

Some foods do not require chewing and are soft and small enough to be reduced by squashing between the tongue and hard palate. These are not subjected to true mastication or chewing cycles involving the teeth. Cycles in which solid foods are reduced to smaller, swallowable particles have three main phases:

- The opening phase. The mandible is depressed, the mouth opens, and the maxillary and mandibular teeth separate.
- The closing phase. The mandible is raised towards the maxilla and tooth–food–tooth contact occurs. In the late part of this phase, when the teeth come into contact with the food, there is a power stroke, in which the food is compressed; this closing phase merges into the next phase.
- The occlusal or intercuspal phase. There is no further vertical movement, but horizontal bucco–lingual movements occur, with the teeth either in contact or separated by a layer of food.

During these three phases, the lips remain closed together, providing an anterior oral seal. Although the main movements described above are vertical and horizontal in bucco–lingual directions, there are also possible movements in horizontal, anteo–posterior and medio–lateral directions.

The chewing cycle can follow on immediately from what has been defined as Stage I transport of food in the mouth. When a piece of food is placed in the mouth or bitten off by the anterior teeth, the lips confine the piece of food and prevent it from leaving the mouth by creating an anterior oral seal. The food is then transported by the tongue to the posterior teeth by a mechanism described as the 'pull-back' process. This takes about a second and is associated with retraction of the hyoid bone and narrowing of the oropharynx. If the food needs to be chewed, then a series of chewing cycles occur, as described above. The number of chewing cycles depends on the consistency of the food. The action of the tongue and other soft tissues in the mouth helps to control the bolus of food. At the end of Stage I transport of the food, the tongue places the bolus on the working side of the mouth, and during the chewing process the bolus is kept on that side by the combination of rhythmic tongue and cheek movements. Sometimes, the tongue will move the bolus from one side of the mouth to the other, thereby switching the working side. In each chewing cycle, the tongue moves forwards and downwards, carrying food on its surface, and this leads to a build-up of food at the front of the mouth. After a time, this swallowable material is moved towards the oropharynx by a process called 'squeeze-back', in which the tongue moves upwards and backwards against the hard palate; this is accompanied by a movement of the hyoid bone.

The final movement of the food distally to the posterior surface of the tongue is called Stage II transport, and the food is finally squeezed through the fauces by the 'squeeze-back' mechanism. The bolus of food to be swallowed accumulates on the pharyngeal surface of the tongue and in the valleculae. During the processing of solid foods, the mouth is continuous with the oropharynx and there is no evidence of a posterior oral seal caused by the lowering of the soft palate on to the posterior surface of the tongue. However, this posterior oral seal may be produced during the ingestion of liquids so as to confine the fluid to the mouth prior to swallowing. Liquids are swallowed from the mouth without Stage II transport, in contrast with solids, which are swallowed from both the mouth and the oropharynx.

The muscles involved in these processes are the so-called muscles of mastication, as well as the muscles of the tongue, lips and cheeks (see above). The muscles of mastication may be classified anatomically and physiologically into two categories:

• Those that lie between the cranium and the mandible and are involved in jaw elevation (closing): namely, the masseter, temporalis and medial pterygoid muscles
• Those that lie between the mandible and the hyoid bone and are involved in jaw depression (opening): namely, the lateral pterygoid, digastric, geniohyoid and mylohyoid muscles.

These muscles are not just involved in vertical jaw opening and closing but also can account for horizontal movements of the mandible with respect to the maxilla. Also, the superior head of the lateral pterygoid muscle is mainly active during elevation of the mandible and in medially directed movements from a laterally displaced position, while the inferior head is active during depression and protrusion of the mandible, as well as in lateral displacements of the mandible. In addition to the above-mentioned muscles of mastication, muscles such as the infrahyoid and facial muscles (e.g. the orbicularis oris and buccinator) play a role in stabilizing the hyoid bone, maintaining an anterior oral seal and controlling the food bolus between the teeth.

The temporomandibular joint (TMJ, see pages 10–12) is the articulation of the mandibular condyle with the mandibular (glenoid) fossa of the cranial temporal bone. The movement of the temporomandibular bone is governed by the occlusion of the teeth, the morphology of the joint, and the attachments of the ligaments and muscles. When relaxed, the teeth are usually a few millimetres apart and the mandibular condyles lie just below the highest part of the mandibular fossa. In the transition from a teeth-together (i.e. an intercuspal) position to a mandibular rest position, there is a small amount of rotation of the TMJ (approximately 2°), as well as a small amount of vertical movement. When the mouth is opened, there is an initial hinge movement or rotation, and further opening is achieved by a forward sliding (translocation) of the condyle on to the articular eminence, together with further rotation. During biting or incising food using the incisors, the mandible protrudes and the condyles are pulled forwards on to the articular eminence; there is a small amount of rotation and the translation component is less than that during mouth opening.

During chewing, the mandible moves from side to side, bringing the maxillary and mandibular posterior teeth on the working side into alignment. The condyle on the working side moves laterally by about 1–5 mm (the so-called Bennett movement) and slightly posteriorly. The condyle on the non-working side moves forwards, downwards and slightly medially.

The masticatory forces generated between the teeth are mainly due to the activation of the jaw elevator muscles. The maximum biting forces in normal human beings have been recorded as being 500–700 N between the molar teeth and 100 N between the incisors. Forces over 1500 N have been reported, with as much as 4345 N seen in a 37-year-old bruxist with hypertrophy of the masseter and temporalis muscles. It has been shown that the maximum molar force is achieved when the mouth is open and at approximately 50% of the maximum gape. However, during mastication the forces developed between the teeth are considerably smaller (range between 70 and 150 N), with the higher values being achieved when eating harder foods (such as peanuts) and the lower forces achieved when eating softer foods (such as cheeses).

Control of mastication

Mastication is regarded as a voluntary process involving the cerebral cortex and motor neurone areas in the trigeminal motor nucleus. However, little conscious effort is involved and mastication is principally an automatic process very similar to breathing and walking. Mastication, breathing and walking are all controlled by their individual neural pattern generators. In the case of mastication, this central pattern generator is to be found in the brain stem. The exact location is not known, but it is thought to lie in the pons, close to the trigeminal motor nucleus, and may be either in the medial reticular formation or within the trigeminal main sensory nucleus itself.

The role of the central pattern generator is to send out a sequence of appropriate signals to the various motor neurones involved in directing the various muscles of mastication. This central pattern generator determines the sequence of muscle actions, the order, the duration and the rhythm of the contractions and relaxations. These basic patterns, in particular the strength and duration of the phases of movement, can be modulated by inputs from the mouth, such as the hardness or softness of the food and the size of the bolus, thereby slowing the frequency of chewing when encountering hard or tough foods or larger boluses. The masticatory rhythm can also be overridden or modulated by voluntary control. Descending pathways from the motor cortex may influence the central pattern generator by switching the process on or off or by altering the duration of the chewing cycles themselves. There is also evidence that signals from higher centres may directly influence the trigeminal motor neurones to achieve a special effect, such as biting hard into food as a purely voluntary act. There is strong evidence that the central pattern generator is also affected by signals from sensory receptors, particularly mechanoreceptors, in and around the mouth. These receptors not only provide feedback to the central pattern generator but also provide sensory information to the somatosensory cortex regarding the physical state of the food in the mouth, and direct inputs into the reflex control of motor neurone activity during chewing.

Reflexes of mastication

The reflexes of mastication are no longer thought to be the major control mechanisms involved in mastication. However, there is no doubt that they play a part in feedback to the central pattern generator described above. In humans, the main jaw reflexes are those involving the jaw elevator muscles: namely, the jaw jerk reflex and the so-called jaw-opening reflexes.

Jaw jerk reflex

The jaw jerk reflex is similar to the knee jerk or stretch reflex seen when a tap is made on the patella tendon. This is the simplest reflex seen in the human body and is termed monosynaptic, as it involves only two neurones (an afferent and an efferent) and one central synapse. The jaw jerk reflex can be elicited by a downward tap to the chin, thus causing a stretch of the jaw elevator muscle spindles (specialized stretch mechanoreceptors that lie in parallel with the extrafusal muscle fibres), which in turn produce a reflex activation of the same muscle in which they lie via their α-motor neurone. Although a tap on the chin is not a normal physiological stimulus, there is evidence that the jaw jerk reflex pathways are present continuously (to a greater or lesser extent) during normal chewing. It can be seen that when the teeth are further apart due to a large bolus or more solid food between the teeth, then the jaw elevator muscles and their muscle spindles will also be more stretched during the closing phase of the chewing cycle, thereby producing a greater excitatory input on to the motor neurone pool. This will in turn assist in the generation of a greater force in order to crush the food. The jaw jerk reflex has been shown to be strongest during the closing phase of the chewing cycle or when there is a resistance to jaw closing.

Jaw opening reflexes

In human beings, when a mechanical or noxious stimulus is applied to the tissues in and around the mouth, the principal resulting reflexes involve the inhibition of activity in the jaw elevator muscles if they are active. It is generally agreed that these inhibitory reflexes involve three or more synapses and so they have been termed polysynaptic. Inhibition of jaw elevator muscles can have the effect of stopping jaw closing and can even produce a reflex jaw opening. Their importance in humans is that they are thought to help prevent overloading of the teeth and muscles during chewing. They may also reduce the likelihood of injury from extremely hard or sharp objects within the food whilst eating.

There is some evidence that the same sort of stimulation, both mechanical and noxious, may, besides producing an inhibitory response, produce an excitatory response in the same muscle. It has been suggested that these responses may, like the jaw jerk reflex, provide a feedback mechanism to the central pattern generator during mastication to allow for different consistencies of food. It has been postulated that these inhibitory or excitatory influences depend on the phase of the chewing cycle (opening, closing or occlusal) at which the stimulus occurs, but so far no clear explanation has been given.

Jaw unloading reflex

The jaw unloading reflex is not a true masticatory reflex in that it occurs during static biting on a hard object. However, it involves an act commonly experienced during the process of eating. This reflex occurs when a hard object is held between the maxillary and mandibular teeth, is bitten upon and then suddenly breaks, thereby 'unloading' the jaw elevator muscles of the resistance against which they were biting. There is a cessation of muscle activity (relaxation) in the jaw elevator (closer) muscles, together with an activation (excitation) of the jaw depressor (opener) muscles. One result of this is that the opposing teeth do not come clashing together and damage one another. Whether this is as a result of the reflex, or because of the physical properties of the jaw elevator muscles, is not known. The exact mechanism is not clear but it is known that, when we bite on something we know will eventually break, we can prepare our jaw opening muscles for activation whilst we stimulate our jaw closing muscles during biting. This leads to an active priming of the depressor muscles during the biting phase of this reflex.

Swallowing

Stages of swallowing

Most textbooks describe swallowing as consisting of three phases: oral, pharyngeal and oesophageal. The first stage is usually described as voluntary and as moving the bolus of food up to the fauces. The second and third stages are usually described as a series of complex reflex responses, elicited by contact of the bolus with the pillars of the fauces, which results in bolus movement through the fauces and then through the pharynx, and its eventual delivery into the oesophagus.

Unfortunately, the human swallow has traditionally been studied as a single isolated event involving a voluntary swallow of a liquid on demand. This involves holding the liquid bolus in the mouth, contained between an anterior oral seal and a posterior oral seal, and then swallowing on command whilst measurements are taken. Swallowing is now regarded as a more complex process comprising a subset of a continuous series of automatic events that transport food from the level of the incisor teeth to the stomach; it also involves, when necessary, a period of chewing of the food between its transportation from incisor to stomach. The swallowing of liquids, in which no chewing takes place, is more like the traditional three-phase account. However, the swallowing of solids or solids mixed with liquids is more complex.

Solids, or solids mixed with liquids, are often chewed and can be transported through the fauces to the posterior part of the tongue before they are swallowed. The food bolus is often not a neat single piece of food but can be smeared over a large area of the mouth and oropharynx at any moment of time during eating. Food collects on the pharyngeal surface of the tongue and accumulates at the back of the tongue. The bolus that is eventually to be swallowed collects in the lower part of the oropharynx and is in turn propelled through the hypopharynx/laryngopharynx, past the laryngeal inlet and relaxed upper oesophageal sphincter, and into the oesophagus. The main difference between swallowing liquids and swallowing solids is that liquids are swallowed from the mouth and there is a true oral phase, but when solids or solids mixed with liquids are swallowed, they are swallowed both from the mouth and/or from the oropharynx in what would best be described as an oral and oropharyngeal phase.

During the so-called pharyngeal phase, liquids are pushed through the oropharynx and hypopharynx into the oesophagus; solids, and solids mixed with liquids, are collected in the oropharynx and pushed through the hypopharynx into the oesophagus. The so-called 'hypopharyngeal transit time' is normally less than 0.5 seconds but is critical, as it is when the food is passing the laryngeal inlet. During this time, breathing is inhibited, the hyoid-laryngeal complex is raised and moves forward, the glottis is closed, the bolus pushes the tip of the epiglottis over the laryngeal inlet, and there is adduction of the vocal folds. All of these mechanisms are designed to prevent food from entering the trachea. As the bolus enters the oesophagus, these changes are reversed; the larynx opens and breathing restarts.

During the oesophageal phase of swallowing, once the bolus has passed through the relaxed upper oesophageal sphincter, the sphincter then closes and the bolus is propelled approximately 25 cm to the stomach by a process called peristalsis. This causes a coordinated series of waves of contractions behind the bolus of the circular and longitudinal muscle layers of the oesophagus. This series of waves forces the food into the stomach following relaxation of the lower oesophageal sphincter. This process can take all of 5 seconds to complete.

Swallowing centre

Like mastication, swallowing is driven by a central pattern generator within the brain stem. This swallowing centre is located in the medulla and consists of two parts, one located dorsally in the medulla (mostly in the nucleus of the solitary tract) and the other more ventrally in the medulla:

- The dorsal medullary pattern generator is largely responsible for receiving inputs that trigger the swallowing process and is responsible for generating the patterns of neuronal activity necessary for the contraction and relaxation of the muscles involved in swallowing.
- The more ventral medullary pattern generator is responsible for the inputs from the dorsal pattern generator and then relays them to the appropriate motor neurones involved in swallowing (motor neurones of the Vth, VIIth, IXth, Xth, XIth and XIIth cranial nerves, as well as motor neurones in the first three cervical segments of the spinal cord).

Swallowing can be inhibited by a voluntary mechanism that originates from the higher centres of the brain, most probably from the cerebral cortex. However, subcortical areas such as the internal capsule, the hypothalamus and the mesencephalic reticular formation have also been implicated in what has been termed voluntary swallowing.

Swallowing reflexes

Swallowing can also be initiated by a series of reflexes, initiated by the stimulation of mechanoreceptors and chemoreceptors at the back of the mouth. These receptors are innervated by the Vth, IXth and Xth cranial nerves. The most important of these receptors seem to be those innervated by the superior laryngeal branch of the vagus nerve (Xth cranial nerve), which is the only one that appears to initiate a swallow if it alone is stimulated. All the others seem to need facilitatory inputs from either higher centres or other peripheral nerves.

The size of the food particles alone does not determine whether a bolus is swallowed or not. Swallowing appears to be more dependent on the physical consistency of the food and whether it is well lubricated by saliva or other fluids.

Four

Self-assessment: questions

True/false statements

Which of the following statements are true and which are false?

a. The mylohyoid muscle, forming the diaphragm for the floor of the mouth, is attached onto the external oblique line of the mandible.

b. The fibrous aponeurosis of the soft palate is derived from the expanded tendon of the levator veli palatini muscles.

c. The tensor veli palatini muscle arises in part from the scaphoid fossa of the sphenoid bone.

d. The depressor labii inferioris muscle arises from the mandible immediately above the mental foramen.

e. The buccinator muscle arises in part from the anterior border of the pterygomandibular raphe.

f. The superior head of the lateral pterygoid muscle arises from the lateral surface of the lateral pterygoid plate.

g. The medial pterygoid muscle takes origin from the inner aspect of the angle of the mandible.

h. The digastric muscle is a weak elevator and retractor of the mandible.

i. The lingual nerve runs between the two heads of the lateral pterygoid muscle.

j. The two heads of the medial pterygoid muscle are separated by fibres of the inferior head of the lateral pterygoid muscle.

k. The masseter muscle is crossed by the parotid duct and by branches of the facial nerve.

l. The attachment of the temporalis muscle is limited above by the superior temporal line.

m. The four primary muscles of mastication are derived embryologically from mesenchyme of the first pharyngeal (branchial) arch.

n. As for the other muscles of mastication, the anterior belly of the digastric muscle is innervated by the mandibular nerve.

o. The masseter is an example of a multipennate muscle.

p. Mastication is necessary for the full absorption of red meats, chicken and vegetables.

q. The term mastication is confined to the process of mechanical reduction of food particles by the act of chewing.

r. Humans are essentially omnivorous and consequently the teeth are heterodont in character, in that they have different anatomical form and function in different parts of the dental arch.

s. Mastication in humans principally involves vertical movements of the jaws.

t. All foods are subjected to at least one chewing cycle before they are swallowed.

u. There are basically two phases of the chewing cycle: the opening and the closing phases.

v. During the early phase of the chewing cycle, the lips remain closed together, thus providing an anterior oral seal; there is a lowering of the soft palate onto the posterior surface of the tongue, thus providing a posterior oral seal.

w. The muscles of mastication include the jaw elevator muscles, the jaw depressor muscles and the muscles of the lips, cheeks and tongue.

x. During chewing, the mandible moves from side to side to bring the maxillary and mandibular teeth on the non-working side into alignment.

y. The maximum force that can be developed between the teeth is when the mouth is opened about 25% of the maximum gape.

z. Mastication is controlled by a central pattern generator that is situated in the medulla oblongata.

aa. Descending pathways from the motor cortex can influence the central pattern generator by switching it on or off, but they cannot influence the rate of chewing or the force of chewing.

ab. The jaw jerk reflex is an example of a polysynaptic reflex involving afferent and efferent neurones and two synapses, a central synapse and the neuromuscular junction.

ac. In human beings, the jaw opening reflexes involve excitation of the jaw depressor muscles and inhibition of the jaw elevator muscles when oral nociceptors or mechanoreceptors are stimulated.

ad. The swallowing of both liquids and solids involves three phases, the first of which is voluntary and the second and third of which constitute a series of complex reflex responses.

ae. The main difference between swallowing a liquid and swallowing a solid is that liquids are mainly swallowed from the mouth, whereas solids can be swallowed from the oropharynx.

af. The hypopharyngeal transit time is normally 1 second and is critical because it is during this time that breathing is inhibited.

ag. During the oesophageal phase of swallowing, the bolus of food is propelled to the stomach by a process of peristalsis.

ah. Swallowing is driven by a central pattern generator located in the medulla oblongata.

ai. Swallowing is initiated by a series of reflexes, brought about by the stimulation of mechanoreceptors and chemoreceptors innervated by the Vth, VIIth and Xth cranial nerves.

aj. Initiation of swallowing is determined by the size of the food particles involved.

Extended matching questions

Theme: The orofacial muscles

Select the most appropriate option to answer items 1–5. Each option can be used once, more than once or not at all.

Self-assessment: questions

Item list

1. The muscle that changes the shape of the lips
2. The muscle that is pierced by the parotid duct
3. The muscle whose posterior (horizontal) fibres retract the mandible
4. The muscle forming the anterior pillar of the fauces at the oropharyngeal isthmus
5. The muscle arising from a fossa just below the genial tubercles (spines)

Option list

A. Buccinator
B. Digastric
C. Genioglossus
D. Hyoglossus
E. Lateral pterygoid
F. Levator anguli oris
G. Levator labii superioris
H. Masseter
I. Medial pterygoid
J. Mylohyoid
K. Orbicularis oris
L. Palatoglossus
M. Styloglossus
N. Temporalis

Picture questions

Figure 4.1

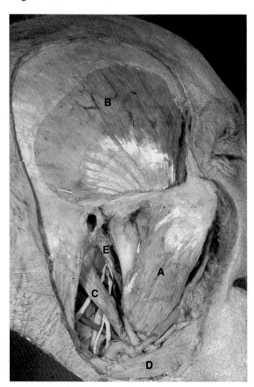

a. Identify the muscles labelled A–D, indicating their nerve supply.
b. Identify structure E and name the muscles attached to it.

Figure 4.2

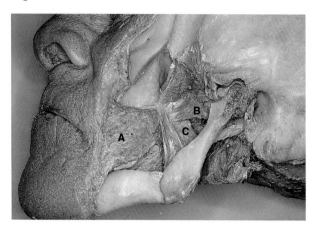

This is a picture of the infratemporal fossa.
a. Identify the muscular structures labelled A–C, indicating their functions.

Figure 4.3

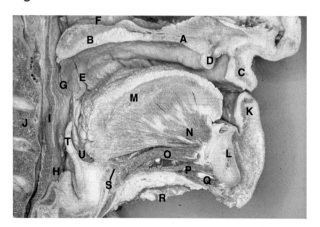

This is a picture of a median sagittal section through the head to show the tongue and the floor of the mouth.
a. Label all the structures labelled A–U.
b. Which nerves innervate the muscles labelled N–Q?
c. What is the function of muscle N?

Self-assessment: questions

Figure 4.4

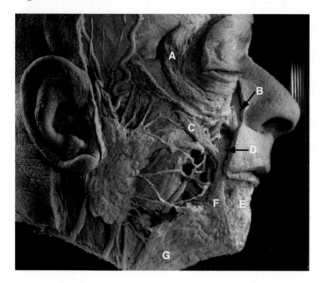

This is a picture of a dissection of the superficial face.
a. Identify the structures labelled A–G, indicating their functions.

Essay questions

1. Describe the muscles that change the shapes and positions of the lips.
2. Relate the movements of the mandible at the temporomandibular joint to the muscles responsible for these movements.
3. Describe the role central pattern generators play in mastication and swallowing.

Self-assessment: answers

True/false answers

a. **False**. The mylohyoid muscle takes origin from the internal oblique (mylohyoid) line of the mandible.

b. **False**. The fibrous aponeurosis of the soft palate is derived from the tendons of the tensor veli palatini muscles.

c. **True**. An additional origin for the tensor veli palatini muscle is the cartilage of the auditory (Eustachian) tube.

d. **False**. The depressor labii inferioris muscle arises below the mental foramen.

e. **True**. The remaining origin of the buccinator muscle is from the alveolar processes of the maxilla and mandible adjacent to the molar teeth.

f. **False**. The superior head of the lateral pterygoid muscle arises from the sphenoid bone in the roof of the infratemporal fossa; the inferior head arises from the lateral surface of the lateral pterygoid plate.

g. **False**. The medial pterygoid muscle arises from the medial surface of the lateral pterygoid plate; the muscle is inserted onto the inner surface of the angle of the mandible.

h. **False**. The digastric muscle depresses and retracts the mandible.

i. **False**. The buccal branch of the mandibular nerve passes between the two heads of the lateral pterygoid muscle.

j. **True**. The two heads of the medial pterygoid muscle are referred to as the superficial and deep heads.

k. **True**. The parotid duct bends sharply at the anterior border of the masseter muscle to pierce the underlying buccinator muscle.

l. **False**. The attachment of the temporalis muscle is limited by the inferior temporal line, the superior temporal line giving origin to the overlying temporal fascia.

m. **True**. Hence the innervation of the muscles of mastication being the nerve of the 1st pharyngeal arch (i.e. the mandibular division of the trigeminal nerve).

n. **True**. The anterior belly of the digastric muscle also is derived from the 1st pharyngeal arch (see answer above). Remember that the posterior belly of the digastric is innervated by the facial nerve and is derived from the 2nd pharyngeal arch.

o. **True**. The multipennate arrangement of the masseter muscle allows the muscle to increase its power.

p. **True**. However, it is not necessary for the full absorption of fish, eggs, rice, bread or cheese.

q. **True**. In the past, all the events that occur from the ingestion of the food to the beginning of the swallow have been termed mastication, but this term is now confined to the process of mechanical reduction of food.

r. **True**. Unlike carnivores or herbivores, which have highly specialized dentitions.

s. **False**. Mastication involves both vertical and lateral (horizontal) movements of the jaws in human beings.

t. **False**. Some foods, particularly those that are soft and small enough to be reduced by squashing between the tongue and palate, do not require chewing.

u. **False**. There are three phases: the opening, closing and occlusal or intercuspal phase.

v. **False**. There is no evidence of a posterior oral seal during the processing of solid foods. However, it does occur during ingestion of liquids.

w. **False**. Although the muscles of the tongue, lips and cheeks are involved in mastication, they are not generally included in the true muscles of mastication.

x. **False**. It is the teeth on the working side that are brought into alignment.

y. **False**. The maximum force is achieved when the mouth is open to about 50% of the maximum gape, the so-called optimal length of the jaw-closing muscles.

z. **False**. Mastication is controlled by a central pattern generator, but it is thought to be situated in the pons and not the medulla.

aa. **False**. Descending pathways not only can switch chewing on or off, but also can influence the duration of the chewing cycle and the force of biting.

ab. **False**. The jaw jerk reflex is an example of a monosynaptic reflex. The neuromuscular junction is not regarded as a true synapse, as it is between nerve and muscle, and not nerve and nerve.

ac. **False**. In humans, the only observable response is the inhibition of the active jaw elevator muscles; excitation of the jaw depressor muscles has only been observed in experimental animals.

ad. **False**. Although this is thought to be true for liquids, the swallowing of solids is now thought to be more complex and to involve a continuous series of automatic events from the level of the incisor teeth to the stomach, rather than the traditional three phases.

ae. **True**. Solids can be swallowed from either the mouth or the oropharynx or both.

af. **False**. The hypopharyngeal transit time is less than 0.5 seconds and not as long as 1 second.

ag. **True**. Peristalsis in the oesophagus involves a coordinated series of waves of contraction behind the bolus.

ah. **True**. The central pattern generator for swallowing is found in two parts: dorsally and ventrally in the medulla.

ai. **False**. It is true that swallowing is initiated by a series of reflexes brought about by stimulation of mechanoreceptors and chemoreceptors, but they are innervated by the Vth, IXth and Xth cranial nerves and not the VIIth cranial nerve.

Self-assessment: answers

aj. **False**. The initiation of swallowing is more dependent on the physical consistency of the bolus and whether or not it is well lubricated, rather than the size of the food particles.

Extended matching answers

Item 1 = Option K. Orbicularis oris (a muscle of facial expression and therefore innervated by the facial nerve) changes the shape of the lips. Muscles like the levator labii superioris and the depressor labii inferioris interdigitate with orbicularis oris and are responsible for moving the lips.

Item 2 = Option A. Buccinator is a muscle of facial expression (therefore innervated by the facial nerve) that lies in the cheek and helps position the bolus of food between the teeth during chewing. The parotid duct passes through the buccinator muscle to end in the cheek intra-orally (usually opposite the maxillary second molar tooth).

Item 3 = Option N. Temporalis is a muscle of mastication (therefore innervated by the mandibular division of the trigeminal nerve). It has anterior (vertical) fibres that elevate the mandible and posterior (horizontal) fibres that retract the mandible.

Item 4 = Option L. The palatoglossus muscle is an extrinsic muscle of the tongue that occupies the anterior pillar of the fauces at the oropharyngeal isthmus. It elevates the back of the tongue during swallowing. Although it is an extrinsic muscle of the tongue, it is derived embryologically with the muscles of the soft palate and is therefore not innervated by the hypoglossal nerve but by the pharyngeal plexus.

Item 5 = Option B. The anterior belly of the digastric is inserted into the digastric fossa at the inferior border of the mandible, beneath the chin and below the genial tubercles.

Picture answers

Figure 4.1

a. A = masseter (innervated by the masseteric branch of the anterior trunk of the mandibular division of the trigeminal nerve). B = temporalis (innervated by the deep temporal branches of the anterior trunk of the mandibular division of the trigeminal nerve). C = posterior belly of digastric (innervated by the digastric branch of the facial nerve). D = platysma (innervated by the cervical branch of the facial nerve).

b. E = styloid process. The structures attached to it are the stylohyoid, styloglossus and stylopharyngeus muscles, as well as the stylohyoid and stylomandibular ligaments.

Figure 4.2

a. A = buccinator (a muscle of the cheek that helps to hold the bolus of food between the teeth during mastication). B = lateral pterygoid (inferior head) (a muscle of mastication that protrudes and depresses the mandible; also involved in side-to-side movements). C = medial pterygoid (a muscle of mastication that protrudes and elevates the mandible; also involved in side-to-side movements).

Figure 4.3

a. A = hard palate. B = soft palate. C = orbicularis oris in upper lip. D = edentulous maxillary alveolar ridge. E = pillars of fauces. F = nasopharynx. G = oropharynx. H = laryngopharynx. I = constrictor muscles of pharynx. J = vertebral column. K = orbicularis oris in lower lip. L = body of mandible. M = tongue. N = genioglossus muscle. O = geniohyoid muscle. P = mylohyoid muscle. Q = anterior belly of digastric muscle. R = platysma muscle. S = hyoid bone. T = epiglottis. U = vallecula.

b. The genioglossus muscle (label N) is innervated by the hypoglossal nerve (XIIth cranial nerve). The geniohyoid muscle (label O) is innervated by fibres from the Ist cervical nerve that accompany the hypoglossal nerve. The mylohyoid muscle (label P) and the anterior belly of the digastric muscle (label Q) are both innervated by the mylohyoid nerve which comes from the inferior alveolar branch of the posterior trunk of the mandibular division of the trigeminal nerve (cranial nerve V_3).

c. The genioglossus muscle (label N) protrudes the tongue. If a clinician believes that there is damage to the hypoglossal nerve (XIIth cranial nerve), a simple test is to ask the patient to protrude her/his tongue. If there is damage to one of the hypoglossal nerves, the tongue will deviate to the affected side on protrusion.

Figure 4.4

a. A = orbicularis oculi (orbital part). This muscle acts as a sphincter of the orbit and closes the orbital fissure tightly ('screwing up' the eye) in bright light. B = levator labii superioris. This muscle, as indicated by its name, raises the upper lip (its nasal slip — the levator labii superioris alaeque nasi muscle — is involved in dilating the nostril). C = zygomaticus major. This muscle is also an elevator of the upper lip (but in a more lateral direction, as in laughing). D = levator anguli oris. This muscle, as indicated by its name, raises the angle/corner of the lip (as in smiling). E = depressor labii inferioris.

Self-assessment: answers

This muscle, as indicated by its name, depresses the lower lip (it is said to provide a facial expression associated with irony). F = depressor anguli oris. This muscle, as indicated by its name, depresses the angle/corner of the lip (as in an expression of grumpiness or grief). G = platysma. This muscle helps in lowering the lower lip and wrinkles the skin over the lower jaw and neck to give 'the look of horror or surprise'.

Outline essay answers

Question 1

The first paragraph should outline, briefly and as a general introduction, the basic morphology and functions of the lips. A listing of the muscles of the lips and a diagram showing the muscles of facial expression in the lips should be provided.

For each of the following muscles, the functions should be stated:

- Orbicularis oris
- Upper lip muscles (levator labii superioris; zygomaticus major and minor; levator anguli oris)
- Lower lip muscles (depressor labii inferioris; depressor anguli oris; mentalis; platysma)
- Muscles at the labial commissures (corners of lips) (risorius; buccinator).

Note that, although not essential, indications of attachments and innervations are helpful.

The final paragraph should provide some clinical scenarios (e.g. facial palsy, cutting the marginal mandibular branch of the facial nerve).

Question 2

The essay should begin with a brief description of the anatomy of the TMJ and of the muscles of mastication. The fact that the TMJ is the major synovial joint of the skull and, because of the intra-articular disc, is both a hinge and a gliding joint should be highlighted. Diagrams of the TMJ and muscles would be appropriate for this essay.

Movements of the TMJ should now be described, such movements being categorized as symmetrical and asymmetrical. Symmetrical movements are those that occur similarly in both TMJs (i.e. protrusion, retraction, depression and elevation of the mandible). Asymmetrical movements are those that occur dissimilarly in the TMJs (i.e. side-to-side movements). Again, diagrams showing these movements should be included in the essay.

The roles of the muscles of mastication (plus digastric and mylohyoid muscles) in symmetrical and asymmetrical movements should now be described (see Table 4.1). Note

Table 4.1 The roles of the muscles of mastication in symmetrical and asymmetrical movements

Type of movement		Muscles involved
Symmetrical movements	Protrusion	Lateral and medial pterygoids on both sides
	Retraction	Temporalis (posterior/horizontal fibres) and digastric
	Depression	Lateral pterygoids and suprahyoid muscles
	Elevation	Medial pterygoids, masseter, temporalis (anterior/vertical fibres)
Asymmetrical movements	Side-to-side	Lateral and medial pterygoids working together but on alternative sides

that retraction only occurs from the protruded position, just as elevation only occurs from the depressed (opened) position. Furthermore, during elevation, masseter muscles may primarily function as the teeth come together to 'put power into the bite'. Other 'complications' include a role for the superior head of the lateral pterygoid muscle in elevation.

The final paragraph should briefly outline the innervations of muscles and, in particular, should emphasize the complexity of the movements of mastication and of the neurological control mechanisms.

Question 3

Mastication is regarded as a voluntary process involving the cerebral cortex and motor neurone areas in the trigeminal motor nucleus. Little conscious effort is involved and mastication is principally an automatic process very similar to breathing and walking. Mastication, swallowing, breathing and walking are all controlled by their individual neural pattern generators. In the case of mastication, the central pattern generator is to be found in the brain stem but its exact location is not known. It is thought to lie in the pons, close to the trigeminal motor nucleus. The role of the central pattern generator is to send out a sequence of appropriate signals to the various motor neurones involved in directing the various muscles of mastication. It determines the sequence of muscle actions, the order, the duration and the rhythm of the contractions and relaxations. These basic patterns, and in particular the strength and durations of the phases of movement, can be modulated by inputs from the mouth such as the hardness or softness of the food and the size of the bolus, thereby slowing the frequency of chewing when encountering hard or tough foods or larger boluses. The rhythm of chewing can also be overridden or modulated by voluntary control. Descending pathways from the motor cortex may influence the central pattern generator by switching

Self-assessment: answers

the process on or off or by altering the duration of the chewing cycles. There is also evidence that signals from higher centres may directly influence the trigeminal motor neurones to achieve a special effect such as biting hard into food as a purely voluntary act. There is strong evidence that the central pattern generator is also affected by signals from peripheral receptors, particularly mechanoreceptors in and around the mouth. These receptors not only provide feedback to the central pattern generator, but also provide sensory information to the somatosensory cortex regarding the physical state of the food in the mouth, and direct inputs into the reflex control of motor neurone activity during chewing.

Like mastication, swallowing is driven by a central pattern generator within the brain stem. This swallowing centre is located in the medulla and consists of two parts, one located dorsally in the medulla, mostly in the nucleus of the solitary tract, and the other more ventrally in the medulla. The dorsal medullary pattern generator is largely responsible for receiving inputs which trigger the swallowing process, and is responsible for generating the patterns of neuronal activity necessary for the contraction and relaxation of the muscles involved in swallowing. The more ventral medullary pattern generator is responsible for the inputs from the dorsal pattern generator and then for relaying them to the appropriate motor neurones involved in swallowing (motor neurones of the Vth, VIIth, IXth, Xth, XIth and XIIth cranial nerves, as well as motor neurones in the first three cervical segments of the spinal cord).

Like mastication, swallowing can be inhibited by a voluntary mechanism which originates from the higher centres of the brain, most probably from the cerebral cortex; however, subcortical areas such as the internal capsule, the hypothalamus and the mesencephalic reticular formation have also been implicated in what has been termed voluntary swallowing.

Swallowing can also be initiated by a series of reflexes, initiated by the stimulation of mechanoreceptors and chemoreceptors at the back of the mouth. These receptors are innervated by the Vth, IXth and Xth cranial nerves.

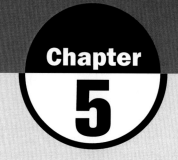

Tongue, flavour, thermoreception and speech

Chapter 5

Introduction	51
Muscles	52
Blood supply	53
Lymphatic drainage	53
Sensory innervation	53
Taste	53
Taste buds	53
Transduction mechanisms	54
Afferent gustatory neurones	55
Common chemical sense	55
Olfaction	55
Olfactory epithelium	55
Odorant membrane receptors	56
Olfactory pathway	56
Thermoreception	57
Cold and warm receptors	57
Thermoreceptive afferent pathway	57
Speech	58
Phonation	58
Articulation	58
Resonance	58
Classification of sounds	58
Pathways and centres for speech	59
Self-assessment: questions	60
Self-assessment: answers	63

Overview

The tongue is a muscular organ which, in addition to moving the food bolus around the mouth during chewing (mastication) and into the pharynx during swallowing (deglutition), is involved in the selection of food for ingestion (via taste) and in speech. This chapter also covers the role of the tongue in gustation and the sensation of flavours (thus including olfaction as well as taste) and thermoreception in the oral cavity as a whole.

Learning objectives

You should:
- have a detailed knowledge of the macroscopic anatomy of the tongue and be able to relate this to function
- have a good knowledge of the physiological mechanisms underlying the sensation of flavours, about thermoreception in the oral cavity, and about the role of the tongue and mouth in speech.

Introduction

The tongue is a muscular organ with its base attached to the floor of the mouth. It is attached to the inner surface of the mandible near the midline and gains support below from the hyoid bone. It functions in mastication, swallowing and speech and carries out important sensory functions, particularly those of taste. The lymphoid material contained in its posterior third has a protective role.

Ventral surface

The ventral surface of the tongue (the inferior surface), related to the floor of the mouth, is covered by a thin lining of non-keratinized mucous membrane that is tightly bound down to the underlying muscles. In the midline, extending onto the floor of the mouth, lies the lingual frenum. Rarely, this extends across the floor of the mouth to be attached to the mandibular alveolus. Such an overdeveloped lingual frenum (ankyloglossa) may restrict movements of the tongue (tongue-tie). Lateral to the frenum lie irregular, fringed folds: the fimbriated folds. Also visible through the mucosa are the deep lingual veins.

Dorsum

The dorsum of the tongue may be subdivided into the anterior two-thirds (palatal part) and the posterior third (pharyngeal part). The junction of the palatal and pharyngeal parts is marked by a shallow V-shaped groove, the sulcus terminalis. The angle (or 'V') of the sulcus terminalis is directed posteriorly. In the midline, near the angle, may be seen a small pit called the foramen caecum. This is the primordial site of development of the thyroid gland. The mucosa of the palatal part of the tongue is partly keratinized and is characterized by the abundance of papillae. The most conspicuous papillae on the palatal surface of the tongue are the circumvallate papillae, which lie immediately in front of the sulcus terminalis. The pharyngeal surface of the tongue is covered with large rounded nodules termed the lingual follicles. These follicles are composed of lymphatic tissue, collectively forming the lingual tonsil. The posterior part of the tongue slopes towards the epiglottis, where three folds of mucous membrane are seen: the median and lateral glosso-epiglottic folds. The anterior pillars of the fauces (the palatoglossal arches) extend from the soft palate to the sides of the tongue near the circumvallate papillae.

The dorsum of the tongue is covered with numerous whitish, conical elevations: the filiform papillae, which are keratinized. Interspersed between the filiform papillae are isolated reddish prominences, the fungiform papillae. These are non-keratinized and contain taste buds. The fungiform papillae are most numerous at the tip of the tongue. The 10–15 circumvallate papillae are considerably larger than either the filiform or fungiform papillae. They lie immediately in front of the sulcus terminalis, do not project beyond the surface of the tongue and are surrounded by a circular 'trench'. The surface of the posterior third of the tongue lying behind the sulcus terminalis is non-keratinized and is covered by a number of smooth elevations produced by underlying lymphoid tissue. Foliate papillae appear as a series of parallel, slit-like folds of mucosa on each lateral border of the tongue, near the attachment of the palatoglossal fold (anterior pillar of the fauces). The foliate papillae are of variable length in humans and are the vestige of large papillae found in many other mammals.

The histological appearance of the mucosa of the tongue is described on page 240.

Muscles

The tongue is composed of intrinsic and extrinsic muscles:

- The intrinsic muscles of the tongue are restricted to the substance of the tongue and change its shape.
- The extrinsic muscles arise outside the tongue and are responsible for bodily movement of the tongue.

Intrinsic muscles

The intrinsic muscles of the tongue can be divided into three fibre groups: transverse, longitudinal and vertical. Rarely can these three groups be distinguished in dissections, but their interlacing gives the tongue its characteristic appearance in cross-section.

- The transverse fibres arise from a sheet of connective tissue called the lingual septum, running longitudinally through the midline of the tongue. These transverse fibres pass laterally from the septum to intercalate with fibres of the other groups of intrinsic muscles.
- The longitudinal fibres may be subdivided into upper and lower groups: the superior and inferior longitudinal muscles of the tongue.
- The vertical fibres pass directly between the upper and lower surfaces, particularly at the lateral borders of the tongue.

Contraction of the vertical fibres would make the tongue thinner (and wider). Contraction of the longitudinal fibres would shorten (and thicken) the tongue. Contraction of the transverse fibres would narrow (and widen) the tongue. The intrinsic muscles receive their motor innervation from the hypoglossal (XIIth) cranial nerve.

Extrinsic muscles

The extrinsic muscles of the tongue arise from the skull and hyoid bone and thence spread into the body of the tongue. The extrinsic musculature is composed of four groups of muscles: genioglossus, hyoglossus, styloglossus and palatoglossus.

Genioglossus

The genioglossus muscle arises from the superior genial tubercle on the medial surface of the body of the mandible. At this level, the two genioglossus muscles cannot be readily separated. As the muscles enter the tongue, a thin strip of connective tissue intervenes between the right and left genioglossus muscles. The bulk of the fibres fan out into the body of the tongue but the superior fibres pass upwards and anteriorly to the tip of the tongue, and some of its inferior fibres insert onto the body of the hyoid bone. The genioglossus muscle is mainly a protractor and depressor of the tongue.

Hyoglossus

The hyoglossus muscle originates from the superior border of the greater horn of the hyoid bone and passes vertically upwards into the tongue. Its function is to depress the tongue. At its origin, the hyoglossus muscle is separated from the attachment of the middle constrictor muscle of the pharynx beneath by the lingual artery.

Styloglossus

Each styloglossus muscle arises from the anterior surface of the styloid process of the temporal bone, from which the muscle runs downwards and forwards to enter the tongue below the insertion of the palatoglossus muscle. At this point, its fibres intercalate with the fibres of the hyoglossus before continuing forwards towards the tip of the tongue. The styloglossus muscle is a retractor of the tongue.

Palatoglossus

Each palatoglossus muscle arises from the aponeurosis of the soft palate and descends to the tongue in the anterior pillar of the fauces, whence its fibres intercalate with the transverse fibres of the tongue. The action of the palatoglossus muscles is to raise the tongue in order to narrow the transverse diameter of the oropharyngeal isthmus. The extrinsic muscles of the tongue are innervated by the hypoglossal nerve (XIIth cranial nerve) (except for the palatoglossus, which is innervated by the cranial part of the accessory nerve (XIth cranial nerve) via the pharyngeal plexus).

Blood supply

The main source of the blood supply to the tongue is the lingual artery. This is a branch of the external carotid artery in the neck. The artery passes into the floor of the mouth deep to the hyoglossus muscle (superficial to the superior constrictor muscle), where it is accompanied by the glossopharyngeal nerve. Dorsal lingual branches supply the dorsum of the tongue and a sublingual branch the floor of the mouth. The terminal branch is the deep lingual artery found running near the lingual frenum on the ventral surface of the tongue. Lingual veins are variable. There is usually a dorsal lingual vein draining the dorsum of the tongue and this becomes the lingual vein that drains into the internal jugular vein in the neck. The deep lingual vein on the ventral surface of the tongue joins the sublingual vein from the sublingual salivary gland to become 'the vein accompanying the hypoglossal nerve' (this also drains into the internal jugular).

Lymphatic drainage

The lymphatic drainage of the tongue is mainly into the submandibular nodes (the lateral lymph vessels draining ipsilaterally but more central vessels draining both ipsilaterally and contralaterally). Lymph from the tip of the tongue drains into the submental nodes. Lymphatics from the posterior third of the tongue drain into the deep cervical chain of nodes (including jugulodigastric nodes) (again the lateral lymph vessels drain ipsilaterally but more central vessels drain both ipsilaterally and contralaterally).

Sensory innervation

Three distinct nerve fields can be recognized on the dorsum of the tongue:

- The anterior part of the tongue, in front of the circumvallate papillae, is supplied by the lingual branch of the mandibular division of the trigeminal nerve (V_3 cranial nerve). However, its accompanying chorda tympani fibres from the nervus intermedius

part of the facial nerve (VIIth cranial nerve) are those associated with the perception of taste. Note that the chorda tympani nerve joins the lingual nerve in the infratemporal fossa and deep to the inferior head of the lateral pterygoid muscle.
- Behind, and including the circumvallate papillae, the tongue is supplied primarily by the glossopharyngeal nerve (IXth cranial nerve), providing both general sensation and taste.
- A small area on the posterior part of the tongue around the epiglottis is supplied by the vagus nerve (Xth cranial nerve), via its superior laryngeal branch.

The mucosa on the ventral surface of the tongue is supplied by the lingual nerve.

The development of the tongue is considered on page 104.

Taste

When we eat and drink we experience a sensation that is commonly called taste, yet eating is a multi-sensory experience involving not only the chemical senses of taste (gustation) and smell (olfaction), but also the senses of texture and touch (mechanoreception), temperature (thermoreception), light (vision), pain (nociception) and even sound (audition). Just think of the combinations of experiences — touch, fizziness, coolness, acidity, colour and exquisite smells, as well as the sound of the popping of the cork — when drinking champagne. Those who like spices in their food derive pleasure from the stimulation of receptors in the sensation of pain (nociceptors). These are stimulated by chemicals found in the common spices, such as chilli peppers, and the resulting sensation is referred to as the common chemical sense.

Taste buds

Taste (gustation) refers to the sensation experienced when chemicals come into contact with the gustatory end organs, the taste buds. Taste buds are embedded in the stratified epithelium of the tongue, soft palate, pharynx, larynx and epiglottis, and are unevenly distributed around these regions. They are innervated by the facial, glossopharyngeal and vagus nerves. The lingual taste buds are associated with three of the four types of papillae (fungiform, foliate and circumvallate), whilst those associated with the other regions of the mouth are found on the smooth epithelial surfaces.

In human beings, the number of taste buds varies from person to person with, on average, a range of 2000–5000, but it can be as low as 500 and as high as 20 000 with no significant age or gender differences. The papillae in the different regions of the tongue have distinctive shapes and characteristic numbers of taste buds associated with them, as well as distinctive innervations related to their position on the tongue.

- Scattered over the main body of the tongue are approximately 200 small, mushroom-shaped, fungiform papillae, which have on average three taste buds each.
- The larger foliate papillae are found on the back and sides of the tongue. They comprise up to nine folds of epithelium and as many as 600 taste buds each.
- About 10–15 larger mushroom-shaped, circumvallate papillae, each surrounded by a circular trough, lie on the back of the tongue in a V-shaped formation. The circumvallate papillae have on average 250 taste buds each.

Each taste bud is connected at its base by terminals of sensory nerve fibres. The nerve supply for most of the taste buds on the soft palate and on the anterior two-thirds of the tongue comes from the chorda tympani branch of the facial nerve, so called because its route to the brain stem passes close to the tympanic membrane in the ear. The glossopharyngeal nerve innervates the taste buds on the posterior third of the tongue and the back of the mouth, whilst branches of the vagus nerve innervate taste buds in the pharynx and epiglottis.

Each taste bud is made up of up to 50–150 neuroepithelial cells arranged like the segments of an orange in a compact pear-shaped structure (intragemmal cells). The taste bud complex is about 70 μm high and 40 μm in diameter, and has a small 2–10 μm opening in the epithelium surface, called the taste pore, which allows direct contact between the chemicals dissolved in the saliva and the small tips of some of the neuroepithelial receptor cells within the taste bud. The exposed parts of the receptor cells are made up of many long, corrugated folds in the membrane called microvilli that provide a large surface area for contact with the chemicals dissolved in the saliva. Saliva is essential for normal taste, as it acts as the solvent for the chemicals as well as a transport medium for the chemicals to reach the receptors. There is a layer of saliva that extends into the taste pore and which constantly bathes the receptor tips. The dissolved chemicals diffuse through this thin layer to reach the microvilli.

There is general agreement that there are four types of intragemmal cell: basal cells (stem cells) that give rise to the receptor cells, type I (dark) cells, intermediate and type II (light) cells. It has been suggested that these different types represent the different stages in the life cycle of the taste receptor cell.

The taste bud complex is an extremely dynamic system in which there is a rapid turnover of receptor cells. The lifespan of an individual receptor cell is approximately 10 days, with cells being continually born through the division of epithelial stem cells (basal cells) within the bud, maturing, performing their gustatory function and then eventually dying.

The receptor cells do not in themselves have an axon or nerve fibre, but the base of each cell has specialized regions that look like terminals of nerve fibres. The cytoplasm at the base of the cell is packed with small vesicles filled with a chemical transmitter substance (possibly serotonin or vasoactive intestinal peptide), which is released when the potential inside becomes more positive (becomes depolarized). In most cases, the depolarization leads to an action potential followed by an increase in intracellular Ca^{2+} within the cell and the subsequent release of the neurotransmitter. In close association with these regions are the endings of the sensory (intragemmal) nerve fibres that make a synaptic-like connection with the receptor cells. The released neurotransmitter elicits generator potentials and hence action potentials in this primary afferent neurone, thereby transmitting impulses into the central nervous system. Each taste bud is innervated by more than one nerve fibre and each single nerve fibre can innervate a number of receptor cells, taste buds and even papillae. This means that there is a high degree of convergence of inputs from taste buds on to the sensory nerve fibres. As there is a rapid turnover of receptor cells, there are also constantly changing connections between the cells and the nerve fibres. The nerves are continually sprouting new processes, forming new synapses with young cells and retracting synaptic connections with dying cells. It has been calculated that, at any one time, fewer than one-third of the cells in a single taste bud are fully innervated. It has been shown that an intact nerve supply is necessary for the normal survival and function of taste buds. If the nerve supply is cut or damaged, the taste buds degenerate and slough off. Following nerve regeneration, the taste buds reappear and can return to normal function.

Transduction mechanisms

Since Aristotle (384–322 BC), there have been attempts to categorize taste into primary or basic qualities of taste. Although many hundreds of different chemicals can stimulate activity in taste receptor cells, the four basic qualities of taste (salt, sour, sweet and bitter) have stood the test of time. A fifth basic quality of taste has been recently identified. This is referred to as umami (delicious taste), which is associated with the amino acid glutamate and some nucleotides.

Gustatory receptor cells have a dual role, namely that of detecting both nutrients and toxins. Because of this, they have to be able to respond, both individually and collectively, to a wide variety of chemicals. These chemicals can be simple ions, such as sodium ions (salt) and hydrogen ions (sour), or the more complex compounds that give the sensations of sweet (glucose), bitter (quinine) and umami (monosodium glutamate).

The transduction mechanisms that convert the chemical stimuli into electrical events in the receptor cell are numerous, varied and sometimes complex. There does not appear to be a unique mechanism for each of the basic tastes; each seems to use several different mechanisms. There may even be similarities of mechanisms for different basic tastes. The way in which we perceive many subtle tastes and distinguish different compounds of the same basic taste category could be explained by the specificity and multiplicity of these mechanisms. However, we do know that simple Na^+ salts depolarize taste cells by Na^+ influx through channels in the apical and lateral cell membrane. Similar channels may be involved in the detection of H$^+$ ions, although the transduction mechanism for this ion shows a marked species variability. Transduction of more complex molecules such as sugars and bitter substances frequently involves membrane receptors linked to G-proteins and second messengers, such as cyclic adenosine monophosphate (cAMP) and inositol trisphosphate (IP$_3$/diacylglycerol (DAG)) that gate ion channels and cause depolarization and action potentials to be initiated. Some artificial sweeteners are known to cause depolarization by modulating ligand-gated ion channels directly. The response to glutamate (umami) is thought to involve N-methyl-D-aspartic acid (NMDA) and metabotropic glutamate receptors, similar to those found in the brain. In most cases, the resultant depolarization leads to an action potential in the receptor cell that in turn is followed by an increase in intracellular Ca^{2+} and the release of the neurotransmitter from the base of the cell associated with the intragemmal nerve ending. Recordings, using tiny electrodes, from individual nerve fibres innervating the taste buds in anaesthetized animals reveal that one does not experience a burst of impulses only when a solution of just one of the basic taste substances is dripped on to the appropriate taste bud or buds. Such selectivity of response is very rare. Most nerves respond to two or more of the basic taste stimuli, the magnitude of the response varying from one taste substance to another (the so-called taste profile). This means that the activity of a single gustatory fibre does not provide unambiguous information to the brain about the quality and intensity of the stimulus. At some point the brain must perform a comparison between the activities in several different nerve fibres in order to determine what the taste actually is.

Afferent gustatory neurones

The primary afferent gustatory neurones have their first synaptic connection within the nucleus of the tractus solitarius (NTS) and it is here that approximately 82% of the neurones respond to three or four basic taste stimuli. There is also convergence here between gustatory and thermoreceptor inputs, with many neurones responding to cooling of the tongue, as well as to chemical stimuli. The second-order neurones in the NTS then project to the most medial part of the ventroposterior medial nucleus of the thalamus. There is a further projection to the brain-stem reticular formation, the parabrachial nuclei and the cranial nerve nuclei involved in the reflexes associated with gestation. The thalamic neurones project to the primary gustatory cortex, which includes an area just anterior to the somatosensory area for the tongue, as well as to the nearby frontal operculum and anterior insular secondary cortex. There is evidence for a secondary gustatory area in the orbitofrontal cortex; studies in primates suggest that neurones at these higher levels of the gustatory pathway respond more selectively, with 25% of the neurones in the primary cortex and 74% of the neurones in the secondary cortex responding to a single basic gustatory stimulus. Neurones in the orbitofrontal cortex that respond to gustatory stimuli are seen to be modulated by hunger and

inputs are reduced when appetite is satiated. The orbitofrontal cortex receives inputs not only from the gustatory neurones, but also from the olfactory, visual and somatosensory pathways, and neurones, have been shown to respond to two or more modalities (touch, vision, smell, taste). This area is thought to be involved in the learning of associations between stimuli: for instance, the association of the taste, smell, texture and sight of food substances, all of which are important in the appreciation of what is termed 'flavour'.

Several textbooks and detailed reviews on taste have, in the past, suggested that different areas of the tongue are more sensitive to the different basic tastes. These so-called tongue maps are now thought to be incorrect, their origin lying in a mistranslation of the early 20th-century work of Hänig. His work referred to thresholds of the basic tastes and not to the exclusive nature of the loci. Subsequent misinterpretations have led to the impression that the tip of the tongue detects sweet, the sides of the tongue detect sour and salt, and the back of the tongue detects bitter tastes. This is clearly not true.

Common chemical sense

The common chemical sense is the sensation caused by stimulation of epithelial or mucosal-free nerve endings by potentially harmful chemicals. The evidence suggests that free nerve endings are polymodal nociceptors that respond to a variety of different modalities of stimuli, such as mechanical, thermal and noxious. In the mouth, the major nerve that contributes to this sense is the trigeminal nerve. This innervates almost all regions of the mouth, the tongue, the hard and soft palate, the mucosa of the lips, and cheek. Free nerve endings are found throughout the oral cavity and amongst the chemicals that are known to stimulate these receptors (besides noxious, damaging chemicals) are alcohol, menthol, peppermint, capsaicin and piperine, the last two found in chilli peppers and black pepper respectively.

Olfaction

The human olfactory organ (the olfactory epithelium) comprises a sheet of cells 100–200 μm thick, situated high in the back of the nasal cavity and on a thin bony partition called the central septum of the nasal passage. This system responds to volatile, airborne molecules that make contact with the olfactory epithelium with the in-out air flow during normal nasal breathing. There is a turbulent air flow in this region because of the turbinate bones in the side walls of the nose (the conchae), and this leads to the odour molecules being distributed over the receptor sheet in an irregular pattern.

Olfactory epithelium

The olfactory epithelium contains olfactory receptors which are specialized, elongated cells. These cells have very fine (0.1–0.4 μm diameter), unmyelinated axons that

Five

run in bundles upwards through perforations in the skull (the cribriform plate of the ethmoid bone) above the roof of the nasal cavity and below the frontal lobes of the brain. These bundles of nerves make up the olfactory nerve (Ist cranial nerve). The olfactory nerve is short and ends in the olfactory bulbs, a pair of small swellings underneath the frontal lobes. The peripheral end of the olfactory receptors points down into the nasal cavity and is extended into a long process ending in small knobs that carry hair-like, non-motile processes called cilia, which are 20–200 μm in length. These cilia are bathed in a 35 μm-thick layer of mucus, which has been secreted by specialized cells in the epithelium and in which the molecules of the odorous substances dissolve. The molecules diffuse through the surface layers of the mucus and interact with olfactory receptor proteins in the cilia membranes. This initiates a cascade reaction inside the cell that leads to a change of frequency of action potentials that pass along the olfactory nerve fibres. Hydrophilic (water-soluble) molecules dissolve readily in the mucus, but the diffusion of less soluble molecules is assisted by odour-binding proteins in the mucus; these proteins are also thought to assist in removing the odour molecules from the receptor cell following stimulation. The mucus layer has been shown to move across the surface of the olfactory mucosa at approximately 10–60 μm min^{-1} towards the nasopharynx. The flow of mucus is increased and becomes more watery in conditions of infection of the nasal cavity. The flow is also thought to assist in the removal of odour molecules from the vicinity of the cilia following stimulation.

In contrast to the limited number of taste sensations, humans can detect 10000 or more different odours. There have been attempts to classify these into a smaller number of basic or primary odours, but there is no universally accepted scheme. Unfortunately, there is no simple relationship between chemical structures and odours. Threshold concentrations of odours can be extremely low, with many substances being detected at picomolar (10^{-12} mol L^{-1}) concentrations.

Odorant membrane receptors

There are thought to be hundreds of different odorant membrane receptors located on the cilia of the olfactory cells. A large family of putative odorant receptor genes (perhaps as many as 1000) have been cloned using oligonucleotide probes targeted to G-protein-binding motifs. Binding of the odorant to the receptor leads to an increased conductance to Na$^+$, and to a depolarizing generator potential, via a GTP-binding protein (G$_{olf}$) and cAMP. Although cAMP appears to be the major second messenger in olfactory transduction, there is increasing evidence for the involvement of phosphoinositide-derived second messengers as well.

Each olfactory receptor neurone spontaneously generates action potentials, with between 3 and 60 impulses per second. When stimulated by a particular odour, they increase their firing frequency. Each receptor cell responds, but not equally, to many different types of odour. Single neurones appear to contain the gene for only one odorant receptor, and are therefore selective for a particular set of odorants, which combine with that receptor. In rodents, it has been shown that neurones containing the same receptor are dispersed within zones in the epithelium, and therefore different regions of the olfactory sheet (consisting of hundreds, if not thousands, of receptor cells) are maximally responsive to particular odours. The overall pattern of activity in the olfactory epithelium can be mapped using electro-olfactograms. Each distinctive odour produces its own fingerprint of activity across the epithelium. This so-called mapping reflects the patterns of activation (expression) of genes that make the receptor proteins in the receptor cell membranes.

Olfactory pathway

As in the gustatory system, the successive nerve cells in the olfactory pathway become more selective, each responding to fewer odours. The special coding of odour quality is transmitted to the first relay of the olfactory pathway, the olfactory bulb. There appears to be a loose topographical projection from the receptor sheet to the bulb. The primary olfactory neurones terminate in the spherical glomeruli (approximately 100–200 μm in diameter), where they synapse with the dendrites of neurones called mitral and tufted cells. Each olfactory neurone projects to only one glomerulus. However, each glomerulus can receive inputs from several thousand olfactory neurones widely dispersed throughout the olfactory epithelium. There is some evidence that each glomerulus may receive inputs from neurones expressing the same receptor, thus making the glomeruli functioning units, responding to a particular group of odorants. The olfactory bulb contains a complex network of nerve cells and is responsible for a considerable amount of sensory processing.

Neurones in the olfactory bulb respond with one distinctive temporal pattern of impulses to one odour and a completely different pattern of impulses to another. Besides the mitral and tufted neurones, the bulb also contains many interneurones (e.g. periglomerular and granule cells). It also receives descending projections from a number of higher brain regions that, together with the interneurones, contribute to the processing of the sensory input. There is evidence of lateral inhibition between neighbouring glomeruli which sharpen olfactory acuity and which is very similar to the process of surround inhibition in other parts of the central nervous system. The mitral and tufted cells send their fibres into the olfactory tract to the thalamus, which in turn sends fibres to the primary olfactory cortex. The primary olfactory cortex includes the anterior olfactory nucleus, the olfactory tubercle and the piriform, periamygdaloid and entorhinal cortices. In addition, there are projections via the anterior commissures, to the contralateral olfactory bulb. From the cortex there are projections to the orbitofrontal cortex. There is evidence that the piriform and the orbitofrontal cortex are involved in odour discrimination and combine with other stimuli to give the perception of flavour.

Olfactory pathways also provide inputs to various regions of the limbic system around the region of the hypothalamus. As the limbic system is thought to be responsible for regulating emotions, this may explain the observation that smells can evoke strong feelings of enjoyment or aversion (the hedonistic component of sensation).

The olfactory system occupies a smaller fraction of the brain in humans than in many other species, and this is part of the evidence for the commonly held belief that our sense of smell is inferior. Studies in other animals, from insects to monkeys, have revealed the importance of olfaction for many basic aspects of behaviour, especially reproduction. However, even in humans, there is growing evidence that olfaction (mainly unconscious) is important in such functions as sexual preferences and recognition of other people.

Thermoreception

The detection of change of temperature is the modality of thermoreception. Receptors within the mouth respond to the temperature of food and drink entering the oral cavity and are subjected to a wide range of temperatures from below 0°C to well above the threshold of pain at 46°C. However, thermal sensation is not a continuous variable but is divided into the sensations of warm and cold. The body surface and oral cavity are not uniformly sensitive to changes in temperature; scattered all over the surface tissues and oral mucosa are small areas (about 1 mm^2) of heightened thermal sensitivity that respond to either warming or cooling of that area, while between these areas are bits of skin or mucosa that are totally insensitive to thermal stimulation. There appear to be about ten times more cold-sensitive areas than warm-sensitive areas. The highest density of both cold and warm areas is found on the face, and in particular the lips, with up to 19 cold areas per square centimetre. The tongue and lips have the highest sensitivity to both cooling and warming within the oral cavity, but overall the oral mucosa appears to be less sensitive to warming than other areas of the face. The sensitivity of different areas is due to the density of the thermoreceptors within the tissues, but it can also be attributed to the thickness and composition of the tissues in which they lie, as well depth of the receptors within that tissue.

Cold and warm receptors

Recordings from thermoreceptors in both skin and oral mucosa have confirmed the two separate types of thermoreceptor: namely, cold and warm receptors. Both receptor types are thought to be free nerve endings, unencapsulated except for a surrounding Schwann cell membrane. The cold receptors are thought to be derived from both small myelinated Aδ and unmyelinated C fibres and lie about 0.18 mm below the surface, whereas the warm receptors are thought to be derived from only unmyelinated C fibres and lie a bit deeper at about 0.22 mm below

the surface. Both types of receptor are spontaneously active, firing impulses at a steady state to the ambient temperature. Cold receptors respond with an increase in discharge frequency on sudden cooling followed by an adaptation of discharge to a new set frequency as long as the stimulus is applied. On warming, the cold receptor responds with a transient inhibition of activity. On the other hand, warm receptors respond with an increase in discharge frequency on sudden warming, followed by an adaptation of discharge to a new set frequency as long as the stimulus is applied. On cooling, the warm receptors respond with a transient inhibition of activity. These increases and decreases of discharge occur irrespective of the initial temperature of the tissues surrounding the free nerve endings. Receptors in the skin are important, not only in detecting these dynamic and static changes in temperature, but also in the maintenance of body temperature, initiating reflexes of sweating and shivering. In the mouth, they are particularly sensitive to sudden changes of temperature, such as when very hot coffee or an iced drink is consumed.

Cold receptors are active over a wide range of surface temperatures (−5 to 43°C), with the maximum static discharge frequency varying from receptor to receptor. Not all cold receptors respond maximally to the same temperature. For a large proportion of cold receptors, the temperature that gives rise to the maximum static discharge frequency of between 5 and 10 impulses per second is variable; it ranges from −5 to 40°C, giving a broad span of temperature ranges within the receptor population. The dynamic response of cold receptors when subjected to transient decreases of temperature results in a higher frequency of discharge, usually discharging in bursts of activity separated by intervals of inactivity.

Warm receptors also have a static spontaneous discharge at ambient temperatures of the tissues in which they lie. The static discharge range begins at about 30°C and reaches a peak frequency when temperatures reach about 46°C. The maximum discharge is higher than that seen in cold receptor fibres at between 10 and 35 impulses per second. The dynamic response of warm receptors when subjected to transient increases of temperature can reach discharge frequencies of 200 impulses per second.

Thermoreceptive afferent pathway

Thermoreceptive afferent neurones from the face and oral cavity form a synapse with second-order neurones in the trigeminal nucleus. These synapses are located in the subnucleus interpolaris and marginal layer (lamina 1) of the medullary dorsal horn. The receptive fields of cold and warm neurones are on the ipsilateral side and cover a larger area than the first-order neurones of between 10 and 100 mm^2, suggesting a degree of convergence at the second-order level. The discharge patterns and static responses of the second-order neurones are similar to those of the first-order neurones, suggesting little if any processing except for a loss of bursting discharge in the second-order cold neurones. The trigeminal thermal neurones ascend further in the trigeminothalamic tract, which terminates in the ventrobasal complex of the thalamus. Here, some of the neurones in the thalamus area respond specifically to cooling, but others are multimodal and respond to touch and taste as well. Again the response characteristics of the cold and warm receptors are preserved at this level. This specificity of peripheral thermal receptors is maintained even within the somatosensory cortex. There are single cortical cells in the oral region of the cortex that only respond to cold stimuli and nothing else. However, there is some degree of evidence for central processing in that the neurones within the central nervous system appear to have a wider range of activity than the individual primary, first-order receptor neurones.

Speech

Speech, and its associated processes of writing and reading, are probably the most complex sensory motor processes involved in the development of humans, and the tongue is an important organ for this activity.

Speech is initiated voluntarily and involves a complex set of muscles around the mouth, the larynx and the throat. It also involves the interruption of breathing and the many muscles of expiration. Sounds are produced during exhalation, initially by the larynx, which acts as a so-called voice box.

Phonation

The production of sound in the larynx is called phonation and involves the co-ordinated movements of abdominal, thoracic and laryngeal muscles. There are a number of ways to produce sounds. One involves using the air pressure provided by the lungs to cause the vocal folds of the larynx to vibrate, and the resulting sound is then altered by the variety of constrictions and openings in parts of the vocal tract. The process of speech production, speech transmission and speech perception is referred to as the 'speech chain', and it is the configuration of the human vocal tract that gives rise to the acoustic properties of speech.

Once the basic sounds are produced in the larynx, they are then modified to become intelligible sounds by the processes of articulation and resonance. The major speech articulators are the lips, jaws, the body itself, the tongue, and the position of the hyoid bone. The position of the hyoid bone sets the height of the larynx and the width of the pharynx.

Articulation

Articulation is the process of producing sounds by means of movement of the lips, mandible, tongue and palatopharyngeal mechanisms in co-ordination with breathing and phonation. The configuration of the speech articulations and their co-ordinated movements generate the sounds that we perceive as language. Phonemes (the consonant and vowel units in a language) are defined as the essential sequential constructive units within a language and therefore they vary considerably between languages.

Resonance

The final quality of the voice depends on the sizes and shapes of the various cavities associated with the nose and mouth. In the nose, these cavities are the nasal cavity itself, the sinuses and the nasopharynx. Of these, only the nasopharynx can be varied by the contractions of the pharyngeal muscles and movement of the soft palate. In the mouth, the cavities involved are the oral cavity itself and the oropharynx. The volume of both of these cavities can be varied by movement of the appropriate muscles. All of these cavities amplify and alter the fundamental sounds produced by the vocal cords; this function is called resonance. The fine balance between the oral and nasal resonance, the movements of the soft palate, larynx, tongue and pharynx, and the position of the fixed structures, such as the teeth, give the unique characteristics of the voice of a particular individual.

Classification of sounds

Sounds may be voiced (i.e. the vocal folds in the larynx vibrate for sound production) or they may be breathed (i.e. the vocal folds do not vibrate). The two main groups of speech sounds are vowels and consonants. Vowel sounds are modified by resonance and are all voiced; they are produced without interruption of the air flow, the air being channelled or restricted by the position of the tongue and lips.

The range of higher harmonics defines or characterizes the vowel sound. Closed vowels are those produced when the tongue is positioned high in the mouth, and open vowels result when the tongue is low in the mouth. Furthermore, front and back vowels are generated when the tongue is located forwards or backwards in the mouth.

A consonant is produced when the air flow is impeded before it is released. Consonants may be voiced (e.g. b, d, z) or breathed (e.g. p, t, s). Consonant sounds are of low amplitude (vowels are created by high-amplitude waves) and are classified in two ways: according to the place of articulation or according to the manner of articulation.

For the classification of sounds based upon the place of articulation, consonants are categorized into bilabial, labiodental, linguodental, linguopalatal and glottal sounds:

- In bilabial sounds (e.g. b, p, m), the two lips are used.
- In labiodental sounds, the lower lip meets the maxillary incisors (e.g. f, v).
- For linguodental sounds (e.g. d, t), the tip of the tongue contacts the maxillary incisors and the adjacent hard palate.

- For linguopalatal sounds, the tongue meets the palate away from the region of the maxillary incisors (e.g. g, k).
- In glottal sounds, sound is produced in the larynx. A glottal stop involves momentary closure of the vocal cords (e.g. in saying uh-uh) or a slightly open glottidis (e.g. h sound in English).

For the classification of consonant sounds based upon the manner of articulation, the degree of stoppage of the air flow is an important criterion. For example, a plosive consonant (e.g. b, p) requires sudden release of air. Note that, although one may describe the position of articulators for a particular vowel or consonant, there are no fixed positions during speech, only continuous movement. The tongue has a significant role during speech, although all oral structures (including the soft palate) are important.

Pathways and centres for speech

Like other patterns of voluntary movement, speech originates in the cerebral cortex. However, several other parts of the brain, such as the cerebellum and the brain stem, together with sensory feedback, can modify and regulate the descending nerve impulses to the motor neurones that activate the various muscles involved in speech. The motor neurones involved are to be found in the brain stem and their axons travel to the muscles of the vocal apparatus. Speech also depends on the co-ordination of the motor neurones in the cervical and thoracic parts of the spinal cord that innervate the muscles that are involved in breathing.

The process of speech involves two main stages of mental activity:

- Firstly, the formation in the mind of thoughts that need to be expressed as well as the choice of words to be used
- Secondly, the motor control of the various pathways and the act of vocalization.

The first stages of speech involve sensory association areas of the brain and in particular a region called Wernicke's area. This lies in the posterior part of the superior temporal gyrus. If Wernicke's area in the dominant hemisphere (the left hemisphere for a right-handed person) is damaged or destroyed, the person has what is termed Wernicke's aphasia, in which he or she is capable of understanding the spoken or written word but unable to interpret the thought that it expresses or formulate the thoughts that are to be communicated.

Another region of the cortex called Broca's area is also involved in speech. This lies in the prefrontal and premotor facial regions of the cortex, about 95% of the time in the left hemisphere. Skilled motor patterns for the control of the larynx, lips, mouth, respiratory system and other accessory muscles involved in speech are all initiated here. Damage of Broca's area leads to the person being capable of deciding what he or she wants to say but unable to make the vocal system emit words instead of incoherent noises. This is called motor aphasia.

Facial and laryngeal regions of the motor cortex activate the muscles involved in articulation, and the cerebellum, basal ganglia and sensory cortex all help to control the sequences and intensities of muscle contractions. Damage to any of these regions can cause either partial or total inability to speak distinctly.

Five

Self-assessment: questions

True/false statements

Which of the following statements are true and which are false?

a. The lingual frenum usually crosses the floor of the mouth to terminate immediately behind the lower incisors.

b. The sulcus terminalis divides the tongue into a smaller anterior part and a larger posterior part.

c. The dorsum of the tongue is characterized by an abundance of papillae, the largest being the circumvallate papillae.

d. The lingual artery, a branch of the external carotid, reaches the tongue by passing across the superficial surface of the hyoglossus muscle.

e. The extrinsic muscles of the tongue alter its shape.

f. All the extrinsic tongue muscles receive their motor innervation from the hypoglossal nerve.

g. Receptor cells in the taste buds on the tongue are innervated by the trigeminal nerve.

h. The filiform papillae do not have taste buds associated with them.

i. Each taste bud comprises four receptor cells and a number of supporting cells.

j. The taste bud complex is a dynamic system in which the lifespan of the receptor cells within the taste bud is 28 days.

k. Receptor cells in the taste bud have synaptic connections with primary afferent neurones and the neurotransmitter is probably acetylcholine.

l. Each taste bud is innervated by more than one nerve fibre and each nerve fibre can innervate more than one receptor cell and taste bud.

m. Umami is the fifth basic taste and is stimulated by monosodium glutamate.

n. The transduction mechanisms that convert chemical stimuli into electrical events in the receptor cells are unique to each of the basic tastes.

o. Primary afferent gustatory neurones have their first synaptic connection within the nucleus of the tractus solitarius and it is here that approximately 50% of the neurones respond to a single basic taste.

p. In the nucleus of the tractus solitarius there is a convergence of gustatory and thermoreceptor neurones onto the second-order neurones.

q. 25% of the neurones in the primary cortex and 74% of the neurones in the secondary cortex respond to a single basic quality of taste stimulus.

r. The area of the brain that is thought to be involved in learning the associations between the modalities of stimuli is called the orbitofrontal cortex.

s. The receptors involved in the common chemical sense are polymodal nociceptors, which are free nerve endings innervated by the facial (VIIth) cranial nerve.

t. Like taste receptor cells, olfactory receptor cells synapse with primary olfactory neurones.

u. As many as 10 000 different odours can be detected by human beings in contrast with only five basic tastes.

v. Primary olfactory neurones synapse in the olfactory bulb with the dendrites of neurones called mitral and tufted cells.

w. Olfactory pathways provide inputs to the limbic system and the hypothalamus, where they are thought to be involved with regulating emotion.

x. Oral thermoreceptors monitor temperature of the oral cavity.

y. Thermoreceptors are divided into two types: warm and cold. They are evenly distributed throughout the oral cavity.

z. Both cold and warm receptors are free nerve endings innervated by Aδ and C fibres.

aa. Motor aphasia, when a person is capable of deciding what he or she wants to say but is unable to say it, is evidence of damage to Wernicke's area of the cortex.

ab. The production of sounds is effected during exhalation of air and is called phonation.

ac. The cavities of the mouth and nose, such as the sinuses, the nasopharynx, the oral cavity and the oropharynx, are all involved in amplifying and altering the fundamental sound produced by the vocal cords and this function is called articulation.

ad. The position of the hyoid bone is one of the major speech articulators, along with the lips, jaws, tongue and the body itself. Its position sets the width of the larynx and the height of the pharynx.

Extended matching questions

Theme: Muscles of the tongue

Lead-in

Select the most appropriate option to answer items 1–5. Each option can be used once, more than once or not at all.

Item list

1. Muscle behind which lies the lingual artery and glossopharyngeal nerve
2. Muscle that protrudes the tongue
3. Muscle that flattens and broadens the tongue
4. Muscle that raises the tongue and floor of mouth in preparation for swallowing
5. Muscle that retracts the tongue so that the food bolus is transported towards the oropharynx during swallowing

Option list

A. Buccinator
B. Genioglossus
C. Geniohyoid
D. Hyoglossus
E. Longitudinal intrinsic muscle fibres
F. Mylohyoid

Self-assessment: questions

G. Palatoglossus
H. Palatopharyngeus
I. Strap muscles
J. Styloglossus
K. Superior constrictor
L. Transverse intrinsic muscle fibres
M. Vertical intrinsic muscle fibres

Theme: Innervation of the tongue

Lead-in

Select the most appropriate option to answer items 1–5. Each option can be used once, more than once or not at all.

Item list

1. Nerve supplying general sensation to most of the posterior third of the dorsum of the tongue
2. Nerve supplying taste fibres associated with the circumvallate papillae
3. Nerve supplying general sensation to the ventral surface of the tongue
4. Motor supply to intrinsic muscles of the tongue
5. Motor supply of the palatoglossus extrinsic muscle of the tongue

Option list

A. Accessory nerve (spinal)
B. Buccal branch of facial nerve
C. Buccal branch of mandibular nerve
D. Chorda tympani
E. Deep petrosal nerve
F. Glossopharyngeal nerve
G. Greater petrosal nerve
H. Hypoglossal nerve
I. Inferior alveolar nerve
J. Lesser petrosal nerve
K. Lingual branch of mandibular nerve
L. Mylohyoid nerve
M. Pharyngeal plexus
N. Vagus nerve

Theme: Taste

Lead-in

Select the most appropriate option to answer items 1–6. Each option can be used once, more than once or not at all.

Item list

1. The chemical stimulus that can lead to a bitter sensation is...
2. The quality of taste, umami, is associated with...
3. The vesicles in the base of the gustatory receptor cells are thought to contain...
4. Stimulation of gustatory receptor cells leads to an increase of intracellular...
5. The chemical stimulus that can lead to a sour sensation is...
6. The transduction of complex molecules such as sugars involves membrane receptors linked to...

Option list

A. The amino acid, glutamate
B. Acetylcholine
C. Hydrogen ions
D. Chlorine ions
E. Calcium ions
F. Sodium ions
G. ATP
H. Sugar
I. Adrenaline
J. G-proteins
K. Quinine
L. Serotonin or vasoactive intestinal peptide

Picture questions

Figure 5.1

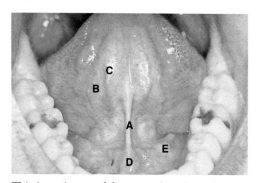

This is a picture of the ventral surface of the tongue.
a. Identify the features labelled A–E.
b. With what anatomical structures are the features labelled D and E associated?
c. What type of mucosa covers this region?
d. How can infections from a mandibular tooth 'pointing' beneath the tongue spread into the submandibular region of the neck?

Self-assessment: questions

Figure 5.2

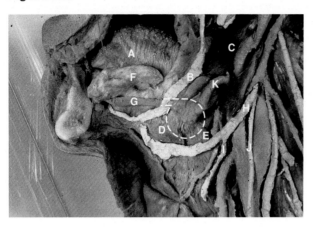

This is a picture of the deep submandibular region.
a. Identify the features labelled A–K.
b. What would be the result of inadvertent section of the structure labelled J?
c. State the specific types of secretion for the two salivary glands in this region.

Figure 5.3

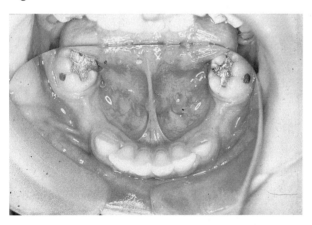

a. What is unusual about the appearance of the floor of the mouth shown here and what signs and symptoms would you expect?

Essay questions

1. Describe the sensory innervation of the mucosa of the tongue, explaining this distribution in terms of the development of the tongue. How would dental local anaesthesia affect the sensory innervation of the tongue?
2. Explain why the tongue is important during mastication, swallowing and speech.
3. List the receptors, with their site, innervation and central pathways, which are involved in detecting that the object in your mouth is a mint with a hole in it.
4. Describe the similarities and differences between the physiological mechanisms involved in taste and smell.

Self-assessment: answers

True/false answers

a. **False**. The lingual frenum usually ends at the sublingual papilla.

b. **False**. The anterior part (palatal part) occupies two-thirds of the dorsum of the tongue.

c. **True**. Other papillae are filiform, fungiform and foliate papillae.

d. **False**. The lingual artery (accompanied by the glossopharyngeal nerve) runs deep to the hyoglossus muscle.

e. **False**. The intrinsic muscles alter the shape of the tongue while the extrinsic muscles alter the position of the tongue in the mouth.

f. **False**. All muscles except palatoglossus are innervated by the hypoglossal nerve. Palatoglossus is a soft palate muscle and is therefore innervated by the pharyngeal plexus.

g. **False**. They are innervated by the facial and glossopharyngeal nerves.

h. **True**. The other three types of papillae (fungiform, foliate and circumvallate) do have taste buds associated with them.

i. **False**. There are between 50 and 150 neuroepithelial cells within each taste bud and four types of cells, basal cells, type I dark cells, intermediate cells and type II light cells.

j. **False**. The lifespan is approximately 10 days.

k. **False**. They do have synaptic connections, although the transmitter substance is not acetylcholine but probably serotonin or vasoactive intestinal peptide.

l. **True**. Each single nerve fibre can even branch to innervate more than one papillae.

m. **True**. Receptors on the taste cells are stimulated by the amino acid glutamate and some nucleotides. Umami is Japanese for 'delicious taste'.

n. **False**. Each basic taste seems to use several different mechanisms and there may even be similarities of mechanisms for different basic tastes.

o. **False**. It is true that they synapse in the nucleus of the tractus solitarius, but more than 80% of the neurones respond to three or more basic taste stimuli.

p. **True**. This can account for the modification of gustatory inputs by the temperature of the food in the mouth.

q. **True**. This is evidence of specialization of neurones as they get higher in the central nervous system.

r. **True**. For instance, the orbitofrontal cortex is involved with the appreciation of flavours combining the inputs of smell, texture and sight of food substances.

s. **False**. They are polymodal nociceptors and they are free nerve endings, but they are innervated by the trigeminal nerve.

t. **False**. Olfactory cells are primary neurones in their own right and synapse in the olfactory bulb.

u. **True**. This accounts for the many different smells humans can detect compared with taste.

v. **True**. The primary olfactory neurones terminate in the spherical glomeruli (approximately 100–200 μm in diameter), where they synapse with these cells.

w. **True**. This may explain the observation that smells can evoke strong feelings of enjoyment or aversion.

x. **False**. Strictly speaking, thermoreceptors do not monitor absolute temperature, but detect changes in temperature in the tissues in which they lie.

y. **False**. There are two types, cold and warm receptors; they are not evenly distributed over the oral cavity and face. There are ten times more cold than warm receptors, and more of both types around the lips and face than in other oral tissues.

z. **False**. Both cold and warm receptors are free nerve endings, but cold receptors are innervated by both Aδ and C fibres, whereas warm receptors appear to be innervated only by unmyelinated C fibres.

aa. **False**. The area affected will be Broca's area, which is found in the prefrontal and premotor facial regions of the cortex. Damage to Wernicke's area leads to the person being capable of understanding the spoken or written word, but being unable to interpret the thought that it expresses or formulate the thoughts that are to be communicated.

ab. **True**. Phonation involves the co-ordinated movements of abdominal, thoracic and laryngeal muscles, resulting in air passing through the vocal folds of the larynx.

ac. **False**. This function is called resonance; articulation is the process of producing the actual sounds by means of the lips, mandible, tongue and palatopharynx in co-ordination with breathing.

ad. **False**. It is true that the position of the hyoid is an important factor when considering the major speech articulators, but its position sets the height of the larynx and the width of the pharynx.

Extended matching answers

Theme: Muscles of the tongue

Item 1 = Option D. The lingual artery and glossopharyngeal nerve lie deep to the hyoglossus muscle, while the lingual nerve, hypoglossal nerve and lingual vein lie superficial to the muscle.

Item 2 = Option B. The genioglossus extrinsic muscles of the tongue arise from the superior genial tubercles and insert into the body and tip of the tongue. They therefore protrude the tongue.

Item 3 = Option L. The transverse intrinsic muscles change the shape of the tongue and will flatten and broaden it. The longitudinal intrinsic muscles will shorten and thicken the tongue.

Item 4 = Option F. The myohyoid muscles form the floor of the mouth. They are able to raise the tongue and floor of the mouth during swallowing.

Self-assessment: answers

· ·

Item 5 = Option J. The tongue moves backwards towards the oropharynx in order to carry the bolus of food for swallowing; this is accomplished by the styloglossus extrinsic muscles of the tongue.

Theme: Innervation of the tongue

Item 1 = Option F. General sensation (and taste) for most of the posterior third of the tongue is associated with the glossopharyngeal nerves. That for the most posterior part of the tongue, close to the epiglottis, is associated with the vagus nerves.

Item 2 = Option F. The circumvallate papillae, although lying in the anterior two-thirds of the tongue immediately in front of the sulcus terminalis, have taste buds innervated by the glossopharyngeal nerves.

Item 3 = Option K. General sensation to the ventral surface of the tongue is associated with the lingual nerves from the anterior divisions of the trigeminal nerves. Note that these nerves also innervate the anterior two-thirds of the dorsum of the tongue (although not for taste) and the mucosa over the floor of the mouth.

Item 4 = Option H. All the intrinsic muscles that change the shape of the tongue are innervated by the hypoglossal nerves.

Item 5 = Option M. The palatoglossus muscle is the exception to the rule that the extrinsic muscles of the tongue are supplied by the hypoglossal nerve. Palatoglossus, being a muscle of the soft palate, is innervated by the pharyngeal plexus.

Theme: Taste

Item 1 = Option K. Complex bitter molecules such as quinine and urea involve membrane receptors linked to G-proteins and second messengers.

Item 2 = Option A. The response to glutamate (umami) is thought to involve N-methyl-D-aspartic acid (NMDA) and metabotropic glutamate receptors, similar to those found in the brain.

Item 3 = Option L. These transmitter substances are released when the potential inside becomes more positive (becomes depolarized). In close association with these regions are the endings of the sensory nerve fibres (intragemmal nerve fibres), which make a synaptic-like connection with the receptor cells. The released neurotransmitter elicits generator potentials and hence action potentials in the primary afferent neurones, thereby transmitting impulses into the central nervous system.

Item 4 = Option E. In most cases, the depolarization of the gustatory cell leads to an action potential followed by an increase in intracellular Ca^{2+} within the cell; there is a subsequent release of the neurotransmitter.

Item 5 = Option C. The movement of simple ions such as hydrogen ions across the receptor membrane leads to the depolarization of the receptor cell. Hydrogen ions are present in all acid fruits.

Item 6 = Option J. Transduction of more complex molecules such as sugars and bitter substances frequently involves membrane receptors linked to G-proteins and second messengers (such as cyclic adenosine monophosphate (cAMP) and inositol trisphosphate (IP_3/diacylglycerol (DAG)), which gate ion channels and cause depolarization and action potentials to be initiated.

Picture answers

Figure 5.1

a. A = lingual frenum. B = fimbriated fold. C = deep lingual vein. D = sublingual papilla. E = sublingual folds.

b. The structure labelled D, the sublingual papilla, has the submandibular ducts (Wharton's ducts) opening on to it. The structure labelled E, the sublingual fold, indicates the position of the sublingual salivary gland and the course of the submandibular duct.

c. The mucosa lining the ventral surface of the tongue has a non-keratinized (lining) stratified squamous epithelium.

d. A sublingual abscess, located above the mylohyoid muscle in the floor of the mouth, may spread to become a submandibular abscess in the suprahyoid region of the neck by passing around the posterior free edge of the mylohyoid muscle. Only rarely would the infection pass through the mylohyoid muscle.

Figure 5.2

a. A = tongue. B = lingual nerve. C = styloglossus muscle. D = hyoglossus muscle. E = outline of deep part of the submandibular salivary gland. F = sublingual salivary gland. G = submandibular duct. H = hypoglossal nerve. I = nerve to thyrohyoid muscle. J = descendens hypoglossi (superior root of ansa cervicalis). K = lingual artery.

b. The descendens hypoglossi (label J) communicates with the ansa cervicalis nerve plexus in the neck. Damage to the descendens hypoglossi would result in partial paralysis of strap (infrahyoid) muscles and some problems for movements of the larynx during and after swallowing.

c. The submandibular salivary gland secretes mixed mucous-serous saliva. The serous acini are much more numerous than the mucous acini (10:1). The sublingual salivary gland also produces a mixed saliva, but with more mucous than serous elements. On occasion, both glands are fused to form a submandibular-sublingual salivary complex.

Self-assessment: answers

Figure 5.3

a. The picture shows a 'tongue-tie'. Normally, the lingual frenum terminates on the sublingual papilla. Here, the frenum extends across the floor of the mouth to become attached to the lingual alveolus behind the mandibular incisors. Tongue-tie may severely limit movements of the tongue and hence could affect speech.

Outline essay answers

Theme: Muscles of the tongue

The essay should be introduced by highlighting the complexity of the innervation of the tongue and the fact that this complexity can be explained by recourse to an understanding of the embryological development of the tongue. A particularly important principle is that a structure/organ maintains its innervation according to its embryological origin.

A description of the embryological development of the tongue should follow (to include diagrams). Mention must be made of the contributions of the first pharyngeal (branchial) arch (distal tongue buds/lateral lingual swellings and median tongue bud/tuberculum impar) and the contributions of 3rd/4th pharyngeal arches (hypobranchial/hypopharyngeal eminence).

It is now appropriate to describe the sensory innervation of the tongue, tying in the embryological development (again to include diagrams):

- For the dorsum of the tongue, general sensation of the anterior two-thirds (palatal part) is from the lingual branch of the mandibular division of trigeminal (the nerve of the 1st pharyngeal arch being the mandibular division of trigeminal).
- Taste for the anterior two-thirds of the tongue is derived from the chorda tympani branch of the facial nerve. The facial nerve is the nerve of the 2nd pharyngeal arch that does not contribute to the development of the tongue. However, the chorda tympani nerve is a pretrematic branch of the facial nerve that invades 1st pharyngeal arch territory.
- The posterior third of the tongue is innervated for both general sensation and taste by the glossopharyngeal and vagus nerves. The glossopharyngeal nerve is the nerve of the 3rd pharyngeal arch and the vagus nerve is the nerve of the 4th pharyngeal arch.
- The ventral surface of the tongue is supplied by the lingual nerve (only general sensation here).

A brief mention could be made of the fact that the muscles of the tongue arise embryologically from occipital myotomes and that these myotomes are associated with the hypoglossal nerve.

For the final paragraph of the essay, the effects of dental anaesthesia on the tongue should be described to complete the answer. Dental anaesthesia in the infratemporal fossa involves 'blocking' the inferior alveolar nerve, the buccal nerve and the lingual nerve. Blocking the inferior alveolar and buccal nerves will have no effect on the tongue. However, blocking the lingual nerve affects both general sensation and taste to the anterior two-thirds of the tongue (dorsal and ventral surfaces). The effects on taste relate to the fact that the chorda tympani nerve joins (and runs with) the lingual nerve.

Theme: Innervation of the tongue

A brief introduction should be provided to highlight the fact that mastication, swallowing and speech are amongst the most complex movements in the body. The criteria for assessing this proposition are:

- the large number and variety of muscles involved
- the significant areas of the higher centres of the brain (cerebral cortex) concerned with the functions of mastication, swallowing and speech
- the large number and variety of nerves involved.

A brief description should be supplied of the intrinsic and extrinsic muscles of the tongue and of their innervations (primarily the hypoglossal nerve, the XIIth cranial nerve).

The role of the tongue in mastication should highlight movements of the food bolus between the teeth and the complementary role played by the buccinator muscles.

The role of the tongue in swallowing should highlight the positioning of the bolus of food in the centre of the tongue and the movement of the tongue backwards towards the oropharyngeal isthmus to expel the food into the oropharynx.

The role of the tongue in speech should highlight the part the tongue plays in articulation of consonant sounds (e.g. in particular linguodentals and linguopalatal sounds).

The final paragraph should return to the criteria for judging the complexity of the tongue's movements by particular reference to areas in the cerebral hemisphere given over to movements of the tongue and mouth (note the motor homunculus and then consider areas associated with speech).

Theme: Taste

Gustatory receptors (taste buds) involved in taste sensation, are found in the stratified epithelium of the tongue, soft palate, pharynx, larynx and epiglottis. They are not evenly distributed throughout these regions. They are innervated by the facial, glossopharyngeal and vagus nerves, depending on where the end organs are situated. All the primary afferent nerve fibres have their first synaptic connection in the nucleus of the solitary tract; the second-order neurones project to most medial part of the ventroposterior medial nucleus of the thalamus, with further projections to the brain-stem reticular formation, the parabrachial nucleus and the cranial nerve nuclei involved in the reflexes associated with gustation. The thalamic neurones project to the primary gustatory cortex, which includes a region just anterior to the somatosensory area for the tongue, as well as to the nearby frontal operculum and anterior insular secondary cortex. There are secondary gustatory areas in the orbitofrontal cortex. These receptors and central pathways will signal the senses of sweet, sour, salt, bitter and umami generated by the object in the mouth.

Olfactory receptors involved in the sensation of smell are to be found in the olfactory epithelium and mucosa in the nasal cavity on a thin bony partition called the central septum of the nasal passage. These specialized, elongated olfactory receptors are innervated by the olfactory nerve. The olfactory nerve is short and ends in the olfactory bulbs, a pair of small swellings underneath the frontal lobes. The primary olfactory neurones terminate in the spherical glomeruli and terminate on so-called mitral and tufted cells. These cells connect to the thalamus via the olfactory tract. The connections from the thalamus are to the primary olfactory cortex (the anterior olfactory nucleus, the olfactory tubercle and the piriform, periamygdaloid and entorhinal cortices). There are additional projections, via the anterior commissures, to the contralateral olfactory bulb. From the cortex there are also projections to the orbitofrontal cortex. The sense of smell will detect the many different constituents of the mint-flavoured sweet, in particular the mint flavouring.

The common chemical sense will also contribute to the overall appreciation of the flavour of the object in the mouth by stimulation of free nerve endings innervated by the trigeminal nerve. These free nerve endings are found throughout the oral cavity and are stimulated normally by noxious chemical stimuli, but are also stimulated by menthol and peppermint. The trigeminal fibres have cell bodies in the trigeminal ganglion and send impulses, via the main sensory nucleus, to the thalamus and the somatosensory cortex.

Receptors involved in mechanoreception will also be involved in sensing the object in the mouth. Mechanoreceptors are involved in the sense of touch and texture whilst eating. The texture (smoothness, crunchiness and firmness) of the mint will be detected by mechanoreceptors in the oral mucosa and the tongue, whilst the tongue moves the object around the mouth. Both slowly adapting and rapidly adapting receptors will be stimulated. The receptors in the tongue will be able to detect the hole in the middle of the mint. Periodontal ligament mechanoreceptors will also detect the hardness of the mint and, if this is bitten, will detect the breaking up of the mint. The majority of the mechanoreceptors in the mouth are innervated by trigeminal nerve. The majority of the cell bodies are again found in the trigeminal ganglion, with a small number of periodontal ligament mechanoreceptor cell bodies in the trigeminal mesencephalic nucleus. Central neuronal connections are located in the trigeminal nuclei, the thalamus and the somatosensory cortex.

Warm and cold thermoreceptors are not likely to contribute to the sensations that detect the mint with a hole in it, as the mint will be at room temperature when placed in the mouth; however, if it were heated up or cooled down before it is placed in the mouth, these receptors would be stimulated accordingly. These are again free nerve endings scattered all around the oral mucosa. Thermoreceptive afferent neurones from the face and oral cavity form a synapse with second-order neurones in the trigeminal nucleus. These trigeminal thermal neurones ascend further in the trigeminothalamic tract, which terminates in the ventrobasal complex of the thalamus and then project further to the somatosensory cortex.

All of these receptor types help the subject detect that the object in the mouth is a mint with a hole in it; this is, of course, appreciated in the light of previous experiences.

Question 4

Both mechanisms involve chemical stimuli which interact with the receptor cell surface proteins and cause local transduction pathways to be initiated. In taste, the chemicals are dissolved in saliva or liquids ingested at the same time as the chemicals. In smell, the molecules of the odorous substance are dissolved in the mucus secreted by specialized epithelial cells in the nasal cavity. The two receptor cell types differ in that taste (gustatory) receptor cells are found in taste buds and are specialized neuroepithelial cells with synaptic connections at their basal end with either the facial, glossopharyngeal and vagus nerves, depending on where the taste bud is situated in the oral cavity. The olfactory receptor cells are specialized, elongated nerve cells of the olfactory nerve with direct connections with the olfactory bulbs.

There are five basic tastes (salt, sour, sweet, bitter and umami) with a number of well-defined transduction mechanisms, whereas in the olfactory system there are hundreds of different odorant membrane receptors located on the cilia of the olfactory cells and humans can detect over 10 000 different odours. The taste receptor cells have microvilli exposed to the oral cavity by the taste pore at the top of the taste bud, whilst the olfactory receptor cells have hair-like, non-motile processes called cilia, which are 20–200 μm in length. These, like the microvilli in the taste receptors, are bathed in fluid; mucus in the case of the olfactory neurones, and saliva or ingested liquids in the case of the taste receptor cells. Both taste receptor cells and olfactory receptor neurones have a limited lifespan (approximately 10 days for taste receptor cells and 60 days for olfactory neurones). Both can regenerate if damaged. Both gustatory and olfactory central neuronal pathways exhibit selectivity as the neurones synapse at higher levels of the central nervous system.

Each olfactory receptor neurone responds, but not equally, to many different odour types. Similarly, in the gustatory system, each neurone responds to more than one basic taste. Both olfactory and gustatory neurones connect to the cortex via neurones in the thalamus and, from the cortex, both systems have neurones that project into the orbitofrontal cortex.

There are, however, thought to be more connections from the olfactory system to the limbic system, which may explain the observation that smells can evoke strong feelings of emotion, such as enjoyment and aversion.

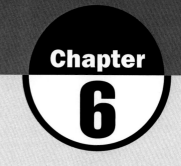

Vasculature, lymphatics and innervation of the orodental tissues

Blood supply to orodental tissues 67
Venous drainage of orodental tissues 68
Lymphatic drainage of orodental tissues 68
Innervation of orodental tissues 69
   Secretomotor innervation of the salivary glands 70
   The trigeminal nerve (maxillary and mandibular divisions) 71
      Self-assessment: questions 73
      Self-assessment: answers 75

Overview

The orodental tissues are well vascularized and well innervated. The high vascularity explains not only the profuse bleeding that occurs with wounds/trauma to the mouth but also, in part, the remarkable potential for healing. The mouth has a sensory, motor and autonomic innervation. The sensory supply includes the special sense related to taste and the autonomic innervation includes the secretomotor supply of salivary glands. The lymphatic drainage of orodental tissues, although variable, is of great importance to the understanding of the spread of pathologies from the mouth through the lymphatic system.

Learning objectives

You are required to:
- have a detailed knowledge of the sources and distribution of blood vessels and nerves supplying the mouth and associated structures (i.e. salivary glands, the musculature of the tongue, palate, floor of mouth, lips and cheeks, and the muscles of mastication), together with functional associations
- have good knowledge of the courses and distribution of the maxillary and mandibular divisions of the trigeminal nerve and also the central connections of the trigeminal nerve
- know the location of the major groups of lymph nodes draining orodental tissues and the tonsillar ring protecting the entrance to the pharynx.

(Note that physiological aspects of taste and thermosensation are dealt with in Chapter 5, in association with an account of the tongue. Mechanoreception in the oral cavity is covered in Chapter 15 in association with an account of the periodontal ligament, and oral pain is dealt with in Chapter 13 in relation to the pulpodentinal complex. Salivation is considered in Chapter 7.)

Blood supply to orodental tissues

Mandibular teeth and periodontium

The face is supplied mainly through the facial artery, a branch of the external carotid artery in the neck. The facial artery first appears on the face as it hooks round the lower border of the mandible, at the anterior edge of the masseter. It then runs a tortuous course between the facial muscles towards the medial corner of the eye. There is a rich anastomosis with the artery of the opposite side and with additional vessels supplying the face (transverse facial branch of the superficial temporal artery; infra-orbital and mental branches of the maxillary artery; dorsal nasal branch of the ophthalmic artery). The main arteries to the teeth and jaws are derived from the maxillary artery, a terminal branch of the external carotid, running in the infratemporal fossa. The alveolar arteries follow roughly the same course as the alveolar nerves.

The inferior alveolar artery, which supplies the mandibular teeth, is derived from the maxillary artery before it crosses the lateral pterygoid muscle in the infratemporal fossa. A mylohyoid branch is given off before the inferior alveolar artery enters the mandibular foramen in the ramus of the mandible. The inferior alveolar artery passes through the mandibular foramen to enter the mandibular canal and terminates as the mental and incisive arteries. Posteriorly, the buccal gingiva is supplied by the buccal artery (a branch of the maxillary artery as it crosses the lateral pterygoid muscle) and by perforating branches from the inferior alveolar artery. Anteriorly, the labial gingiva is supplied by the mental artery and by perforating branches of the incisive artery. The lingual gingiva is supplied by perforating branches from the inferior alveolar artery and by the lingual artery, a branch of the external carotid artery.

Maxillary teeth and periodontium

The posterior superior alveolar artery arises from the maxillary artery in the pterygopalatine fossa. Occasionally, the posterior superior alveolar artery is derived from the buccal artery. It courses tortuously over the maxillary tuberosity before entering bony canals to supply molar and premolar teeth. The artery also gives off branches to the adjacent buccal gingiva, maxillary sinus and cheek.

The middle superior alveolar artery, when present, arises from the infra-orbital artery (which is itself a branch of the third part of the maxillary artery in the pterygopalatine fossa). The middle superior alveolar artery runs in the lateral wall of the maxillary sinus, terminating near the canine tooth where it anastomoses with the anterior and posterior superior alveolar arteries.

The anterior superior alveolar artery also arises from the infra-orbital artery and runs downwards in the anterior wall of the maxillary sinus to supply the anterior teeth. Like the superior alveolar nerves, the superior alveolar arteries form plexuses. The buccal gingiva around the posterior maxillary teeth is supplied by gingival and perforating branches from the posterior superior alveolar artery and by the buccal artery. The labial gingiva of anterior teeth is supplied by labial branches of the infra-orbital artery and by perforating branches of the anterior superior alveolar artery. The palatal gingiva around the maxillary teeth is supplied primarily by branches of the greater palatine artery, a branch of the third part of the maxillary artery in the pterygopalatine fossa.

Palate, cheek, tongue and lips

The palate derives its blood supply from the greater and lesser palatine branches of the maxillary artery. The greater palatine artery anastomoses with the nasopalatine artery at the incisive foramen. The cheek is supplied by the buccal branch of the maxillary artery, and the floor of the mouth and the tongue by the lingual arteries. The lips are mainly supplied by the superior and inferior labial branches of the facial arteries.

Venous drainage of orodental tissues

Teeth and periodontium

The venous drainage of this region is extremely variable. The facial vein is the main vein draining the face. It begins at the medial corner of the eye by confluence of the supra-orbital and supratrochlear veins and passes across the face behind the facial artery. Below the mandible, it joins with the anterior branch of the retromandibular vein. This union is sometimes referred to as the common facial vein.

Small veins from the teeth and alveolar bone pass into larger veins surrounding the apex of each tooth, or into veins running in the interdental septa. In the mandible, the veins are then collected into one or more inferior alveolar veins, which themselves may drain anteriorly through the mental foramen to join the facial veins or posteriorly through the mandibular foramen to join the pterygoid plexus of veins in the infratemporal fossa. In the maxilla, the veins may drain anteriorly into the facial vein or

posteriorly into the pterygoid plexus. No accurate description is available concerning the venous drainage of the gingiva, though it may be assumed that the buccal, lingual, greater palatine and nasopalatine veins are involved; apart from the lingual veins which pass directly into the internal jugular veins, these veins run into the pterygoid plexuses.

Palate, cheek, tongue and lips

The veins of the palate are rather diffuse and variable. However, those of the hard palate generally pass into the pterygoid venous plexus, and those of the soft palate into the pharyngeal venous plexus. The buccal vein of the cheek drains into the pterygoid plexus. Venous blood from the lips drains into the facial veins via the superior and inferior labial veins. The veins of the tongue follow two different routes. Those of the dorsum and sides of the tongue form the lingual veins, which, accompanying the lingual arteries, empty into the internal jugular veins; those of the ventral surface form the deep lingual veins, which ultimately join the facial, internal jugular or lingual veins.

Lymphatic drainage of orodental tissues

As with the venous system, the lymphatic drainage is extremely variable.

Lymphatics from the lower part of the face generally pass through, or around, the buccal lymph nodes to reach the submandibular lymph nodes. However, lymphatics from the medial portion of the lower lip drain into the submental nodes.

The lymph vessels from the teeth usually run directly into the submandibular nodes on the same side, although lymph from the mandibular incisors drains into the submental nodes. Occasionally, lymph from the molars passes directly into the jugulodigastric group of nodes. The lymph vessels of the labial and buccal gingivae of the maxillary and mandibular teeth unite to drain into the submandibular nodes, although in the labial region of the mandibular incisors they may drain into the submental nodes. The lingual and palatal gingivae drain into the jugulodigastric group of nodes, either directly or indirectly through the submandibular nodes.

Lymphatics from most areas of the palate terminate in the jugulodigastric group of nodes. Vessels from the posterior part of the soft palate terminate in pharyngeal lymph nodes. Lymph from the floor of the mouth region can drain directly to the jugulodigastric nodes.

Lymphatics from the anterior two-thirds of the tongue may be subdivided into two groups: marginal and central vessels. The marginal lymphatic vessels drain the lateral third of the dorsal surface of the tongue and the lateral margin of its ventral surface. The remaining regions drain into the central vessels. The marginal vessels pass to the submandibular lymph nodes of the same side. The central vessels at the tip of the tongue pass to the submental lymph nodes. Central vessels behind the tip drain into ipsilateral and contralateral submandibular lymph nodes. Some marginal and central lymph vessels pass directly to the jugulodigastric group of nodes (or even the jugulo-omohyoid nodes). Lymphatics from the posterior third of the tongue drain into the deep cervical group of nodes, vessels centrally draining both ipsilaterally and contra-laterally. Knowledge of the ipsilateral and contralateral drainage from the tongue is important clinically where, for example, a tumour near the central part of the tongue may be associated with spread into lymph nodes on both sides.

At the oropharyngeal isthmus lie the palatine tonsils between the pillars of the fauces and the lingual tonsils on the pharyngeal surface of the tongue. These tonsils form part of a ring of lymphoid tissue known as Waldeyer's tonsillar ring. The other components are the tubal tonsils and adenoid tissue (pharyngeal tonsils) located in the nasopharynx.

Innervation of orodental tissues

Excepting regions around the oropharyngeal isthmus, the sensory innervation of the oral mucosa is derived from the maxillary and mandibular divisions of the trigeminal nerve. The trigeminal nerve also supplies the teeth and their supporting tissues (see Table 6.1). Both the major and the minor salivary glands are supplied by secretomotor parasympathetic fibres from the facial and glossopharyngeal nerves.

The motor innervation of the muscles of the jaws and oral cavity is from the trigeminal, facial, accessory and hypoglossal nerves.

All three divisions of the trigeminal nerve are involved with the cutaneous innervation of the face:

• The ophthalmic division supplies the upper part of the face, forehead and scalp.

Table 6.1 Nerves supply to the teeth and gingivae

Maxilla	Nasopala-tine nerve	Greater palatine nerve		Palatal gingiva
	Anterior superior alveolar nerve	Middle superior alveolar nerve	Posterior superior alveolar nerve	Teeth
	Infraorbital nerve	Posterior superior alveolar nerve and buccal nerve		Buccal gingiva
	1 2 3 4 5 6 7 8			Tooth position (Zsigmondy system)
	Mental nerve	Buccal nerve and perforating branches of inferior alveolar nerve		Buccal gingiva
Mandible	Incisive nerve	Inferior alveolar nerve		Teeth
	Lingual nerve and perforating branches of inferior alveolar nerve			Lingual gingiva

• The maxillary and mandibular divisions essentially supply the upper and lower jaw regions respectively.

Knowledge of these areas, and of the specific branches involved, is important clinically for assessing the effects of nerve damage and for an understanding of the successful anaesthetization of the buccal, infra-orbital and inferior alveolar (mental) nerves during dental treatment. The areas supplied by the three divisions of the trigeminal nerve also relate to aspects of the development of the face.

Inferior alveolar nerve

The inferior alveolar nerve courses through the mandible in a mandibular canal. Close to the premolar teeth, and after giving molar branches to the molar teeth, the inferior alveolar nerve divides into a mental branch and an incisive branch:

• The mental nerve is a sensory nerve to the skin and mucosa of the lower lip region.
• The incisive nerve supplies the anterior mandibular teeth.

The distribution of nerves to the mandibular premolars and molars is variable, dental branches coming either directly from the inferior alveolar nerve by short or long branches or indirectly through several alveolar branches. In rare instances, the nerve to the mandibular third molar may arise from the inferior alveolar nerve before it enters the mandibular canal. Communications between the inferior alveolar nerve and nerves from the temporalis and lateral pterygoid muscles have been described, the nerves penetrating the mandible through foramina in the region of muscle attachments. It has been suggested that such nerve connections might explain why, in approximately 5% of patients, the teeth may not be anaesthetized after the main trunk of the inferior alveolar nerve has been blocked at the mandibular foramen by the injection of local anaesthetic solution. It is said that, in any one individual, the mandibular canal remains in a relatively fixed position with respect to the lower border of the mandible. The canal is often closely related to the roots of the mandibular molars. Indeed, the roots of lower third molars may even be perforated by the mandibular canal.

In the premolar region, the main trunk of the inferior alveolar nerve divides into mental and incisive nerves. The mental nerve runs for a short distance in a mental canal before leaving the body of the mandible at the mental foramen to emerge on to the face. In about 50% of cases, the mental foramen lies on a vertical line passing through the mandibular second premolar. In an adult with a full dentition, the mental foramen usually lies midway between the upper and lower borders of the mandible. During the first and second years of life, as the prominence of the chin develops, the opening of the mental foramen alters in direction, from facing forwards to facing upwards and backwards. As well as supplying the skin of the lower lip, the mental nerve provides fibres to an incisor plexus, which innervates the labial periodontium of the mandibular incisors.

The incisive nerve runs forwards in an intraosseous incisive canal. This nerve primarily supplies the incisors and canines but may also supply the first premolar. In some instances, the canine may be supplied directly from the inferior alveolar nerve.

Superior alveolar nerves

Supplying the maxillary dentition there are usually three superior alveolar nerves.

The posterior superior alveolar nerve arises from the maxillary nerve in the pterygopalatine fossa, whence it passes through the pterygomaxillary fissure to descend on the posterior wall (tuberosity) of the maxilla. The dental branches of the nerve enter the maxilla and run in narrow posterior superior alveolar canals above the roots of the molar teeth. A gingival branch does not enter the bone, however, but runs downwards and forwards along the outer surface of the maxillary tuberosity. The dental branches of the posterior superior alveolar nerve may arise from a common nerve trunk within the bone or on the tuberosity before entering bone, or alternatively may appear as separate nerve trunks from the main trunk of the maxillary nerve in the pterygopalatine fossa.

The middle superior alveolar nerve is found in about 70% of subjects. It generally arises from the infra-orbital nerve in the floor of the orbit/roof of the maxillary air sinus, although it may arise from the maxillary nerve in the pterygopalatine fossa. The nerve may run in the posterior, lateral or anterior walls of the maxillary sinus. It terminates above the roots of the premolar teeth.

The anterior superior alveolar nerve arises from the infra-orbital nerve within the infra-orbital canal, generally as a single nerve, but occasionally as two or three small branches. The nerve leaves the infra-orbital canal near its termination and then, diverging laterally from the infra-orbital nerve, runs in the anterior wall of the maxillary sinus. It terminates near the anterior nasal spine after giving off a small nasal branch.

Note that the posterior superior alveolar nerve has an extrabony course that permits anaesthesia of the nerve trunk(s) as it passes across the maxillary tuberosity, whereas the middle and anterior superior alveolar nerves are entirely intrabony in their course and cannot be 'blocked' with an anaesthetic injection. The superior alveolar nerves form a plexus above the root apices of the maxillary teeth. From this plexus nerves pass to the teeth, although it is difficult to trace the precise innervation of the teeth from specific superior alveolar nerves. As a general rule, however, the incisors and canines are supplied by the anterior nerve, the molars by the posterior nerve, and intermediate areas by the middle nerve.

Sensory nerves to oral cavity

The sensory nerve supply to the palate is derived from the maxillary division of the trigeminal nerve via branches of the pterygopalatine ganglion. A small area behind the incisor teeth is supplied by terminal branches of the nasopalatine nerves. These nerves emerge onto the palate at the incisive foramen. The remainder of the hard palate is supplied by the greater palatine nerves emerging onto the palate at the greater palatine foramina. The soft palate is supplied by the lesser palatine nerves emerging onto the palate via the lesser palatine foramina. Although the maxillary division of the trigeminal nerve supplies most of the palate, there is evidence to suggest that some areas supplied by the lesser palatine nerves may also be innervated by fibres from the facial nerve. The posterior part of the soft palate and the uvula are also supplied by the glossopharyngeal nerve, providing the anatomical basis for the gag reflex.

The sensory and motor innervation of the tongue is considered on pages 52–53.

The mucosa of the upper lip is supplied by the infra-orbital branch of the maxillary division of the trigeminal nerve. That of the lower lip is supplied by the mental branch of the mandibular division of the trigeminal nerve. The mucosa of the cheeks is supplied by the buccal branch of the mandibular division of the trigeminal. The mucosa on the floor of the mouth is innervated by the lingual branch of the mandibular division of the trigeminal nerve. The mucosa over the pillars of the fauces (the oropharyngeal isthmus) is supplied by the glossopharyngeal nerve.

Secretomotor innervation of the salivary glands

Parotid gland

The secretomotor supply of the parotid gland is derived through the otic parasympathetic ganglion. This ganglion is situated in the roof of the infratemporal fossa, close to the foramen ovale and the mandibular division of the trigeminal nerve. Like other parasympathetic ganglia in the head, three types of nerve fibre are associated with it: parasympathetic, sympathetic and sensory. However, only the parasympathetic fibres synapse in the ganglion. The preganglionic parasympathetic fibres to the otic ganglion originate from the inferior salivatory nucleus in the brain stem and pass with the glossopharyngeal nerve via its lesser petrosal branch. The sympathetic root of the otic ganglion is derived from postganglionic fibres from the superior cervical ganglion and reaches the otic ganglion via the plexus around the middle meningeal artery in the infratemporal fossa. The sensory root is derived from the auriculotemporal branch of the mandibular division of the trigeminal nerve. The postganglionic parasympathetic fibres (with sensory and sympathetic fibres) reach the parotid gland through the auriculotemporal branch of the mandibular nerve.

Submandibular and sublingual glands

The secretomotor supply of the submandibular and sublingual glands is derived through the submandibular parasympathetic ganglion. This ganglion is situated, with the lingual nerve, on the hyoglossus muscle in the floor of the mouth above the deep part of the submandibular gland. The preganglionic parasympathetic fibres to the ganglion originate from the superior salivatory nucleus in the brain stem and pass with the nervus intermedius of the facial nerve, and subsequently its chorda tympani branch, to reach the lingual nerve in the infratemporal fossa. It is via the lingual nerve that the preganglionic fibres are conveyed to the submandibular ganglion. The sympathetic root of the ganglion is derived from postganglionic fibres from the superior cervical ganglion and reaches the submandibular ganglion via the plexus around the facial artery. The sensory root is derived from the lingual nerve. The postganglionic parasympathetic fibres (with sensory and sympathetic fibres) pass directly to the adjacent submandibular gland, but reach the sublingual gland after re-entering the lingual nerve.

Innervation of the oral musculature

The functions of mastication, swallowing and speech are amongst the most complex in the body. This is reflected in the number and variety of muscles found around the mouth and by the range of cranial nerves that innervate them. Table 6.2 summarizes the innervation of the oral musculature.

The trigeminal nerve (maxillary and mandibular divisions)

Maxillary division

The maxillary division of the trigeminal nerve contains only sensory fibres. It supplies the maxillary teeth and their supporting structures, the palate, the maxillary air sinus, much of the nasal cavity, and the skin overlying the middle part of the face. The nerve emerges into the pterygopalatine fossa through the foramen rotundum of the sphenoid bone. Its subsequent branches can be subdivided into branches from the main nerve trunk and branches from the pterygopalatine ganglion:

- From the main trunk come the meningeal, ganglionic, zygomatic, posterior superior alveolar and infra-orbital nerves. The infra-orbital nerve gives rise to the middle and anterior superior alveolar nerves.
- The branches arising from the ganglion are the orbital, nasopalatine, posterior superior nasal, greater and lesser palatine, and pharyngeal nerves. The branches of the maxillary nerve that arise via the pterygopalatine ganglion contain a mixture of sensory, parasympathetic (secretomotor) and sympathetic (vasomotor) fibres.

Thus, the branches supplying the teeth and their supporting structures and the palate and the upper lip are the posterior, middle and anterior superior alveolar nerves, the nasopalatine and the greater and lesser palatine nerves, and the infra-orbital nerve.

Mandibular division

The mandibular division of the trigeminal nerve is the largest division of the trigeminal nerve. It is the only division that contains motor fibres as well as sensory fibres.

Table 6.2 Innervation of the oral musculature

Region	Muscle	Nerve
Lips	Orbicularis oris	Facial
Cheeks	Buccinator	Facial
Tongue (intrinsic musculature)	Transverse	
	Longitudinal Vertical	Hypoglossal
Tongue (extrinsic musculature)	Genioglossus	
	Hyoglossus Styloglossus	Hypoglossal
	Palatoglossus	Accessory (cranial part)
Floor of mouth	Mylohyoid	Mandibular division of trigeminal
	Geniohyoid	Hypoglossal (C1 fibres)
Palate	Tensor veli palatini	Mandibular division of trigeminal
	Levator veli palatini	
	Palatoglossus	Accessory (cranial part)
	Palatopharyngeus Musculus uvulae	

- Its sensory fibres supply the mandibular teeth (and their supporting structures), the mucosa of the anterior two-thirds of the tongue and the floor of the mouth, the skin of the lower part of the face, and parts of the temple and auricle.
- Its motor fibres supply the muscles of mastication, the mylohyoid, anterior belly of the digastric, and the tensor veli palatini and tensor tympani muscles.

The mandibular nerve emerges into the infratemporal fossa through the foramen ovale of the sphenoid bone. It lies deep to the lateral pterygoid muscle, where it gives off all its branches, dividing into anterior (mainly motor) and posterior (mainly sensory) trunks. Proximal to this division, it gives off the meningeal branch and the nerve to the medial pterygoid. The meningeal branch passes back into the middle cranial fossa through the foramen spinosum of the sphenoid bone (accompanied by the middle meningeal artery). The nerve to the medial pterygoid muscle passes through the otic ganglion (without synapsing) and, after supplying the muscle, continues on to supply the tensor veli palatini and tensor tympani muscles. The anterior trunk gives motor branches to the masseter, temporalis and lateral pterygoid, and the sensory buccal nerve. The posterior trunk gives off the sensory auriculotemporal, lingual and inferior alveolar nerves, and the motor mylohyoid nerve. Note that the chorda tympani branch of the facial nerve joins the lingual nerve and that postganglionic fibres from the otic parasympathetic ganglion run with the auriculotemporal nerve to provide secretomotor fibres to the parotid gland.

Central connections

Central connections of the trigeminal nerve are complex, as befits a nerve with such important functions and range of distribution. The trigeminal nerve conveys discriminative tactile information from the ipsilateral half of the face and the top of the head; the axons of the trigeminal ganglion cells pass to the principal sensory nucleus and to the pars oralis of the spinal tract of the trigeminal nerve. Proprioceptive information from the ipsilateral muscles of mastication and the temporomandibular joint reach the mesencephalic nucleus of the trigeminal. However, recent evidence suggests that proprioceptive information from the teeth also passes to the principal sensory nucleus. Direct and indirect connections of these nuclei form the basis of cranial nerve reflexes. Signals from the principal sensory and mesencephalic nuclei are transmitted mainly via the contralateral ventral trigeminothalamic tract (trigeminal lemniscus) and the ipsilateral dorsal trigeminothalamic tract to the nucleus ventralis posterior medialis of the thalamus. Axons from this nucleus pass through the posterior limb of the internal capsule to the inferior part of the postcentral gyrus and frontoparietal operculum. The nucleus of the spinal tract of the trigeminal nerve is subdivided into the pars oralis, pars interpolaris and pars caudalis:

- The pars oralis deals mainly with tactile signals.
- The pars interpolaris receives cutaneous and proprioceptive information and sends fibres to the cerebellum.
- The pars caudalis deals particularly with nociceptive signals (but also with tactile and thermal information).

Fibres from the nucleus of the spinal tract pass to the reticular formation (for cranial nerve reflexes). Some fibres run near the medial lemniscus in the contralateral ventral trigeminothalamic tract to reach the various thalamic nuclei. The motor nucleus of the trigeminal nerve lies close to the principal central nucleus in the central part of the pons. It receives fibres from the other sensory trigeminal nuclei, the reticular formation, the cerebellum and the cerebral cortex via bilateral corticonuclear fibres.

Self-assessment: questions

True/false statements

Which of the following statements are true and which are false?

a. The inferior alveolar nerve is derived from the anterior trunk of the mandibular division of the trigeminal nerve.

b. The lingual nerve in the infratemporal fossa lies anterior to, and slightly deeper than, the inferior alveolar nerve.

c. The otic parasympathetic ganglion is secretomotor to the parotid gland.

d. The nerve to the medial pterygoid muscle is derived from the posterior trunk of the mandibular division of the trigeminal nerve.

e. The sensory supply of the temporomandibular joint is derived primarily from the great auricular nerve.

f. With the exception of palatopharyngeus, all muscles of the soft palate are supplied by the pharyngeal plexus of nerves.

g. To anaesthetize the gingivae around a permanent maxillary first molar tooth it is necessary to anaesthetize the buccal branch of the mandibular nerve and the lesser palatine nerve.

h. In order to surgically remove (extract) a permanent mandibular first molar tooth, it is only necessary to anaesthetize the inferior alveolar nerve.

i. In order to surgically remove (extract) a permanent mandibular incisor tooth, it is only necessary to anaesthetize the mental nerve.

j. Nerve fibres from a tooth synapse in the trigeminal (Gasserian) ganglion on the floor of the middle cranial fossa.

k. The facial artery supplies labial branches to upper and lower lips.

l. The artery supplying the mandibular teeth arises from the maxillary artery in the pterygopalatine fossa.

m. The arterial supply to the muscles of mastication arises from the 2nd part of the maxillary artery in the infratemporal fossa.

n. The pterygoid venous plexus extracranially communicates with the cavernous sinus intracranially via emissary veins though the sphenoid bone in the roof of the infratemporal fossa.

o. The facial vein drains into the retromandibular vein in the parotid gland.

Extended matching questions

Theme: Nerves associated with orodental structures

Lead-in

Select the most appropriate option to answer items 1–5. Each option can be used once, more than once or not at all.

Item list

1. Sensory nerve supplying the maxillary molar teeth
2. Sensory nerve supplying the soft palate
3. Nerve carrying preganglionic parasympathetic fibres to the submandibular ganglion
4. Motor nerve to the anterior belly of the digastric muscle
5. Motor nerve to the muscle of the cheek

Option list

A. Anterior superior alveolar nerve
B. Auriculotemporal nerve
C. Buccal branch of facial nerve
D. Buccal branch of mandibular nerve
E. Chorda tympani
F. Glossopharyngeal nerve
G. Greater palatine nerve
H. Inferior alveolar nerve
I. Infra-orbital nerve
J. Lesser palatine nerve
K. Lingual nerve
L. Mylohyoid nerve
M. Nasopalatine nerve
N. Posterior superior alveolar nerve

Theme: Blood vessels associated with orodental structures

Lead-in

Select the most appropriate option to answer items 1–5. Each option can be used once, more than once or not at all.

Item list

1. Venous system in the infratemporal and pterygopalatine fossae
2. Venous structure having close relationships with cranial nerves III, IV, V_1, V_2 and VI
3. Artery crossing the inferior border of the mandible anterior to the attachment of the masseter muscle
4. The origin of the transverse facial artery
5. A branch of the 1st part of the maxillary artery that runs close to the neck of the mandibular condyle

Option list

A. Cavernous venous sinus
B. Deep facial vein
C. Lingual veins
D. Maxillary vein
E. Ophthalmic veins
F. Pterygoid venous plexus
G. Deep temporal artery
H. Facial artery
I. Greater palatine artery
J. Inferior alveolar artery
K. Lingual artery

Self-assessment: questions

L. Maxillary artery
M. Middle meningeal artery
N. Superficial temporal artery

Picture questions

Figure 6.1 (Courtesy of Professor M. C. Dean)

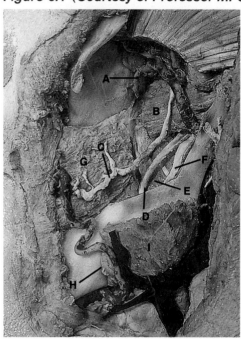

In this view of the infratemporal fossa:
a. Identify the structures labelled A–I.
b. What is the function of structure D?
c. What is the origin of structure A and where does it terminate?

Figure 6.2

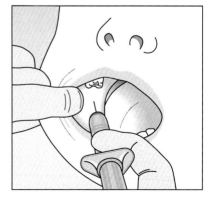
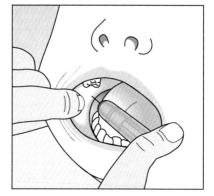

In order to anaesthetize the inferior alveolar nerve in the infratemporal fossa, it is often necessary to approach the nerve indirectly by a two-stage technique (Figure 6.2).
a. What are the anatomical reasons for this?

Essay questions

1. Describe the course and distribution of the mandibular division of the trigeminal nerve, highlighting, wherever possible, the clinical significance.
2. Give an account of the pterygoid venous plexus and indicate how the connections of this plexus have clinical importance.
3. From your knowledge of the anatomy of the infratemporal fossa, describe the complications that may follow an inferior alveolar nerve block.

Self-assessment: answers

True/false answers

a. **False**. The inferior alveolar nerve is derived from the posterior trunk of the mandibular division of the trigeminal nerve. The posterior trunk gives mainly sensory branches (except the motor nerve to mylohyoid), while the anterior trunk is mainly motor (except the sensory buccal branch of the mandibular nerve).

b. **True**. This relationship is important when inserting a needle into the infratemporal fossa to deliver local anaesthetic around nerves supplying orodental structures.

c. **True**. The preganglionic parasympathetic fibres are derived from the lesser petrosal branch of the glossopharyngeal nerve. Postganglionic fibres pass to the parotid gland with the auriculotemporal branch of the mandibular nerve.

d. **False**. The nerve to the medial pterygoid muscle is derived from the mandibular division of the trigeminal nerve before it divides into anterior and posterior trunks. After supplying the medial pterygoid muscle, the nerve goes on to provide the motor innervation for the tensor veli palatini and tensor tympani muscles. Note that the anterior trunk of the mandibular nerve supplies all other muscles of mastication.

e. **False**. The sensory supply of the temporomandibular joint is derived primarily from the auriculotemporal (and masseteric) nerve.

f. **False**. Most muscles of the soft palate (including palatopharyngeus) are supplied by the pharyngeal plexus of nerves. However, the tensor veli palatini muscle is supplied by the mandibular nerve (see d. above).

g. **False**. The buccal gingivae around a permanent maxillary first molar tooth are supplied by a buccal branch from the posterior superior alveolar nerve and the palatal gingivae are supplied by the greater palatine nerve.

h. **False**. While the permanent mandibular first molar tooth itself is supplied by the inferior alveolar branch of the mandibular nerve, to remove this tooth painlessly it is necessary also to anaesthetize the buccal and lingual nerves supplying the gingivae.

i. **False**. While it is true that the labial gingivae around a permanent mandibular incisor tooth are supplied by the mental nerve, the inferior alveolar and lingual nerves will also have to be anaesthetized.

j. **False**. Sensory nerve fibres from a tooth are bipolar and have their cell bodies in the trigeminal (Gasserian) ganglion on the floor of the middle cranial fossa.

k. **True**. The facial artery crosses the face at the lower border of mandible and then runs a tortuous course through the slips of muscles of facial expression, close to the lips, and towards the inner canthus of the eye.

l. **False**. The artery supplying the mandibular teeth is the inferior alveolar artery and it arises from the 1st part of the maxillary artery in the infratemporal fossa.

m. **True**. The arterial supply to the muscles of mastication does arise from the 2nd part of the maxillary artery in the infratemporal fossa, the first part being before crossing the lateral pterygoid muscle, the 2nd part being as the maxillary artery crosses (superficially or deep to) the lateral pterygoid muscle, and the 3rd part being in the pterygopalatine fossa.

n. **True**. The communication between the pterygoid venous plexus in the infratemporal fossa and the cavernous sinus intracranially (via emissary veins) is clinically important because of the possibility of spread of infection intracranially (thrombophlebitis) from the infratemporal fossa.

o. **False**. The facial vein receives the anterior retromandibular vein before draining into the internal jugular vein. Note that the anterior retromandibular vein has left the parotid gland to approach the facial vein as it runs in the neck.

Extended matching answers

Theme: Nerves associated with orodental structures

Item 1 = Option N. The maxillary molars receive their sensory innervation from the posterior superior alveolar nerves; the maxillary premolars from the middle superior alveolar nerves (although these are absent in 30% of persons); the maxillary canines and incisors from the anterior superior alveolar nerves. All the superior alveolar nerves are branches of the maxillary divisions of the trigeminal nerves (although the middle and anterior nerves arise from the infra-orbital branch of a maxillary nerve).

Item 2 = Option J. The soft palate receives its sensory innervation from the lesser palatine branches of the maxillary divisions of the trigeminal nerves. The lesser palatine nerve arises indirectly from the maxillary nerve and via the pterygopalatine parasympathetic ganglion, thereby picking up postganglionic parasympathetic fibres and sympathetic fibres in addition to its sensory fibres. The parasympathetic fibres supply minor salivary and mucus glands in the soft palate, and the sympathetic fibres supply blood vessels.

Item 3 = Option E (K). The submandibular parasympathetic ganglion is in the floor of the mouth (on the hyoglossus muscle) and gives postganglionic secretomotor fibres to the submandibular and sublingual salivary glands. Preganglionic fibres come from the chorda tympani nerve (a branch of the facial nerve; VIIth cranial nerve), although the chorda tympani nerve joins the lingual branch of the mandibular division of the trigeminal to reach the floor of mouth.

Self-assessment: answers

Item 4 = Option L. The digastric muscle has a dual innervation. The posterior belly (being derived embryologically from the 2nd pharyngeal arch) is innervated by the facial nerve. The anterior belly (being derived embryologically from the 1st pharyngeal arch) is innervated by the mandibular division of the trigeminal nerve via the branch that supplies the mylohyoid muscle (a branch from the inferior alveolar nerve just before it enters the mandibular canal).

Item 5 = Option B. The parotid gland receives its secretomotor innervation from the otic parasympathetic ganglion. Preganglionic fibres arise from the lesser petrosal branch of the glossopharyngeal nerve. Postganglionic fibres are conveyed to the gland via the auriculotemporal branch of the mandibular division of the trigeminal nerve (ostensibly a sensory nerve).

Theme: Blood vessels associated with orodental structures

Item 1 = Option F. The pterygoid venous plexus is found in the infratemporal and pterygopalatine fossae. It is so named because it is particularly prominent around the lateral pterygoid muscle. It drains via the deep facial vein to the facial vein and the maxillary vein to the retromandibular vein. The plexus has clinically important connections via emissary veins to the cavernous sinus intracranially (thus enabling spread of infection — thrombophlebitis).

Item 2 = Option A. The cavernous sinus lies in the middle cranial fossa and, as indicated in the answer immediately preceding, can become infected from the pterygoid venous plexus. If this happens, the consequences can be very significant, not just because of its intracranial location, but because important cranial nerves (oculomotor, trochlear, ophthalmic, maxillary and abducens) run through its walls. Thus, there will be problems associated with movements of the extra-ocular muscles and with the sensory distribution associated with the ophthalmic and maxillary divisions of the trigeminal nerve.

Item 3 = Option H. The facial artery comes from the external carotid artery in the neck. Having come to lie close to the superficial part of the submandibular gland, it runs tortuously beneath the inferior border of the mandible before crossing on to the face just at the anterior margin of the masseter muscle. Incisions running along the inferior border of the mandible are to be avoided, not only because of this location of the facial artery, but also because of the relationships with the facial vein and the (marginal) mandibular branch of the facial nerve that is going to supply the muscles of the lower lip.

Item 4 = Option N. The transverse facial artery arises from the superficial temporal artery, one of the terminal branches of the external carotid artery.

Item 5 = Option M. The middle meningeal artery arises from the maxillary artery in the infratemporal fossa before it crosses the lateral pterygoid muscle (i.e. the 1st part of the maxillary artery). It passes through the foramen spinosum to become one of the major arteries of supply of the middle cranial fossa. In its course, it is in danger of being damaged by fracture of the mandibular condyle, with the consequence that there might be marked intracranial haemorrhage.

Picture answers

Figure 6.1

a. A= maxillary artery. B = lateral pterygoid (lower head). C = buccal branch of mandibular division of trigeminal nerve. D = lingual nerve. E = medial pterygoid muscle. F = inferior alveolar nerve. G = buccinator muscle. H = facial blood vessels. I = masseter muscle.

b. The lingual nerve carries fibres of general sensation for the anterior two-thirds of the tongue, floor of mouth and lingual gingivae for the mandibular teeth. In addition, the chorda tympani nerve joins it. This nerve carries taste fibres for the anterior two-thirds of the tongue, as well as parasympathetic secretomotor fibres that synapse in the submandibular ganglion, subsequently reaching the submandibular and sublingual salivary glands.

c. The maxillary artery is a terminal branch of the external carotid artery. It arises within the substance of the parotid gland at the level of the neck of the mandibular condyle. After crossing the infratemporal fossa, it enters the pterygopalatine fossa to give its terminal branches.

Figure 6.2

a. The inferior alveolar nerve in the infratemporal fossa lies close to the sphenomandibular ligament and behind the posterior edge of the medial pterygoid muscle. It enters the mandible through the mandibular foramen, situated approximately halfway up the vertical dimension of the ramus of the mandible (and hence the infratemporal fossa). Thus, to approach the nerve directly for local anaesthesia would involve placing the needle of the anaesthetic syringe through the medial pterygoid muscle. Furthermore, because of the lateral 'flanging' of the ramus relative to the line of the body of the mandible, an indirect, two-staged approach to the inferior alveolar nerve not only avoids the medial pterygoid muscle, but also allows the needle to pass easily around the protecting 'buttress' of bone produced by angulation of the ramus.

Self-assessment: answers

Outline essay answers

Question 1

The introductory paragraph should briefly relate the mandibular nerve to the other divisions of cranial nerve V (trigeminal) and should state that it is the only division with motor fibres. Mention should also be made of the distribution of the mandibular nerve to the region of the lower jaw/inferior third of the face. A statement about the mandibular nerve having considerable importance for successful dental treatment should end this paragraph.

Although the essay could now describe the course of the mandibular nerve from the periphery to the central nervous system, it is often by convention dealt with the other way round. In this case, the mandibular nerve first appears as a division of the trigeminal nerve at the trigeminal (Gasserian) ganglion. The location of this ganglion (a sensory ganglion containing the cell bodies of bipolar sensory nerve fibres) in the floor of the middle cranial fossa (trigeminal depression; trigeminal cavum) should be described. Information should also relate this ganglion to trigeminal neuralgia and its treatment.

There should then follow a description of the passage of the mandibular nerve from the trigeminal ganglion to the foramen ovale and into the infratemporal fossa. Information concerning the union of sensory and motor components of the nerve at, or near, the foramen ovale should be provided and again issues relating to trigeminal neuralgia should be raised. The location of the mandibular nerve in the infratemporal fossa (i.e. deep to the lateral pterygoid muscle) should be mentioned.

There can then follow a description of the branches of the mandibular nerve, mentioning that all arise deep to the lateral pterygoid muscle. The initial branches are the sensory meningeal branch (previously known as the nervus spinosus) and the motor nerve to the medial pterygoid muscle that passes hence to innervate tensor veli palatini and tensor tympani muscles. Subsequently, the mandibular nerve divides into two trunks — an anterior trunk (mainly motor) and a posterior trunk (mainly sensory).

Branches of the anterior trunk are as follows:
- Temporal nerve
- Masseteric nerve
- Nerve to lateral pterygoid muscle
- Buccal nerve (only sensory branch of anterior trunk).

The clinical importance to dentistry of the buccal nerve should be emphasized (i.e. it needs to be anaesthetized when treating the cheek region and the buccal gingivae around the mandibular teeth).

Branches of the posterior trunk are as follows:
- Auriculotemporal nerve (also conveying postganglionic fibres from the otic ganglion to the parotid gland)
- Lingual plus chorda tympani (a branch of cranial nerve VII)
- Inferior alveolar nerve (should also include the sensory mental branch and the motor mylohyoid branch).

The importance of anaesthetizing the lingual and inferior alveolar nerves should obviously be highlighted. Mention should also be made of the proximity of the lingual nerve to the mandibular third molar tooth (and thus the possibility of its damage during surgical removal of the tooth) and of the relationships of the inferior alveolar and mental nerves to the teeth (and the possibility of their damage during dental surgery).

The final paragraph should briefly summarize the clinical importance of the mandibular nerve and the need to have a good working knowledge of the infratemporal fossa.

Question 2

In the introduction to the essay the location of the pterygoid venous plexus in the infratemporal fossa (mainly around lateral pterygoid muscle) and in the pterygopalatine fossa should be described and the importance of this plexus for the venous drainage of these regions should be emphasized.

Then should follow an account of the connections of the plexus:
- Deep facial vein to the facial vein
- Maxillary vein to the parotid and the retromandibular veins
- Emissary veins (passing through the foramen ovale, the foramen spinosum and the sphenoidal emissary foramen intracranially to the cavernous dural venous sinus)
- Other connections (for example, inferior alveolar veins).

The final part of the essay should be related to applied clinical aspects, in particular:
- the fact that the veins of the plexus have no valves; mention should therefore be made of spread of infections (thrombophlebitis) intracranially
- damage to the plexus leading to bleeding and haematomas; if extensive, these can lead to infections
- trismus (difficulty in opening the mandible).

Question 3

In anaesthetizing the teeth during various dental procedures, local infiltration techniques are usually adequate where the surrounding alveolar bone is thin (such as in the maxilla and anterior region of the mandible). However, when treating the mandibular cheek teeth, which are surrounded by thicker bone, it is necessary to anaesthetize the inferior alveolar nerve in the infratemporal fossa, before it enters the mandibular canal. This involves placing the needle in the pterygomandibular space in a procedure known as an inferior alveolar

Self-assessment: answers

nerve block (see above, Question 2). From a knowledge of the anatomy of the infratemporal fossa, the following common complications may arise following an inferior alveolar nerve block:

- If the needle (and anaesthetic solution) is injected too far medially, it may penetrate the medial pterygoid muscle; if placed too far laterally, it may penetrate the temporalis muscle. In either case, there will be an absence of anaesthesia that may be followed by trismus (painful spasm of the muscle).
- If the needle is advanced too deeply, the facial nerve may be affected and a temporary unilateral facial palsy may result.
- The needle may rupture a vein(s) associated with the pterygoid venous plexus, resulting in a haematoma.
- If the needle directly encounters the inferior alveolar nerve, the patient may experience the sensation of an 'electric shock'. The needle must be withdrawn before injecting the anaesthetic solution.
- Local anaesthetic solution may pass into the pterygomandibular space and thence into the inferior orbital fissure. The closest nerve is the abducent nerve, which may be temporarily anaesthetized resulting in diplopia (double vision) due to paralysis of the lateral rectus muscle.

- The needle may penetrate the inferior alveolar artery, but to prevent the consequences of injecting anaesthetic solution directly into the artery, the needle should always be aspirated first.

If a careful aseptic technique is not followed during anaesthesia, the possibility arises of introducing infective agents into the pterygomandibular space. From here, infection may spread to adjacent tissue spaces, including, rarely, the cavernous sinus via emissary veins from the pterygoid venous plexus.

Even if a correct inferior alveolar nerve block is administered to anaesthetize a molar tooth, pain may still be felt by a patient undergoing a clinical procedure. This 'escape from anaesthesia' may be related to anatomical variation. For example, a nerve branch supplying the tooth may arise high up from the parent inferior alveolar nerve in the infratemporal fossa and be unaffected by the normal nerve block injection given lower down. Occasionally, additional branches supplying the tooth pass with the buccal or temporal branches of the mandibular nerve. Additional local infiltration of anaesthetic solution around the tooth may solve the problem.

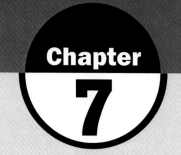
Salivary glands, saliva and salivation

Gross anatomy	79
Parotid gland	79
Submandibular gland	80
Sublingual gland	80
Physiology and biochemistry of salivary glands and saliva	80
Composition of saliva	80
Formation of saliva	81
Reflex activity	82
Histology of the salivary glands	83
Parotid gland	84
Submandibular gland	84
Sublingual gland	85
Minor salivary glands	85
Self-assessment: questions	86
Self-assessment: answers	89

Overview

In producing saliva, the exocrine salivary glands are essential for the maintenance of oral health. Although it is over 99% water, the small content of other elements (such as bacteriocidal agents and growth factors) allows the saliva to undertake many functions. There are both major and minor salivary glands, and serous, mucous or mixed glands; secretion is under the control of the autonomic nervous system. The primary saliva produced by the parenchymal cells undergoes modification within striated ducts as it passes along the duct system. Reduction in salivary flow in older patients, often as a side-effect of drugs, can give rise to dry mouth (xerostomia).

Learning objectives

You should:
- know the formation, composition and functions of saliva and how its secretion is controlled
- be able to describe the gross anatomy and relationships of the major salivary glands and the situation of the groups of minor salivary glands
- understand the histology of the salivary glands both in terms of the parenchymal cells (mucous and serous) and the nature of the duct system, and be able to appreciate the differences between the three pairs of major salivary glands
- be aware of how such knowledge is relevant to the clinical situation.

Salivary glands are compound, tubuloacinar, merocrine, exocrine glands whose ducts open into the oral cavity. The term compound refers to the fact that a salivary gland has more than one tubule entering the main duct; tubuloacinar describes the morphology of the secreting cells; merocrine indicates that only the secretion of the cell is released; exocrine describes a gland that secretes fluid on to a free surface. The many functions of saliva include:

- lubrication for mastication, swallowing and speech
- bringing substances in solution for taste
- acting as a buffer to maintain the integrity of enamel
- limiting the activity of bacteria
- promoting the health of the oral mucosa.

Salivary glands may be classified according to size (major and minor) and/or the types of secretion (mucous, serous or mixed). The three, paired, major salivary glands are the parotid, the submandibular and the sublingual glands. The numerous minor salivary glands are scattered throughout the oral mucosa and include the labial, buccal, palatoglossal, palatal and lingual glands.

Gross anatomy

Parotid gland

The parotid gland is serous and is the largest of the major salivary glands. It occupies the region between the ramus of the mandible and the mastoid process. The parotid is pyramidal in shape; its apex extends beyond the angle of the mandible and the base is closely related to the external acoustic meatus. The deep surface of the gland rests anteriorly on the ramus and masseter. The gland is surrounded by an unyielding tough fibrous capsule, the parotid capsule. The parotid duct appears at the anterior border of the gland and passes horizontally across the masseter muscle before piercing the buccinator to terminate in the oral cavity opposite the maxillary second molar. Lying with the duct on the masseter may be an accessory parotid gland.

Within the parotid gland are found the external carotid artery, the retromandibular vein and the facial nerve. Branches of the facial nerve are seen emerging from the anterior and inferior margins of the gland. Appearing at the superior border of the gland are the superficial temporal vessels and the auriculotemporal nerve. From the inferior border of the gland may be seen the anterior and posterior branches of the retromandibular vein. Lymph nodes are also associated with the parotid gland.

The parasympathetic innervation of the parotid gland is from the lesser petrosal branch of the glossopharyngeal nerve. The preganglionic fibres synapse in the otic ganglion, and postganglionic fibres reach the gland by travelling with the auriculotemporal branch of the mandibular nerve.

Submandibular gland

The submandibular gland is a mixed gland but is primarily serous. A large part it (the superficial part) is visible just beneath the inferior border of the mandible, where it lies on the mylohyoid muscle. The gland has an important relationship with the mylohyoid muscle, wrapping around the free posterior border (not unlike the letter C). This gives rise to the smaller deep portion of the gland that lies on the hyoglossus muscle. The submandibular duct appears from the deep part of the gland and wraps around the lingual nerve as it crosses the hyoglossus muscle to terminate on the sublingual papilla in the floor of the mouth.

Sublingual gland

The sublingual gland is the smallest of the three major salivary glands. It is a mixed gland but has a preponderance of mucous elements. The sublingual gland is not a single unit like the parotid and submandibular glands, but is made up of one large segment (the major sublingual gland) with a main duct that either joins the submandibular duct or drains directly on to the sublingual papilla, and a group of 8–30 mixed, minor salivary glands, each having its own duct system emptying into the sublingual fold in the floor of the mouth. The major sublingual gland is a mixed gland with a preponderance of mucous elements. The sublingual gland lies between the hyoglossus and mylohyoid muscles and lies against the sublingual fossa of the mandible.

The parasympathetic innervation of both the submandibular and sublingual glands is from the chorda tympani branch of the facial nerve. Preganglionic fibres are carried via the lingual nerve to the submandibular ganglion. Postganglionic fibres pass from this ganglion to the submandibular and sublingual glands.

Physiology and biochemistry of salivary glands and saliva

Saliva has a number of major functions, being important in mastication, swallowing, digestion, maintenance of oral hard and soft tissues, control of oral microbial population, and voice and speech articulation. Lubrication of the oral cavity is important in that it enhances the movement of the tongue and lips, and aids in cleansing the oral cavity of food debris and bacteria. Mastication, bolus formation and swallowing depend on a moist, lubricated oral mucosa and fluid

to wet the bolus. Digestive enzymes are present in saliva and aid in the initial process of digestion. Saliva has a protective function, maintaining an effective barrier to external insults. Saliva calcium and phosphorus are in supersaturated concentrations in the saliva and play a role in the remineralization of the teeth. Also a neutral pH in the oral cavity is maintained by the buffering capacity of the saliva.

Composition of saliva

About 99% is water, with the remaining 1% being made up of ions and organic constituents. It is most often hypotonic when compared with plasma; however, it has the ability to be isotonic and even hypertonic under physiological control mechanisms. The important ions in saliva are the cations Na^+ and K^+, and the anions Cl^- and bicarbonate (HCO_3^-). Other electrolytes present in saliva are calcium phosphate, fluoride, thiocyanate, magnesium sulphate and iodine. Saliva is derived from blood plasma but is not an ultrafiltrate of plasma.

Organic constituents

The organic constituents consist of proteins, carbohydrates, lipids and small organic molecules.

Proteins and glycoproteins

Saliva contains a variety of proteins and glycoproteins, including the serum proteins γ-globulins, albumin and α/β globulins. The proteins synthesized in the glands are:

- IgA (analogous to serum proteins)
- enzymes, including amylase, lysozyme, peroxidase, kallikrein and small amounts of many others (e.g. acid phosphatase, RNAase, cholinesterase, lipase)
- glycoproteins that contribute to viscosity of saliva, enhancing and facilitating its lubricating and agglutinating properties
- various small N-containing compounds.

In general, the parotid gland will synthesize more protein than glycoprotein, so parotid saliva has a lower carbohydrate content, whereas the submandibular and sublingual glands synthesize and secrete greater amounts of glycoprotein than protein, and saliva from these two glands is higher in carbohydrate content. This is observed histologically, where the parotid gland contains high levels of secretory granules (protein-rich) but no secretory droplets (mucin-rich), which are present in the submandibular and sublingual glands.

The function of the salivary proteins can be related to their structural features; in general they facilitate the lubricating properties of the saliva, essential for healthy mucosal tissue and antimicrobial protection. The presence of the enzymes such as amylase highlights the digestive role played by saliva, whereby complex starch present in food can be broken down (amylase hydrolyses α1–4 glycosidic linkages) prior to the food bolus entering the stomach. Lysozyme, acid phosphatases and peroxidases may well facilitate the protective role saliva plays in maintaining a balanced oral microflora, as these enzymes have anti-microbial properties. Lysozyme functions by cleaving β-N-acetylmuramic acid residues in bacterial cell walls and aggregates bacterial cells in suspension. It can also enhance the activity of immunoglobulins. Salivary peroxidase catalyses the reaction of bacterial metabolic products, hydrogen peroxide with salivary thiocyanate to oxidized derivatives. Salivary carbonic anhydrase increases the buffering capacity of saliva by producing bicarbonate. The secretory immunoglobulin IgA is produced as a specific response to contact with an antigen. It is synthesized by immune cells and translocated to the surface by epithelial cells. Lactoferrin binds ferric iron (Fe^{3+}), an essential microbial nutrient, and therefore demonstrates some antibacterial activity (nutritional immunity) but can have direct bactericidal effects on some micro-organisms.

Salivary mucins are a large family of glycoproteins existing with differing oligosaccharide chains and a protein core. Two main mucin subfamilies have been identified: namely, MG1 (high molecular weight and high carbohydrate content) and MG2 (lower molecular weight and lower carbohydrate content). These mucins form superstructures through electrostatic bonds and formation of covalent disulphide bonds. The main functions of salivary mucins relate to:

- lubrication (due to the high negative charge of salivary mucin, superstructures adopt an expanded structure aiding lubrication)
- hydration (as mucins exhibit negative charges that help bind water)
- pellicle formation and remineralization (MG1 helps in binding Ca^{2+} and hydroxyapatite)
- facilitating the direct removal of bacteria (MG2 can interact with bacteria).

Saliva contains a number of small molecular weight proteins that are generally phosphorylated and non-glycosylated. These include the proline-rich peptides, which have a negatively charged amino terminal that is phosphorylated and a positively charged carboxy terminal. These function by inhibiting calcium phosphate crystal growth; they may also have a role in remineralization of enamel. They also exhibit selective interaction with oral bacteria and other pellicle proteins, demonstrating a role in pellicle formation. Statherin, a tyrosine-rich protein, has a negative amino terminal (phosphorylated) and hydrophobic carboxy terminal. These molecules function by maintaining supersaturated levels of Ca^{2+} and PO_4^{4-} whilst inhibiting mineral formation in the salivary glands and oral cavity. The histatins are histidine-rich proteins and are inhibitors of *Candida albicans* and *Streptococcus mutans* growth in the oral cavity.

Growth factors

Growth factors (epidermal growth factor and nerve growth factor) and other regulatory peptides are also present in saliva, though the precise role of these has not been determined with certainty.

Formation of saliva

As mentioned earlier, saliva is mostly a hypotonic secretion. Its formation is dependent upon the stimuli mediated by both the parasympathetic and sympathetic parts of the autonomic nervous system. Parasympathetic cholinergic stimuli provide the principal stimulus for fluid secretion; however, it is most likely that under reflex control mechanisms, cholinergic, adrenergic and peptidergic neurotransmitters are involved in the secretion of saliva.

Primary stage of salivary secretion

Saliva is formed in the acinar cells of the glands and is delivered into the mouth through a series of ductal trees. Salivary secretion is essentially a two-stage process. The primary stage of salivary secretion results in the formation of an isotonic primary secretion by the acinar cells; this is later rendered hypotonic by the removal of Na^+ and Cl^- as it flows through the ductal system with little loss of fluid volume. When the parasympathetic nerves are stimulated, acetylcholine (ACh) binds to the muscarinic ACh receptors and causes an increase in inositol trisphosphate (IP_3) levels. This rise in IP_3 levels leads to an increase in Ca^{2+} release from intracellular stores and, in turn, these higher Ca^{2+} levels lead to an increase of fluid secretion from the cells. The mechanisms brought into play by this increase in Ca^{2+} are as follows:

- Cl^-, which is concentrated within the acinar cells, is released across the apical membrane of the acinar cell.
- This leads in turn to a secretion of Na^+.
- The combined NaCl secretion takes water across the cells by osmosis.

Water crosses the epithelium by two possible routes, moving:

- through the tight junctions between the cells via paracellular transport
- through the acinar cells through both the apical and basolateral membranes via transcellular transport.

Second stage of salivary secretion

The second stage of salivary secretion involves the modification of the isotonic saliva secreted by the acini into the hypotonic saliva secreted from the salivary ducts into the mouth. This ductal modification of the primary, acinar-derived isotonic solution is effected by apical Cl^- and Na^+ channels, along with Cl^-/HCO_3^- and Na^+/H^+ exchanges. These allow movement of Na^+ and Cl^- along a concentration gradient into the striated duct cells and then drive them out of the cell across the basolateral membrane. As the striated duct cells are impermeable to water, there is no osmotically driven reabsorption of water and so the saliva in the duct becomes hypotonic. Since the fluid secretory process in the acinar cells has a greater capacity than the electrolyte reabsorption process in the ductal cells, there can be large composition changes of the saliva entering the mouth. At low, resting flows, saliva moves slowly through

Seven

the ducts and the striated epithelium cells are able to modify the composition of the saliva substantially by absorbing Na^+ and Cl^-. However, at high, stimulated flows the saliva passes rapidly through the ducts with much less alteration of electrolyte concentrations. Thus, the electrolyte concentrations of saliva at high rates of flow are more similar to the primary saliva concentrations produced by the acinar cells.

Bicarbonate secretion

Salivary bicarbonate ions (HCO_3^-) are important in buffering plaque acid within the mouth. HCO_3^- can pass through Cl^- channels and so are secreted along with Na^+ and Cl^- into the ductal lumen by the acinar cells and possibly the intercalated duct cells close to the acinar cells. At low salivary flow rates HCO_3^- is reabsorbed by the striated duct cells and so very little will get into the mouth; however, at high flow rates there is less reabsorption of HCO_3^- and therefore higher concentrations reach the mouth when needed during eating.

Protein secretion

Whilst the secretions of water and electrolytes are a secretory modality called 'hydrokinetic', the secretion of proteins is termed 'proteokinetic'. Both these functions do not occur synchronously but are influenced by which nerves are firing, the impulse frequency and also the type of cell that is being stimulated. In general, the bulk of the fluid flow is generated by parasympathetic nerve activity. The amount of protein secreted tends to be low when impulse frequencies are low and higher when the stimulus is greater. The flow of saliva is usually less with sympathetic nerve stimulation but it does cause a greater concentration of proteins and this can lead to greater outputs for short periods of time. It is thought that sympathetic activity is usually superimposed on parasympathetic activity rather than in isolation and thus produces synergistic effects on flow and protein outputs. Proteins are secreted in two possible ways:

- Firstly, by 'exocytosis' of pre-packaged proteins from secretory granules in specialized exocrine cells
- Secondly, by a process called 'constitutive secretion' from the movement of Golgi-derived vesicles to the surface of the cells in all glandular cells.

It has been shown that similar-looking cells in different glands produce quite different proteins, and similar mucins may be differently glycosylated in different glands.

Reflex activity

Reflexes are automatic, predictable, reproducible and goal-directed responses to stimuli. Most are innate and almost all involve the central nervous system. Salivary secretion is dependent on reflex activity. Resting flows are present throughout the day and night and keep the mouth and oropharynx moist, lubricated and protected. However, in human beings large increases in secretion over short periods of time are seen during eating and these increases are attributed, in varying degrees, to stimulation of a number

of sensory receptors, including chemoreceptors involved in gustation and olfaction, mechanoreceptors and nociceptors.

The parotid, submandibular, sublingual and minor salivary glands all contribute to what is termed whole-mouth saliva. Not only does the secretion from the different glands vary in composition and volume to a given stimulus, but also the saliva produced by a single gland is variable. Therefore, the mixed whole-mouth saliva can vary considerably in its volume and composition depending on the type, amplitude and duration of the stimuli applied. The control of salivation depends on reflex nerve impulses. These reflexes involve afferent limbs, salivary nuclei within the medulla, and efferent limbs comprising both the sympathetic and parasympathetic secretomotor nerves supplying the various glands. Eating is the main cause of an increase of salivary flow above that of resting levels of flow. A variety of receptors are stimulated before, during and following the ingestion of food and drink; amongst these are gustatory, masticatory, olfactory, psychic, visual, thermoreceptive and possibly nociceptive. Inevitably, the afferent inputs during normal eating will comprise combinations of all these stimuli in variable amounts and lead to a complex reflex response. However, most studies have been done on the individual reflexes and very few on the combinations of inputs and their responses. There are also a number of reflex responses in which salivary secretion occurs, which are not normally associated with eating, such as nausea, vomiting and pain.

Whole-mouth saliva flow rates vary from resting with a mean of 0.3 ± 0.22 ml min^{-1}. When stimulated, the whole-mouth salivary flow will rise to a mean of 1.7 ± 2.1 ml min^{-1}. The daily flow rates lie between 500 and 1000 ml per day. The contribution to the whole-mouth saliva made by the different glands varies according to whether the gland is at rest or stimulated:

- The parotid gland provides only 20% of the saliva when rested and as much as 50% when stimulated.
- The submandibular gland provides over 65% of resting whole-mouth saliva, but only 30% of stimulated saliva.
- The sublingual and minor salivary glands supply the remaining saliva equally in both rest and stimulated conditions.

Gustatory-salivary reflex

Stimulation of gustatory receptors, mainly found in the taste buds, leads to the reflex secretion of saliva (gustatory-salivary reflex). All five basic tastes (salt, sour, sweet, bitter and umami) will cause a reflex salivary secretion. The volume and composition of saliva depend on the quality of the stimulus. There is common agreement that sour stimuli will evoke a maximal secretory response from most salivary glands. Lower concentrations of acid, along with all other basic gustatory stimuli, give variable degrees of salivary responses; however, all are considerably smaller than the maximum flow seen with, for instance, 5% citric acid. Very few foods contain an acid concentration as high as 5% citric acid; it therefore follows that concentrations as high as these cannot be regarded as normal (physiological) gustatory stimuli. The gustatory stimulus that evokes the greatest salivary response is sour, followed by umami, salt, sweet and bitter. Contrary to some suggestions, fats do not cause a salivary reflex response, suggesting that there are no specific fat receptors on the taste receptor cells in the taste buds.

The transduction of a chemical stimulus to an electrical event within the taste bud receptor cell leads to the initiation of action potentials, which are transmitted by the afferent limb of the reflex to the salivary nuclei. It is thought to be the pattern of these impulses and the type and location of the gustatory receptors, and not the perception of the taste, that lead to a reflex salivary flow. The perception must be a parallel response.

There is evidence that, not only does the individual gustatory stimulus produce different volumes of saliva, but also it can produce saliva with different overall compositions unrelated to the fact that the rate of salivary flow through the ducts affects the concentrations of some electrolytes. In some animals sweet stimuli have been shown to produce low flows of parotid saliva with a high protein content and, in human beings, it has been shown that salt stimuli produce parotid secretions higher in proteins than do other basic stimuli at the same flows.

Masticatory-salivary reflex

There is now considerable evidence that mastication causes a reflex salivary secretion (masticatory-salivary reflex). When one chews on one side of the mouth, there is greater flow of saliva from the parotid gland on that side than from the gland on the opposite non-chewing side. It appears that 'each gland seems to be most intimately associated with the receptors on its own side' (Lashley 1916). It has been shown that the output of saliva from the parotid gland is directly proportional to the masticatory forces and there is now substantial evidence that intra-oral mechanoreceptors, and in particular periodontal ligament mechanoreceptors, contribute to this reflex. The role of mucosal mechanoreceptors in the reflex cannot be excluded, as the reflex is still present in edentulous subjects and flow is considerably reduced when the oral mucosa underlying the dentures is anaesthetized with a topical anaesthetic ointment.

Olfactory-salivary reflex

Since the classical work of Pavlov in the late 1920s, on the conditioned reflex, it has been assumed that the smell of food causes salivation in human beings (olfactory-salivary reflex). Many textbooks state the existence of an olfactory-salivary reflex and significant increases in whole-mouth salivary flow have been recorded in response to olfactory stimulation. Over the years there has been some confusion as to whether olfactory stimuli cause secretion in all the major glands. Recently it has been shown that in human beings a true olfactory-parotid salivary reflex does not exist when normal pleasant food odours are presented to the olfactory epithelium. When the same pleasant food odours are presented to the olfactory epithelium and flow recordings made from the submandibular/sublingual glands, there are, however, significant increases in flow of saliva. This suggests that, whilst olfactory stimuli do cause a reflex secretion of

saliva in human beings, this reflex involves the submandibular/sublingual glands and not the main parotid glands.

Visual and psychic salivary reflexes

It is widely believed that the thought and sight of food act as a strong stimulus to the production of saliva (visual and psychic salivary reflexes), despite the lack of evidence in the literature. There is no convincing evidence that a non-conditioned salivary reflex in response to the sight or thought of food exists. It is possible that, when individuals think about or see food, not only do they perform anticipatory mouth movements, but also they become more aware of the presence of saliva in the mouth. The evidence for a conditioned reflex salivation in human beings, similar to that seen by Pavlov in dogs, is very weak; if such a reflex exists, it is extremely small and extinguished very rapidly. It is highly unlikely that normal individuals, going about their daily lives, experience an increased salivary flow when subjected to the sight and thought of food.

Oral nociceptor-salivary reflexes

In a small number of studies in human beings in which noxious stimuli have been applied to the oral tissues using solutions such as capsaicin (a substance found in chilli peppers), an increase above resting levels of parotid salivary flow has been recorded (oral nociceptor-salivary reflexes). It is suggested that this is brought about by the stimulation of the so-called common chemical sense, with stimulation of the trigeminal afferent nociceptive fibres.

Oesophageal-salivary reflex

When patients with gastro-oesophageal reflux suffer from heartburn, they often experience the 'waterbrash phenomenon', which is characterized by a sudden filling of the mouth with fluids (oesophageal-salivary reflex). This is thought to be similar to the increased salivation experienced with nausea and is believed to be due to higher levels of acid in the oesophagus.

One conclusive thought: The question of how the additive and/or synergistic effects of all these various stimuli impact on the total salivary flow or its composition remains unanswered at present.

Histology of the salivary glands

Salivary glands consist of two main elements:

- The glandular secretory tissue (the parenchyma)
- The supporting connective tissue (the stroma).

From the stroma of the capsule surrounding and protecting the gland pass septa that subdivide the gland into major lobes; lobes are further subdivided into lobules. Each lobe contains numerous secretory units consisting of clusters of grape-like structures (the acini) or more tubular structures positioned around a lumen. A secretory acinus may be serous, mucous or mixed. Serous acini can be distinguished from mucous acini according to the nature of the secretion produced and, in structural terms, the morphology of their secretory granules. Serous cells secrete more protein and less carbohydrate than mucous cells. The acinus, via its lumen, empties into an intercalated duct lined with cuboidal epithelium, which in turn joins a larger striated duct lined by columnar cells. Both the intercalated and striated ducts are intralobular and affect the composition of the secretion passing through them. The striated ducts empty into the collecting ducts, which are mainly interlobular. Basal cells are present and are sparsely distributed in the striated ducts, and are more densely distributed in the collecting ducts. The collecting ducts join until the main duct is formed at the hilum of the gland. The main duct carries the saliva to the mucosal surface and may be lined near its termination by a layer of stratified squamous epithelial cells.

The connective tissue septa carry the blood and nerve supply into the parenchyma. Apart from fibroblasts and collagen, the connective tissue also contains fat cells. Plasma cells (which secrete the immunoglobulins) are found in the stroma of the gland around the intralobular ducts. Unlike endocrine glands, whose secretion is controlled by the activity of hormones, the secretion of saliva by the salivary glands is under the control of the autonomic nervous system.

Parotid gland

Serous cells

The parotid gland is comprised entirely of serous acini. The cells have a wedge-shaped outline, the basal surface being broader, and a characteristic granular appearance, resulting from the numerous refractile granules in the luminal portion of the cell. The prominent nucleus is round and is located in the basal third of the cell, which also contains rough endoplasmic reticulum; capillaries are seen in close approximation to the basal surface. The basal part of each serous cell is delineated from the surrounding connective tissue by a basal lamina. The luminal part of the cell contains dense, round, secretory granules. Adjacent cell membranes contact at desmosomes, gap junctions and tight junctions. The appearance of serous cells varies with the levels of secretory activity. Following the synthesis of secretory products, resting (unstimulated) serous cells will contain numerous secretory granules. With reflex stimulation of salivary flow during mastication at mealtimes, the number of granules will be severely depleted after being discharged into the lumen by exocytosis. Both parasympathetic and sympathetic fibres innervate the acini and act collaboratively in the production of saliva during eating.

Duct system
Intercalated duct

The smallest (and most distal) of the ducts is the intercalated duct. This leads from the serous acini into the striated duct. It is lined by cuboidal epithelial cells. The nuclei in the duct cells appear prominent owing to the relatively scanty cytoplasm and there are only small amounts of the organelles normally associated with protein synthesis. In the parotid gland, intercalated ducts are characteristically long, narrow and branching.

Striated ducts

The striated ducts are intralobular and form a much longer and more active component of the duct system than the intercalated ducts. The cells of the striated ducts have a large amount of cytoplasm and a large, spherical, centrally positioned nucleus. The cells of the striated duct are highly polarized. The basal (abluminal) surface shows numerous striations in the light microscope. Ultrastructurally, the striations correspond to multiple infoldings of the plasma membrane at the base of the cell. Vertically aligned mitochondria are packed between the infoldings. The striated ducts are the site of electrolyte resorption (especially of sodium and chloride) and secretion (potassium and bicarbonate) without the loss of water. The effect is to convert an isotonic or slightly hypertonic fluid (with concentrations similar to those in the plasma) into a hypotonic fluid.

Collecting ducts

The striated ducts lead into the collecting ducts. In addition to the columnar layer (which now lacks striations), the collecting ducts may have an additional layer of basal cells and are situated in the interlobular region. The basal cells have been implicated as potential stem cells during turnover and/or cell regeneration in salivary glands. As it enlarges, the main parotid duct may have an outer connective tissue adventitia. Near its termination, the lining of the main duct becomes stratified as it merges with the stratified squamous epithelium of the surface oral epithelium.

Myoepithelial cells

Myoepithelial cells are of neural crest (ectomesenchymal) origin and lie between the basal lamina and the basal membranes of the acinar secretory cells and the intercalated duct cells. Myoepithelial cells are dendritic cells, consisting of a stellate-shaped body containing the nucleus and a number of tapering processes radiating from it. Ultrastructurally, the cell contains numerous contractile actin microfilaments about 7 nm in diameter and has desmosomal attachments with underlying parenchymal cells. Myoepithelial cells contain cytokeratin intermediate filament 14. They are stimulated by the autonomic nervous system and help increase salivary flow.

Submandibular gland

In the submandibular gland, the serous cells are similar to those in the parotid gland. However, the gland also contains about 20% of mucous acini.

Mucous cells

The mucous cells within the submandibular gland are readily distinguished in the resting gland from the darker-staining and granular serous cells, as they are paler (their mucin content does not readily take up routine stains). In addition, their nuclei tend to be compressed into the basal part of the cell. Small, crescent-shaped collections of serous cells may be found in routine sections at the most distal ends of the mucous acini; these are referred to as serous demilunes (although this has been shown to be the result of an artefact of preparation).

The mucous cell can be distinguished from the serous cell at the ultrastructural level as it has a more conspicuous Golgi apparatus (because of the greater amount of carbohydrate that is added to the secretory protein). At a later phase of its secretory cycle, the mucous cell exhibits numerous round and isolated secretory granules which are paler than those seen in a serous cell.

Duct system

The duct system of the submandibular gland is similar to that of the parotid. The intercalated ducts are shorter, however, while the striated ducts are longer.

Sublingual gland

The sublingual gland is a mixed gland, but is composed primarily (about 80% or more) of mucous acini.

Duct system

The duct system is much less well developed than in the other major salivary glands and striated ducts are usually absent. The acini sometimes lead to intercalated ducts, however these may be absent and the acini then lead directly to collecting ducts, which are usually rich in mitochondria but lack the basal striations that characterize striated ducts. The sublingual saliva is, therefore, rich in sodium. The major sublingual gland usually drains into a main duct, and the minor sublingual glands drain independently through many smaller ducts.

Minor salivary glands

The minor salivary glands are classified by their anatomical location: buccal, labial, palatal, palatoglossal and lingual. It has been estimated that they may number between 450 and 750. They are primarily mucous, except for the serous glands of von Ebner that drain into the trench of the circumvallate papillae. Whereas the sympathetic innervation appears to be important in evoking reflex protein secretion from major glands, such nerves do not innervate the secretory tissue of minor mucous glands and so mucus secretion is entirely mediated by parasympathetic nerve impulses.

Changes with ageing

With age, the major salivary glands show a reduction in the secretory acini and an increase in the stroma and in the amount of adipose tissue. However, there is no comparable reduction in salivary flow. The greater frequency of dry mouth (xerostomia) reported in older populations is associated with the increasing drug usage, many having side-effects that result in reduced salivary secretion.

Seven

Self-assessment: questions

True/false statements

Which of the following statements are true and which are false?

a. Salivary glands are classified as holocrine glands.
b. Within the substance of the parotid gland, the facial nerve lies deep to the external carotid artery.
c. The superficial and deep parts of the submandibular gland are separated by the hyoglossus muscle.
d. The posterior portion of the sublingual gland drains via numerous ducts on to the sublingual fold.
e. The secretomotor nerve supply to the parotid gland is derived via the greater petrosal nerve.
f. The minor salivary glands in the hard palate are serous.
g. In serous cells, the endoplasmic reticulum is concentrated mainly at the basal end of the cells.
h. Striated duct cells exhibit numerous infoldings lined by mitochondria on their basal surfaces.
i. Myoepithelial cells lie between the basal lamina and the basal cell membrane of acinar secretory cells.
j. The luminal cells of the intercalated and striated ducts contain cytokeratins 4 and 13.
k. All three major pairs of salivary glands exhibit striated ducts.
l. Myoepithelial cells contain cytokeratin intermediate filament 14.
m. The digestive enzymes in saliva are thought to play little role in digestion, as they are denatured by the stomach acid.
n. Parasympathetic stimulation causes an increase in salivary secretion, and sympathetic stimulation causes a decrease in salivary secretion and a dry mouth.
o. At high flow rates bicarbonate is reabsorbed rapidly by the striated duct cells, so little bicarbonate gets into the mouth.
p. Striated epithelial duct cells are impermeable to water.
q. At high stimulated flow rates of saliva it is possible for the saliva entering the mouth to be isotonic with plasma.
r. In human beings salivary secretion is dependent on conditioned reflex activity.
s. Masticatory, gustatory, olfactory, psychic and visual stimuli all contribute to the reflex production of saliva into the mouth.
t. Nausea, vomiting and pain can contribute to a reflex salivation in human beings.
u. The parotid glands contribute the highest percentage of saliva to whole-mouth saliva in both the resting and stimulated states.
v. There is no true reflex olfactory salivary secretion in humans.

Extended matching questions

Theme: Salivary glands

Lead-in

Select the most appropriate option to answer items 1–6. Each option can be used once, more than once or not at all.

Item list
1. Parotid gland
2. Minor salivary glands
3. Striated duct
4. Intercalated duct
5. Myoepithelial cells
6. Serous cells

Option list
A. It is innervated via the lesser petrosal nerve
B. These cells lie adjacent to striated ducts
C. Striated ducts are generally absent
D. Its luminal surface has numerous infoldings (brush border)
E. These cells can be identified using antibodies to contractile actin filaments
F. These cells have a haemopoietic origin
G. Its granules are most numerous soon after stimulation
H. Parasympathetic drive in these cells causes fluid formation
I. They are considered endocrine glands
J. Their secretion is considered holocrine
K. These are the smallest of the salivary ducts
L. Their activity significantly changes the composition of saliva

Theme: Saliva

Lead-in

Select the most appropriate option to answer items 1–6. Each option can be used once, more than once or not at all.

Item list
1. 3 ml per minute
2. Sympathetic nerve stimulation causes
3. Parasympathetic nerve stimulation causes
4. Saliva from the parotid gland
5. Salivary carbonic anhydrase increases the buffering capacity of saliva by producing
6. Salivary mucins aid

Option list
A. The release of acetylcholine, which stimulates nicotinic receptors
B. Has a higher carbohydrate content than saliva from the submandibular gland

Self-assessment: questions

C. Would be regarded as a normal stimulated whole-mouth saliva flow rate
D. Amylase
E. A dry mouth
F. Hydration because of their positive charge which helps bind water
G. Remineralization by binding hydroxyapatite
H. A greater concentration of proteins to be secreted in saliva
I. Is the major contributor to whole-mouth saliva during eating
J. The release of acetylcholine which stimulates muscarinic receptors
K. Would be regarded as a resting whole-mouth saliva flow rate
L. Bicarbonate

Picture questions

Figure 7.1 (Courtesy of Dr J. D. Harrison)

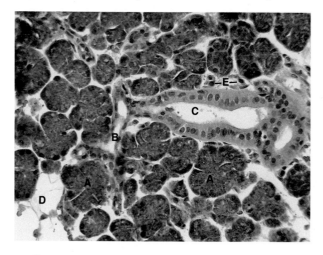

This is a micrograph of the parotid gland.
a. Identify structures A–D.
b. What probable blood cells found in the stroma are labelled E and what is its function in this gland?

Figure 7.2 (Courtesy of Mr P. F. Heap)

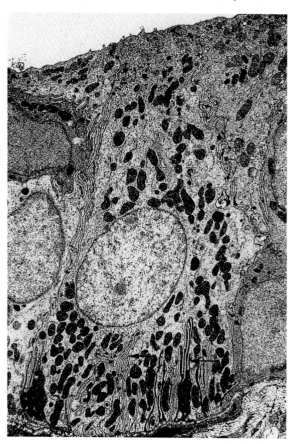

This is a transmission electron micrograph of a duct cell within the parotid gland.
a. Identify the type of duct, giving your reasons.

Figure 7.3 (Courtesy Dr A. W. Barrett)

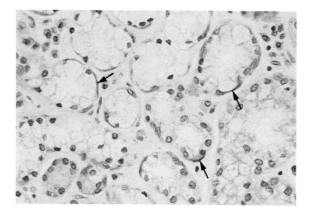

This is a micrograph of the submandibular gland.
a. Identify the cells arrowed.

Self-assessment: questions

b. What kind of antibody can be used to identify these cells?
c. What controls their activity?

Figure 7.4 (Courtesy of Dr J. D. Harrison)

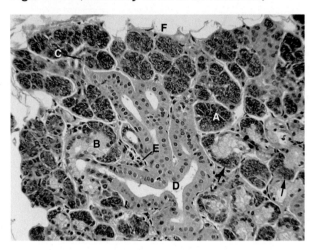

This is a section of the submandibular gland.
a. Identify structures A–E.
b. Account for the appearance of the structures arrowed.
c. Would any differences exist in structure D in the sublingual gland?

Figure 7.5 (Courtesy of Dr J. D. Harrison)

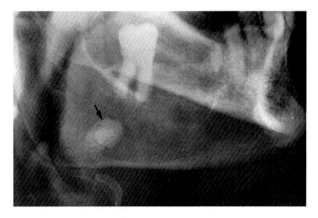

This is a radiograph of a 55-year-old male patient.
a. Give the most likely diagnosis of the radiopaque structure arrowed.
b. What symptoms might the patient complain of to confirm your diagnosis?
c. What clinical test might be carried out to confirm your diagnosis?

Figure 7.6 (Courtesy of Dr J. Potts)

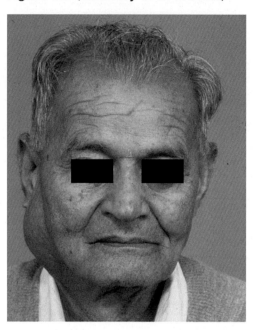

This picture shows a slow-growing, non-tender encapsulated tumour on the right side of the head.
a. In terms of the topographical anatomy of the head, in which region does the tumour lie?
b. Is the tumour likely to be benign or malignant?
c. The tumour in this region is non-tender and has therefore not affected the nerves located there. Assuming the presence of other lesions which do affect the innervation, what peripheral nerves might become involved?
d. How may the tumour spread to involve the palate and be associated with dysphagia (difficulty in swallowing)?

Essay questions

1. Describe the duct system of the parotid gland. How does it differ from that of the sublingual gland?
2. Give some examples of how a knowledge of salivary glands can impact on the clinical situation.
3. Salivary secretion is essentially a two-stage process. Highlight the mechanisms of these two stages.
4. Describe the structural features and functions of the salivary glycoproteins.

Self-assessment: answers

True/false answers

a. **False.** Salivary glands are merocrine glands (i.e. only the secretion of the cell is released) and not holocrine glands (where secretions are produced within the cell followed by the rupture of the plasma membrane, thus releasing all the cellular contents into the lumen, as in sebaceous glands).

b. **False.** The facial nerve is superficial to the external carotid artery.

c. **False.** The two parts of the gland are continuous around the posterior border of the mylohyoid muscle.

d. **True.** The ducts from the anterior part of the gland may unite to form a larger duct (Bartholin's duct), which either joins the submandibular duct or drains directly into the floor of the mouth at the sublingual papilla.

e. **False.** It is derived from the lesser petrosal nerve and therefore is associated with the glossopharyngeal nerve and not the facial nerve.

f. **False.** These minor salivary glands are mucous. In the palate of patients who smoke heavily, the orifices of the ducts of the mucous glands may present as red spots against the more whitish appearance of the oral mucosa resulting from a more pronounced ortho-keratinized layer being present due to the chronic irritation.

g. **True.** The secretory granules are concentrated at the distal end of the cell adjacent to the lumen. Initially, the immature granules are of pale electron density, but as they move to the luminal plasma membrane they become more electron-dense as the protein content is concentrated.

h. **True.** Active transport occurs at this surface, and the fluid in the duct is transformed into a hypotonic one by reabsorption of sodium and chloride ions.

i. **True.** These myoepithelial cells (of neural crest origin) are contractile and also surround the intercalated duct.

j. **False.** Cytokeratins 4 and 13 characterize stratified squamous lining epithelium. The luminal cells of the intercalated and striated ducts contain the low-molecular-weight cytokeratin intermediate filaments 7, 8, 18 and 19.

k. **False.** The sublingual gland lacks striated ducts.

l. **True.** Myoepithelial cells exhibit desmosomes and hemidesmosomes.

m. **False.** Amylase and lipase are thought to initiate digestion in the mouth and oesophagus before the bolus reaches the stomach and within the bolus in the stomach before stomach acids reach the inner parts of the bolus.

n. **False.** Both parasympathetic and sympathetic stimulation cause increases in salivary flow, but secretion is less with sympathetic stimulation; however, it does cause a greater concentration of proteins to be secreted. It is thought that they can both act synergistically with one another rather than in isolation.

o. **False.** This statement is truer at low flow rates rather than high flow rates as there is more time for the bicarbonate ions to be reabsorbed.

p. **True.** This leads to a retention of fluid volume as saliva travels through the ducts.

q. **True.** This is because of the lack of time for absorption of various ions.

r. **False.** Salivary secretion is dependent on reflex activity, not by conditioned reflexes but by innate reflexes.

s. **False.** There is strong evidence for masticatory and gustatory salivary reflexes, and some evidence for an olfactory-submandibular gland reflex, but there is little or no evidence for psychic or visual stimuli causing salivary secretion in human beings.

t. **True.** These stimuli are not normally associated with eating but all three can cause the release of saliva into the mouth.

u. **False.** The submandibular glands contribute the highest percentage at rest (approx 65%) and the parotid glands contribute the highest percentage when stimulated (approx 50%).

v. **False.** There is no true reflex olfactory-parotid salivary secretion but there is a reflex olfactory-submandibular/sublingual salivary secretion.

Extended matching answers
Theme: Salivary glands

Item 1 = Option A. The lesser petrosal nerve is a branch of the glossopharyngeal nerve and synapses in the otic ganglion.

Item 2 = Option C. The absence of striated ducts may not remove much salt, so that the final saliva released from them may not be as hypotonic as that from the major salivary glands, which possess striated ducts.

Item 3 = Option L. The striated ducts are the site of electrolyte resorption (especially of sodium and chloride) and secretion (potassium and bicarbonate) without loss of water.

Item 4 = Option K. For this reason, intercalated ducts are not easily demonstrated in routine light microscopy when compared with the larger striated and collecting ducts.

Item 5 = Option E. Myoepithelial cells also contain cytokeratin intermediate filament 14 which, together with actin, can be used to help identify them using immunocytochemistry.

Item 6 = Option H. Parasympathetic drive causes fluid formation by the secretory units; sympathetic drive usually increases the output of preformed components from the cells. Both pathways cause contraction of the myoepithelial cells, which helps direct fluid from the acinar lumen out along the duct system.

Self-assessment: answers

Theme: Saliva

Item 1 = Option C. Whole-mouth saliva flow rates vary from resting with a mean of 0.3 ± 0.22 ml min^{-1}. When stimulated, the whole-mouth salivary flow will rise to a mean of 1.7 ± 2.1 ml min^{-1}.

Item 2 = Option H. Sympathetic stimulation causes a small increase in saliva production with a higher concentration of protein, whereas parasympathetic stimulation causes a higher flow of saliva with a smaller concentration of protein.

Item 3 = Option J. The membrane receptors on the acini are muscarinic receptors and not nicotinic as in other tissues.

Item 4 = Option I. During rest the submandibular contributes the major component of whole-mouth saliva (over 65%).

Item 5 = Option L. At low salivary flow rates bicarbonate is reabsorbed by the striated duct cells and so very little will get into the mouth; however, at high-flow rates there is less reabsorption and therefore higher concentrations reach the mouth when needed during eating.

Item 6 = Option G. Mucin's properties are chiefly related to its negative charge, which particularly aids hydration.

Picture answers

Figure 7.1

a. A = serous acinus (due to its darker granular appearance). B = intercalated duct. C = striated duct. D = fat cell.
b. The cells labelled E are likely to be plasma cells. It is a cell of the immune system and secretes antibodies, predominantly IgA, that pass into the duct system.

Figure 7.2

a. This is a cell from a striated duct. It is from a single layer of columnar cells with a centrally placed nucleus and a considerable amount of cytoplasm. There is evidence of cell polarization; the basal (abluminal) surface at the bottom shows many infoldings with numerous mitochondria. If it were from an intercalated duct, this would be a low, cuboidal cell with no obvious polarization or infoldings of the basal cell membrane, and lacking the high number of mitochondria. If it were from a collecting duct, although the cells would be columnar, it would again lack the infoldings of the basal cell membrane. Collecting ducts are generally larger and may consist of two layers of cells (and are interlobular rather than intralobular).

Figure 7.3

a. Myoepithelial cells. These cells are derived from neural crest cells.
b. These cells can be highlighted by antibody stains for actin or cytokeratin 14.

c. Their contraction, which helps expel saliva from the duct system, is controlled by the autonomic nervous system, both parasympathetic and sympathetic.

Figure 7.4

a. A = serous acini. B = mucous acini. C = intercalated duct. D = part of striated duct. E = fat cells.
b. In very carefully fixed material, serous cells in the submandibular gland align with mucous cells in mixed acini to surround a common lumen, leaving no demilune structure. However, with routine fixation, the mucous cells are distended and displace adjacent serous cells towards the basal portion of the acinus to form the serous demilunes arrowed, which must therefore represent an artefact of fixation.
c. In the sublingual gland, the predominant mucous acini sometimes lead to intercalated ducts but these may be absent and the acini lead directly to collecting ducts, striated ducts being absent. These collecting ducts are usually rich in mitochondria but lack the basal striations that characterize striated ducts. The sublingual saliva is therefore rich in sodium.

Figure 7.5

a. The patient has a sialolith (stone) at the proximal end of the submandibular duct, which is radio-opaque and is visible on the radiograph within the outline of the mandible.
b. The patient may notice that the floor of the mouth on the affected side becomes swollen at mealtimes, giving him/her some discomfort. This is due to the stone obstructing the flow of saliva. If blockage is incomplete, this swelling may gradually recede. The patient may also complain of a bad taste in the mouth. This is due to the fact that the sialolith predisposes to infection and the presence of pus. On examination, there is often evidence of inflammation around the opening on the sublingual papilla.
c. A radio-opaque dye can be injected into the submandibular duct (to produce a sialogram). It should normally pass freely into the submandibular duct and outline the whole duct system of the normal gland. If a large sialolith is present, this will be prevented and the obstruction indicated.

Figure 7.6

a. The tumour lies in the parotid region.
b. The tumour is likely to be benign because it is well defined, has a capsule and is slow-growing.
c. The parotid gland is itself innervated (secretomotor) by postganglionic parasympathetic fibres from the optic ganglion which travel to the gland via the

Self-assessment: answers

auriculotemporal branch of the glossopharyngeal nerve. There is some evidence that the secretomotor supply may also be derived from the chorda tympani branch of the facial nerve. The sympathetic supply to the gland initially comes from the superior cervical sympathetic ganglion. From here, the innervation reaches the gland via the plexus around the middle meningeal artery, the otic ganglion and, eventually, the auriculotemporal nerve. Sensory fibres to the connective tissue within the parotid gland are derived directly from the auriculotemporal nerve. The parotid fascia covering the gland receives a sensory innervation from the great auricular nerve of the cervical plexus, and the skin overlying the gland receives its nerve supply from the great auricular nerve and the auriculotemporal and buccal branches of the mandibular nerve. If the facial nerve is involved, a paralysis may follow.

d. A parotid tumour may spread inwards from the deep portion of the gland, which is situated at the posterior boundary of the infratemporal fossa. From this site, the tumour can spread to extend into the palate and the pharynx, and thus be associated with dysphagia.

Outline essay answers

Question 1

Three types of duct are found in the parotid gland: the intercalated, striated and collecting ducts. The most distal and smallest of these is the intercalated duct and this is usually compressed between the serous acini of the gland. It is lined by cuboidal epithelial cells. The nuclei in the duct cells appear prominent, owing to the relatively scanty cytoplasm. At the ultrastructural level, both luminal and basal surfaces of the intercalated duct cells are smooth and desmosomes unite adjacent cells. There are only small amounts of the organelles normally associated with protein synthesis. However, the cells sometimes contain apical secretory granules and thus appear to make a small contribution to the primary secretion. Several acini drain into each intercalated duct. In the parotid gland, intercalated ducts are characteristically long, narrow and branching.

The intercalated duct leads into the striated duct. The striated ducts are intralobular and form a much longer and more active component of the duct system than the intercalated ducts. The cells of the striated ducts have a large amount of cytoplasm and a large, spherical, centrally positioned nucleus. The cells of the striated duct are highly polarized. Their luminal surfaces have short microvilli. The duct's basal (abluminal) surface, adjacent to the basal lamina separating it from the adjacent connective tissue, shows numerous striations at the light microscope level. Ultrastructurally, the striations correspond to multiple infoldings of the plasma membrane at the base of the cell. Vertically aligned mitochondria are packed between the infoldings.

Adjacent cells are intertwined in a complex pattern and anchored together by desmosomes. This large surface area, supplied with high levels of energy, is clearly involved in active transport. The striated ducts are the site of electrolyte resorption (especially of sodium and chloride) and secretion (potassium and bicarbonate) without loss of water. As this resorption is against a concentration gradient, it requires substantial amounts of energy: hence the large number of mitochondria. The effect on the material in the lumen is to convert an isotonic or slightly hypertonic fluid (with concentrations similar to those in the plasma) into a hypotonic fluid. The cells of the striated duct exhibit small secretory granules on the luminal side that may contain epidermal growth factor, lysozyme, kallikrein and secretory IgA.

The striated duct leads into the collecting duct. Whereas the intercalated and striated ducts modify the composition of the saliva (as well as transport it) and may be termed secretory ducts, the collecting ducts only transport it into the mouth, where the opening of the parotid duct lies in the cheek adjacent to the maxillary second molar tooth. In addition to the columnar layer (which now lacks striations), the collecting ducts may have a layer of basal cells and are situated in the interlobular region. As the ducts enlarge and merge, the main parotid duct appears like many excretory passages and contains two layers: the mucosa and the outer connective tissue adventitia. Near its termination, the lining of the main duct becomes stratified as it merges with the stratified squamous epithelium of the surface oral epithelium.

The luminal cells of the intercalated, striated and collecting ducts contain the low-molecular-weight cytokeratin intermediate filaments 7, 8, 18 and 19. However, the epithelium of the main parotid duct, when stratified, contains keratin intermediate filament types typical of stratified epithelium in the oral mucosa (i.e. types 4 and 13).

The duct system of the sublingual gland is less well developed than that of the parotid glands and striated ducts are usually absent. The acini sometimes lead to intercalated ducts, but these may be absent and instead the acini lead to collecting ducts, which are usually rich in mitochondria but lack the basal striations that characterize striated ducts. The sublingual saliva is therefore rich in sodium. The major sublingual gland usually drains into a main duct, and the minor sublingual glands drain independently through many smaller ducts. Both sets of ducts drain into the floor of the mouth in the region of the sublingual fold, the main sublingual duct draining into the submandibular duct.

Question 2

a. Xerostomia

Older patients frequently complain of a dry mouth (xerostomia), with all the unpleasant symptoms one might expect from a consideration of the important functions of saliva. This condition was once thought to be a reflection

Self-assessment: answers

of decreased salivary production associated with the ageing process. However, this is not the case, as there is no evidence that salivary flow decreases with age. It is more likely that the decreased salivary production reflects increased use of medication (many drugs depress salivary production, sometimes centrally as well as peripherally, with unstimulated salivary flow rates falling from approximately 0.3 ml/min to less than half this value). Loss of salivary tissue is also a consequence of radiotherapy treatment for certain tumours in the region of the jaws, or of Sjögren's syndrome, where there is invasion and destruction of the parenchyma by lymphoid tissue. As saliva is important in the maintenance of oral health, decreased secretion from the salivary glands can result in an increased incidence in oral conditions such as periodontal disease, dental caries and candidal infections ('thrush'), as well as halitosis and problems with taste and speech. Partial relief may be obtained by the frequent administration of artificial salivas. Dentures may be constructed with compartments capable of holding saliva substitutes that may be released slowly into the mouth.

b. Sialolith

Blockage of the main collecting duct of a major salivary gland may occur. The cause is usually a sialolith (stone or calculus) generally affecting the submandibular duct (but occasionally the parotid). The site of the submandibular duct may relate to its slightly tortuous nature and to the presence of mixed saliva with its more viscous mucin content. Sometimes blockage is associated with an anatomical anomaly such as a stricture or dilatation. The lack of access to the mouth caused by the blockage results in swelling of the gland, especially at mealtimes, together with a possible inflammatory discharge and pain. An incomplete blockage will allow the gradual discharge of saliva.

c. Mucoceles and ranulas

Damage to the ducts of mucus-containing salivary glands may result in the extravasation of mucus into the surrounding soft tissues. When a minor salivary gland is affected, the lesion is more likely to persist and is termed an extravasation mucocele. In the case of the sublingual gland, it is also termed a ranula because the swelling it causes to the floor of the mouth somewhat resembles the belly of a frog. When a ranula is situated above the mylohyoid muscle (oral ranula), it produces a painless swelling that may displace the tongue. If it penetrates the mylohyoid (cervical ranula), it produces a swelling in the neck. Treatment of these conditions may necessitate the surgical removal of the affected sublingual gland.

d. Sialomicroliths

These are small, hard masses (concrements) that are only evident microscopically in salivary glands and may occur in the parenchymal cells, in the lumina or in the stroma.

They contain variable amounts of both mineral (in the form of calcium phosphates that include hydroxyapatite), as well as non-mineralized components in the form of condensed organic secretory material. Sialomicroliths are present in all normal submandibular glands and 20% of normal parotid glands. This frequency appears to relate to the higher concentration of calcium in the submandibular gland. Sialomicroliths are rare in sublingual glands and minor salivary glands where secretion is continuous and stagnation is less likely. They may eventually be associated with chronic submandibular sialadenitis (inflammation of the submandibular gland that may produce symptoms of pain, swelling and discharge from the gland).

e. Staphne's cavity (cyst)

A portion of the submandibular gland may invaginate into the lingual surface of the mandible, typically in the region of the ramus below the mandibular canal, near the angle of the ramus. On a radiograph, this will give the appearance of a well-circumscribed, unilateral radiolucent lesion with a radio-opaque border. It can be distinguished from other lesions by careful computed tomography and by sialography, when a radiolucent dye injected in the submandibular duct will spread into the radiolucency. A similar but rarer radiolucency can occur in the anterior region of the mandible, where it is due to an invagination related to the sublingual gland.

f. Tumours in salivary glands

Tumours within salivary glands constitute by far the most common site for tumours in the head and neck. The range of presentation to the oral pathologist is also considerable due to the diversity of the number of cells present. Tumours may range from the benign to the malignant. When malignant, they may spread to other parts and may also involve the facial nerve that is located within the parotid gland itself.

g. Age changes

These need to be taken into account when examining the salivary glands histologically in clinical diagnosis. This is particularly so when biopsies of lower labial salivary glands are examined in an attempt to diagnose Sjögren's syndrome, in which there are characteristic changes in the parotid and, to a lesser extent, other salivary glands that involve an infiltration by lymphocytes. However, there is an infiltration by lymphocytes to form lymphocytic foci in salivary glands that increases with age and may be as great as what has been considered to be diagnostic of Sjögren's syndrome in the lower labial glands.

h. Tissue engineering and salivary gland regeneration

Salivary glands have some capacity for regeneration. There is considerable proliferation in the presence of noxious

Self-assessment: answers

stimuli, such as in chronic sialadenitis, which is the biological basis for the encouraging results of the conservative treatment of this disease (rather than surgical removal of the gland). It had been assumed that this regeneration was essentially the property of the basal cell population associated with the striated and collecting ducts, as these showed the highest proliferative index (approximately 3%). However, recent research has shown the presence of a low baseline proliferation of mature acinar, intercalated ductal and myoepithelial cells, indicating that these cells also have the capacity to contribute to parenchymal regeneration. As with other dental tissues, investigations are being undertaken in the hope of increasing salivary gland regeneration following the loss of parenchymal tissue associated with tumours and other disorders by injecting grafting stem-cell populations into the glandular remains.

Question 3

In the first stage, saliva is formed as an isotonic primary secretion by the acinar cells of the salivary glands. It then becomes a hypotonic solution due to the removal of Na^+ and Cl^- as it flows through the ductal system; during this process there is little loss of the fluid volume since striated epithelial duct cells are impermeable to water. Acetylcholine (ACh) binds to the muscarinic ACh receptors following parasympathetic nerve stimulation and this causes an increase in inositol trisphosphate (IP_3) levels. This rise in IP_3 levels leads to an increased Ca^{2+} release from intracellular stores, and in turn this stimulates greater fluid secretion from the cells.

The increase in Ca^{2+} leads to the release of Cl^-, which is concentrated within the acinar cells, across the apical membrane of the acinar cell; this leads in turn to a secretion of Na^+ and this combined NaCl secretion takes water across the cells by osmosis. Water crosses the epithelium by two possible routes, either through the tight junctions between the cells via paracellular transport mechanisms, or through the acinar cells through both the apical and basolateral membranes via transcellular transport mechanisms.

Bicarbonate ions (HCO_3^-) can pass through Cl^- channels, and so are secreted along with Na^+ and Cl^- into the ductal lumen by the acinar cells and possibly the intercalated duct cells close to the acinar cells.

The second stage of salivary secretion involves the modification of the isotonic saliva secreted by the acini into the hypotonic saliva secreted from the salivary ducts into the mouth. This modification of the primary, acinar-derived isotonic solution by the ducts is effected by apical Cl^- and Na^+ channels, along with Cl^-/HCO_3^- and Na^+/H^+ exchanges which allow movement of Na^+ and Cl^- along a concentration gradient into the striated duct cells and then drive them out of the cell across the basolateral membrane. The striated duct cells are impermeable to water; therefore there is no osmotically driven reabsorption of water and because of this the saliva within the duct becomes hypotonic.

Because the fluid secretory process in the acinar cells has a greater capacity than the electrolyte reabsorption process in the ductal cells, there can be large volume and composition changes in the saliva entering the mouth. At low, resting flows, saliva moves slowly through the ducts; the striated epithelium cells are able to absorb more Na^+ and Cl^- and thereby substantially modify the composition of the saliva. However, at higher, stimulated, flows, the saliva passes rapidly through the ducts with much less alteration of their electrolyte concentrations. Thus, the electrolyte concentrations of saliva at high rates of flow are more similar to the primary saliva concentrations produced by the acinar cells. At low salivary flow rates HCO_3^- is reabsorbed by the striated duct cells and so very little will get into the mouth. However, when eating, there are higher stimulated flow rates, there is less reabsorption of HCO_3^- by the ducts and therefore higher concentrations reach the mouth.

Question 4

The salivary mucins are a large family of glycoproteins existing with differing oligosaccharide chains and a protein core. Two main mucin subfamilies exist, MG1 (high molecular weight and high carbohydrate content) and MG2 (lower molecular weight, lower carbohydrate content). These mucins form superstructures through electrostatic bonds and formation of covalent disulphide bonds. Their general function in saliva is to confer protection on the oral tissues. They also have a role in lubrication; due to the high negative charge of salivary mucin, the superstructures adopt an expanded structure, aiding lubrication. Conversely, they are important in regulating hydration. Mucins exhibit negative charges which help bind water. They are also important in pellicle formation and remineralization (MG1) by binding Ca^{2+} and hydroxyapatite. They also facilitate direct removal of bacteria (MG2), as they can directly interact with them. Saliva contains a number of low molecular-weight proteins, which are generally phosphorylated and are non-glycosylated. The proline-rich peptides, which have a negatively charged amino terminal that is phosphorylated and a positively charged carboxy terminal, function by inhibiting calcium phosphate crystal growth. They may have a role in the formation of the enamel pellicle and remineralization of enamel. They also exhibit selective interaction with oral bacteria and other pellicle proteins influencing pellicle formation. Statherin has a negative amino terminal (phosphorylated) and hydrophobic carboxy terminal. These molecules function by maintaining supersaturated levels of Ca^{2+} and PO_4, and inhibit mineral deposition in the salivary glands and oral cavity. Histatins are histidine-rich proteins and inhibit *Candida albicans* and *Streptococcus mutans* growth in the oral cavity, again conferring protection on the oral tissues.

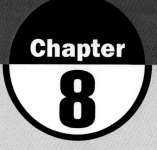

Investing organic layers on enamel surfaces

Chapter 8

Soft tissues covering an erupting tooth	94
The erupted healthy tooth	94
Dental plaque	94
Calculus	96
Self-assessment: questions	98
Self-assessment: answers	100

Overview

Throughout its life, the crown of a tooth is covered by an organic layer or integument. Before the tooth erupts into the oral cavity the crown is covered by the overlying oral mucosa, the coronal part of the dental follicle, and the vestiges of the enamel organ (plus its associated primary enamel cuticle). After emerging into the mouth, parts of the integument of enamel organ origin are lost by degeneration of its epithelial component and by attrition or abrasion of the underlying cuticular component. In the region of the gingival crevice or sulcus, the primary (or pre-eruptive) enamel cuticle acquires additional matter from the lining epithelium and, coronal to the gingival margin, from saliva. The salivary layer is known as the acquired pellicle. Oral bacteria adhere initially to the enamel cuticle and later to the acquired pellicle, to form the dental plaque. Dental plaque may mineralize to form dental calculus.

Learning objectives

You should:
• know the origins of the acquired pellicle
• understand the mechanisms of attachment of bacteria and proteins to the acquired pellicle, leading to plaque formation
• appreciate how different dietary carbohydrates influence plaque matrix and how that matrix affects cariogenicity
• know how dental calculus is formed.

Soft tissues covering an erupting tooth

The soft tissues covering an erupting tooth comprise oral mucosa and the subjacent connective tissue of the dental follicle. Between the dental follicle and the enamel is an epithelial layer that is the remains of the enamel organ — the reduced enamel epithelium; a basal lamina (primary enamel cuticle) is interposed between the enamel surface and the reduced enamel epithelium. The reduced enamel

epithelium and the primary enamel cuticle comprise Nasmyth's membrane.

The erupted healthy tooth

A number of organic layers cover the erupted healthy tooth.

Primary enamel cuticle

The original reduced enamel epithelium is lost, leaving the primary enamel cuticle initially covering the exposed enamel. This cuticle immediately acquires an organic element of salivary origin, the acquired pellicle. The primary enamel cuticle is in intimate contact with the underlying organic enamel matrix. Generally approximately 30 nm thick, the cuticle acquires accretions in the region of the gingival crevice, which derive from crevicular epithelium and from plasma and may increase the cuticle to about 5 μm thick.

Acquired pellicle

Where the enamel surface is exposed to wear, either by attrition or abrasion, the vestigial enamel organ is worn away, but the enamel rapidly acquires a layer of acquired pellicle. Indeed, this pellicle always forms a protective coat following any wear. This acellular layer is derived mainly from salivary proteins, but includes elements from crevicular fluid and bacteria.

Dental plaque

Dental plaque is the combination of bacteria embedded in a matrix of salivary proteins and bacterial products superimposed on the acquired pellicle. Dental plaque is an example of a biofilm, a term used to describe communities of microbes attached to surfaces. Early plaque is composed of mainly Gram-positive, facultative, anaerobic cocci and filaments. With time, the deposit will thicken, although in non-pathological, supragingival situations its microfloral composition is unlikely to vary greatly. Plaque can be described as a soft, adherent, predominantly microbial mass which accumulates on the tooth surface in the absence of oral hygiene measures. Although it contains a large variety of micro-organisms, it is also composed of a rich organic matrix, derived from saliva, foodstuffs and microbial metabolism.

Mechanisms of plaque formation

It is clear that there are distinct stages to the formation of plaque:

- Firstly, there is the initial transport of bacteria to tooth surface.
- This is followed by reversible adsorption of the bacteria on to the pellicle surface.
- Less reversible attachment of bacteria to tooth surface then occurs.
- These stages are repeated, forming new layers of bacterial adherence.
- Finally, there is growth of the attached organisms, leading to the formation of a 'climax' community.

The transport of micro-organisms to the pellicle-coated tooth is via passive means, and local variations in the chemical composition of the pellicle can influence the pattern of microbial deposition.

Attachment of bacteria

Initial reversible attachment of bacteria to the tooth surface involves the formation of long-range, physicochemical interactions between micro-organisms and pellicle proteins. Such interactions include electrostatic interactions (ionic and hydrogen bonds), Van der Waals forces (induced dipole formation) and hydrophobic bonds. As micro-organisms are generally negatively charged due to nature of the cell surface molecules and acidic proteins are present in acquired pellicle, these interactions usually involve the formation of calcium bridging between the pellicle proteins and bacterial membranes for successful interaction. Less reversible attachment of bacteria to tooth surface involves short-range interactions between adhesins on the microbial surface and receptors in the acquired pellicle. These are usually specific and irreversible.

Bacteria–host interactions

Examples of bacteria–host interactions include:

- lectin-like bacterial proteins interacting with carbohydrates, or with oligosaccharides within salivary glycoproteins
- hydrophobic fimbriae with hydrophobic portions within salivary proteins
- specific protein–protein interactions by antigenically and functionally distinct fimbriae.

Macromolecules and bacterial adherence

A function of salivary macromolecules is in the aggregation and subsequent removal of bacteria. For plaque formation to proceed, it is necessary that not all bacteria aggregate in saliva before they reach the tooth surface. Conformational changes of proteins on adsorbed surfaces allow for the binding of specific proteins. Examples of this include the removal of sialic acid by bacterial neuraminidase facilitating the adherence of certain bacteria.

As plaque formation continues, there is multiplication of attached organisms to produce confluent growth and a biofilm is formed. The production of proteases by bacteria removes inhibitors of growth (e.g. IgA, histatin) and provides nutrients for further microbial growth. Growth of a pioneer population creates conditions suitable for colonization of bacteria with more demanding growth requirements (dependent on nutrient supply, O_2 tension, pH, ionic concentration, toxins within plaque fluids) and organisms within the plaque begin to synthesize extracellular polymers.

Where the plaque is associated with chronic inflammatory periodontal disease and becomes subgingival, a more complex flora develops with anaerobic Gram-negative organisms predominating, to include cocci, rods, filaments and many motile forms (particularly spirochaetes). The microbial composition of dental plaque will vary, not only with the stages of maturity of the deposit, but also from individual to individual, from tooth to tooth, from site to site and from surface to surface. Plaque can be seen on all tooth surfaces that are not subject to constant abrasion, especially in areas that are difficult to clean such as occlusal pits and fissures, interproximal regions and the gingival margin.

Plaque matrix and extracellular polysaccharides

Plaque matrix and extracellular polysaccharides are as important in the functions of plaque as the microorganisms. The plaque matrix is the intercellular material between bacteria. It can be directly related to the diet consumed and be a key source of carbohydrate for acid production during caries. The matrix consists of carbohydrates from foodstuffs as well as polysaccharides produced by bacterial metabolism. It also contains salivary proteins and glycoproteins that have precipitated out of solution. The plaque matrix is directly related to the diet consumed and its consistency, and composition may vary with the presence or absence of diet. In the absence of diet (e.g. stomach tube feeding), the plaque matrix is thin and porous and composed mainly of precipitated salivary glycoproteins. These are incorporated onto the tooth surface and into the plaque as they have a strong negative charge due to terminal sialic acid sugars on side chains and thus low pI. In more mature plaque, acid production by bacteria may cause some precipitation of salivary glycoproteins and incorporation into the matrix. High levels of calcium in plaque may also help precipitation.

Plaque matrix during diet

Plaque matrix during diet is related to the type of carbohydrate consumed. If the carbohydrate source is primarily glucose the plaque is thin, whereas if the carbohydrate is sucrose the plaque is much thicker and gelatinous with sticky properties. This thick and sticky matrix is far more cariogenic due to extracellular polysaccharides produced by the plaque bacteria. Extracellular polysaccharides increase the bulk of plaque and may play a role in caries by aiding bacteria to stick or agglutinate within the matrix, and also by acting as a source of carbohydrate for bacterial acid production.

These extracellular polysaccharides improve the structural integrity of plaque and are formed by bacterial glucosyltransferases or fructosyltransferases, which are found in bacterial cell walls and are cell wall enzymes. Action of these enzymes on sucrose gives rise to dextrans/glucans, which are polymers of glucose, or levans/fructans, which are polymers of fructose.

n-sucrose **glucosyltransferase** (glucan)$_n$ + n-fructose

n-sucrose **fructosyltransferase** (fructan)$_n$ + n-glucose

Soluble dextrans

The soluble dextrans produced by the action of bacterial glucosyltransferases contain a higher proportion of alpha 1–6 linked dextrans, whilst insoluble dextrans contain predominantly alpha 1–3 linked dextrans. These help consolidate bacterial attachment. It is worth noting that *Streptococcus mutans* also produces a specific highly insoluble polymer (mutan). Fructosyltransferases convert sucrose to fructans; these polymers are labile, generally soluble and readily broken down, and are therefore not involved in plaque adhesion. They may act as extracellular storage compounds for other plaque bacteria and can be used by plaque bacteria as an energy source.

Intracellular polysaccharides

Intracellular polysaccharides produced by plaque bacteria are energy stores for bacteria during times of carbohydrate deprivation and do not contribute to the plaque matrix. These intracellular polysaccharides are usually polymers of 1–4 linked glucose units and can be formed from a variety of sugars as they are synthesized through high-energy phosphate intermediates such as glycogen. They can be metabolized to acid like any sugar and tend to be formed when sugar is in excess.

Calculus

Mineralization of plaque leads to the formation of calculus. This mineralization is through the precipitation of calcium and phosphate, which is present in the saliva. Saliva is supersaturated with minerals (such as calcium and phosphate) that have the potential to mature newly erupted enamel, protect exposed tooth surfaces from acid action and remineralize areas in the early stages of demineralization. Salivary inhibitors prevent precipitation and crystallization of minerals in saliva, but bacterial enzymes can degrade these inhibitors. Thus, under suitable conditions (e.g. with high concentrations of minerals derived from saliva), precipitation and crystallization may occur within dental plaque.

Composition of dental calculus

Approximately 20% dry weight of calculus is organic and includes a range of proteins, carbohydrates and lipid, most associated with the plaque matrix. The remaining 80% dry weight is inorganic mineral, of which only 50% is hydroxyapatite. Whereas the mineral in enamel consists of carbonated hydroxyapatite, that in dental plaque consists of a number of different mineral forms due to the variety of local factors associated with its formation. There is thus regional variation in the Ca/P ratio of dental calculus. Early calculus formation includes deposition in the matrix of poorly crystalline calcium phosphate types, including dicalcium phosphate dehydrate (brushite) and octacalcium phosphate, together with dying bacterial cells. With time, more structured crystalline elements, including carbonated hydroxyapatite and whitlockite, are formed. In supragingival calculus, hydroxyapatite and octacalcium phosphate are most abundant, whilst in subgingival calculus, whitlockite is most abundant, with little brushite being present. Supragingival plaque is less mineralized than subgingival plaque (approximately 40% v. 60%).

Formation of calculus

Numerous factors are involved in the formation of calculus. The presence of the oral fluids (saliva/gingival crevicular fluid) is essential, as the calcium and phosphate required for mineralization of the plaque are present to some extent in these fluids. The oral bacteria may also produce substances which facilitate the mineralization of plaque. Although this mineralization is regarded as pathological, there is a need for seeding/nucleating molecules to allow the process to occur. The presence of such molecules (such as acidic proteins discussed in Chapter 11) will also encourage mineralization of the organic plaque. The possibility that an individual's diet may have a possible role in calculus formation cannot be ignored.

The mechanisms of calculus formation are not fully understood. It is a pathological calcification so no specific mechanism exists. It is likely to be a combination of simple precipitation and heterogenous nucleation. A rise in oral pH and an increase in concentrations of ions by evaporation both encourage precipitation of calcium and phosphate, leading to mineral deposition. As mentioned above, the presence of various nucleation molecules (acidic proteins, glycosaminoglycans (GAGs)) will mediate these processes, increasing mineralization.

Classification of calculus

Dental calculus can be classified into:

- supragingival (above the free gingival margin and attached to enamel)
- subgingival (below the free gingival margin and therefore attached to cementum).

Supragingival dental calculus is cream-coloured and is found adjacent to the opening of the ducts of the major salivary glands. Thus it is seen predominantly on the lingual surfaces of the anterior mandibular teeth, near the opening of the submandibular and sublingual glands, as well as on the buccal surfaces of the maxillary molars (near the openings of the parotid glands). Subgingival calculus is darker in colour and can occur throughout the dentition from minerals in the inflammatory exudate associated with periodontal disease.

The different distribution of supra- and subgingival calculus deposits relates to the causes of mineralization. Supragingivally, a rise in salivary pH, due to evaporation of dissolved CO_2 on entering the mouth (together with the greater viscosity and higher Ca/P ratio of the saliva coming out from the submandibular duct), promotes calculus formation; on the other hand, subgingival calculus formation, promoted by formation of alkaline bacterial waste products within periodontal pockets, may occur anywhere in the mouth.

As calculus is hard, large removal forces are required to detach it. A number of anti-tartar agents that are present in oral hygiene products either act as inhibitors of mineralization or slow down crystal growth. These include pyrophosphate, zinc salts and polyphosphates.

Self-assessment: questions

True/false statements

Which of the following statements are true and which are false?

a. The content of plaque matrix formed in high dietary glucose is thick, gelatinous and sticky.

b. Interactions leading to reversible attachment of bacteria to the tooth surface tend to involve calcium bridging.

c. Plaque matrix is not linked to diet.

d. Nasmyth's membrane is an alternative name for the reduced enamel epithelium.

e. Throughout its life, the crown of a tooth is covered by an organic integument.

f. The types of bacteria found in plaque are relatively constant.

g. Early plaque is composed of mainly Gram-negative bacteria.

h. Plaque bacteria may produce proteases to remove inhibitors of growth, facilitating their growth within the plaque.

i. The majority of calcium phosphate precipitate in dental calculus is carbonated hydroxyapatite.

j. Supragingival plaque is more mineralized than sub-gingival plaque.

k. Subgingival calculus can occur throughout the dentition.

Extended matching questions

Theme: Integuments, plaque and calculus

Lead-in

Select the most appropriate option to answer items 1–6. Each option can be used once, more than once or not at all.

Item list

1. Ionic and hydrogen bonds
2. Thin and porous
3. Subgingival plaque
4. Precipitated salivary glycoproteins
5. Bacterial glucosyltransferases
6. An acellular layer derived mainly from salivary proteins

Option list

A. Is the plaque matrix formed in the absence of diet

B. Is known as the acquired pellicle

C. Are important in the formation of extracellular polysaccharides

D. Are interactions leading to reversible attachment of bacteria to the pellicle

E. Is known as Nasmyth's membrane

H. Is associated with chronic inflammatory periodontal disease

I. Is the plaque matrix formed when the carbohydrate source is sucrose

J. Has whitlockite as the most abundant mineral

K. Is associated with the ducts of major salivary glands

L. Are important in the formation of intracellular polysaccharides

Picture questions

Figure 8.1 (Courtesy of Professor H. N. Newman)

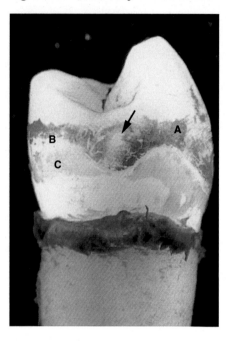

a. If the relatively clear zone labelled B in this extracted, recently erupted, premolar tooth is at the level of the gingival crevice, account for the staining seen above (zone A) and below it (zone C). (The stain used is Alcian blue-aldehyde fuchsin.)

Figure 8.2 (Courtesy of Professor H. N. Newman)

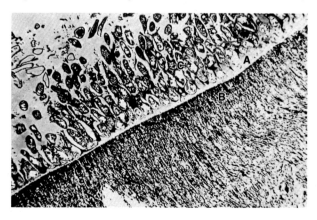

a. Identify structures A–C in this electron micrograph.

Self-assessment: questions

Essay question

1. Discuss the formation of bacterial extracellular poly-saccharides and how diet can influence them; briefly outline their role in the structure of plaque and its potential cariogenicity.

Self-assessment: answers

True/false answers

a. **False**. The plaque matrix is thin and porous.

b. **True**. Micro-organisms and acidic proteins in the pellicle are generally negatively charged; calcium bridges overcome this apparent repulsion.

c. **False**. Components of the diet are present in the plaque matrix and are an essential component of it, especially the dietary sugar source.

d. **False**. Nasmyth's membrane consists of the reduced enamel epithelium plus the primary enamel cuticle.

e. **True**. Before eruption it is covered by Nasmyth's membrane; after eruption it is covered by the acquired pellicle.

f. **False**. The bacterial composition of dental plaque will vary, not only with the stages of maturity of the deposit, but also from individual to individual, from tooth to tooth, and from surface to surface.

g. **False**. Early plaque is composed mainly of Gram-positive bacteria.

h. **True**. Bacteria may produce proteases such as histatins and IgA to allow growth of their populations.

i. **False**. Only 50% of calcium phosphate precipitate in calculus is carbonated hydroxyapatite. The remainder is a mixture of octacalcium phosphate, whitlockite and brushite amongst others.

j. **False**. Supragingival plaque is less mineralized than subgingival plaque (40% v. 60%).

k. **True**. Subgingival calculus does occur throughout the dentition, as mineral salts are present in the inflammatory exudate associated with periodontal disease.

Extended matching answers

Item 1 = Option D. Initial reversible attachment of bacteria to the tooth surface involves the formation of long-range physicochemical interactions between micro-organisms and pellicle proteins, and include electrostatic interactions.

Item 2 = Option A. In the absence of diet, the carbohydrate source is minimal and the plaque matrix is composed from salivary glycoproteins and bacterial agglutination. There is a lack of extracellular polysaccharide within the matrix; hence it is thin.

Item 3 = Option H. Where the plaque is associated with chronic inflammatory periodontal disease, it becomes subgingival and contains components from inflammatory exudate. A more complex flora develops, with anaerobic Gram-negative organisms predominating.

Item 4 = Option A. In the absence of diet, the plaque matrix contains little exogenous carbohydrate source and little, if any, extracellular polysaccharides are produced by the bacteria. It is mainly composed of salivary glycoproteins.

Item 5 = Option C. Extracellular polysaccharides are formed by bacterial glucosyltransferases or fructosyltransferases, which are bacterial cell wall enzymes.

Item 6 = Option B. The acquired pellicle forms a protective coat on the enamel and is an acellular layer derived mainly from salivary proteins, but includes elements from crevicular fluid and bacteria.

Picture answers

Figure 8.1

a. The zone labelled A, above the gingival sulcus, stains because of the accumulation of dental plaque. Zone B, adjacent to the gingival crevice, is virtually plaque-free because of the close apposition of the gingiva to the tooth, limiting plaque to the gingival margin. The paler-staining zone C, below the gingival crevice, is related to the presence of cells of the junctional epithelium.

Figure 8.2

a. A = primary enamel cuticle and pellicle. B = enamel. C = plaque with colonizing bacteria.

Outline essay answers

Question 1

Extracellular polysaccharides are produced by bacteria as a consequence of metabolism of carbohydrate from the diet. The carbohydrate may be sucrose and these extracellular polymers are stored outside the bacterial cell and within the plaque matrix. They are formed by bacterial glucosyltransferases of fructosyltransferases, which are found in the bacterial cell wall

n-sucrose **glucosyltransferase** $(glucan)_n$ + n-fructose

n-sucrose **fructosyltransferase** $(fructan)_n$ + n-glucose

Diet is a key source of carbohydrate for acid production by plaque. If the carbohydrate source is glucose, limited extracellular polysaccharides are produced by the bacteria; the plaque matrix is not complex and does not grow very thick, so there is less bacterial agglutination on plaque and a limited sugar source for bacteria to use in the production of acid. More complex sugars, such as sucrose, lead to larger breakdown products and far thicker and gelatinous plaque, which has sticky properties. Due to the metabolism of sucrose by bacteria, the plaque matrix formed contains more extracellular polysaccharides, and this aids further bacterial agglutination onto plaque and provides a larger carbohydrate source for bacteria to metabolize to produce acid. These extracellular polysaccharides increase the bulk of the plaque matrix and the incidence of anaerobic bacteria within the matrix, contributing to the structural integrity of the plaque matrix and acting as extracellular storage compounds for other plaque bacteria. They play a role in caries, as they may facilitate agglutination of bacteria and are a source of carbohydrate for bacterial acid production.

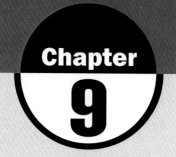

Chapter 9

Development of the craniofacial complex

Development of the face 101
Development of the palate 102
Development of the jaws 102
Development of the tongue 104
Development of the thyroid gland 104
Self-assessment: questions 105
Self-assessment: answers 109

Overview

Craniofacial development is here defined as the development of the face, palate, jaws and tongue. Much of this development is related to derivatives of the pharyngeal (branchial) arches. However, many different mechanisms are involved, from the merging of mesenchymal facial processes to the intramembranous calcification around the cartilage of the 1st pharyngeal arch to form the body of the mandible to the hydration of palatal shelves to produce shelf elevation necessary for the formation of the definitive palate. Craniofacial development is clinically important since craniofacial anomalies are amongst the most common congenital anomalies found in humans.

Learning objectives

You should:
- be able to describe the mesenchymal facial processes around the developing mouth (stomodeum) and understand how these contribute to the formation of the upper and lower lip regions
- be able to describe the ectodermal placodes on the developing face and know their derivatives
- be able to give an account of the development of the primary and secondary palates and understand the processes and mechanisms responsible for the elevation and fusion of the lateral palatal shelves
- be able to describe the prenatal and postnatal development of the mandible and the maxillae
- be able to give an account of the development of the tongue and relate this to the innervation of the tongue once fully formed
- know the origin of development of the thyroid gland
- be able to understand, for all aspects of craniofacial development, how disturbances in normal development can result in common congenital abnormalities (e.g. clefts of the lip and palate).

Development of the face

During early development (4 weeks in utero), the primitive oral cavity (stomodeum) is bounded by five facial swellings, produced by proliferating zones of mesenchyme lying beneath the surface ectoderm — the frontonasal, mandibular and maxillary processes. The frontonasal process lies above, the two mandibular processes lie below, and the two maxillary processes are located at the sides. The maxillary and mandibular processes are derived from the 1st pharyngeal (branchial) arches. At this early stage, a membrane (the oropharyngeal membrane) separates the primitive oral cavity from the developing pharynx. The oropharyngeal membrane is composed of an outer ectodermal layer and an inner endodermal layer. This membrane soon breaks down to establish continuity between the ectodermally lined oral cavity and the endodermally lined pharynx.

In a 5-week-old embryo, localized thickenings of ectoderm give rise to the nasal and lens placodes. These placodes will form the olfactory epithelium and the lenses of the eyes respectively. The nasal placodes sink into the underlying mesenchyme, forming two blind-ended nasal pits (the primitive nasal cavities). Proliferation of mesenchyme from the frontonasal process around the openings of the nasal pits produces the medial and lateral nasal processes. The nasal pits continue to deepen until eventually they approach the roof of the primitive oral cavity, being partitioned from it by oronasal membranes. By the end of the fifth week, these membranes rupture to produce communications between the developing nasal and oral cavities.

In the 6-week-old embryo, the two mandibular processes fuse in the midline to form the tissues of the lower jaw. The mandibular processes and maxillary processes meet at the angle of the mouth, thus defining its outline. From the corners of the mouth, the maxillary processes grow inwards beneath the lateral nasal processes and towards the medial nasal processes of the upper lip. Between the merging maxillary and the lateral nasal processes lie the naso-optic furrows. From each furrow a solid ectodermal rod of cells sinks below the surface and canalizes to form the nasolacrimal duct. The maxillary processes subsequently 'replace' the medial nasal processes to meet in the midline and thus contribute all the tissue for the upper lip. Fusion of the facial processes ultimately produces the region known as the 'intermaxillary segment'. It is from this area that the primary palate will develop (see page 102).

Development of the palate

The definitive palate (or secondary palate) appears in the human fetus between the sixth and eighth weeks of intrauterine life. Palatogenesis is a complex event and, while the events and mechanisms responsible for the development of the palate have been much studied, some controversy remains.

By the sixth week of development, the primitive nasal cavities are separated by a primary nasal septum and are partitioned from the primitive oral cavity by a primary palate. Both the primary nasal septum and the primary palate are derived from the frontonasal process. The stomodeal chamber is divided at this stage into the small primitive oral cavity beneath the primary palate and the relatively large oronasal cavity behind the primary palate. During the sixth week of development, two lateral palatal shelves develop behind the primary palate from the maxillary processes. A secondary nasal septum grows down from the roof of the stomodeum behind the primary nasal septum, thus dividing the nasal part of the oronasal cavity into two.

During the seventh week of development, the oral part of the oronasal cavity becomes completely filled by the developing tongue. Growth of the palatal shelves continues such that they come to lie vertically. During the eighth week of development, the stomodeum enlarges, the tongue 'drops' and the vertically inclined palatal shelves become horizontal. On becoming horizontal, the palatal shelves contact each other (and the secondary nasal septum) in the midline to form the definitive or secondary palate. The shelves contact the primary palate anteriorly so that the oronasal cavity becomes subdivided into its constituent oral and nasal cavities. After contact, the medial edge epithelia of the two shelves fuse to form a midline epithelial seam. Subsequently, this degenerates so that mesenchymal continuity is established across the now intact and horizontal secondary palate. Fusion of the palatal processes is complete by the twelfth week of development. Behind the secondary nasal septum, the palatal shelves fuse to form the soft palate and uvula.

Several mechanisms have been proposed to account for the rapid movement of the palatal shelves from the vertical to the horizontal position. Although it was once thought that extrinsic forces might be responsible (e.g. forces derived from the tongue or jaw movements), research has primarily focused on the search for a force intrinsic to the palatal shelf. It has been proposed that the intrinsic shelf elevation force might develop as a result of hydration of extracellular matrix components (principally hyaluronan) in the shelf mesenchyme, or as a result of mesenchymal cell activity. Present evidence favours the former hypothesis.

Once the palatal shelves have elevated, they contact each other (initially in the middle third of the palate) and adhere by means of a 'sticky' glycoprotein, which coats the surface of the medial edge epithelia of the shelves. The epithelial cells develop desmosomes and consequently an epithelial seam is formed. The adherence of the medial edge epithelia is specific, as palatal epithelia will not fuse with epithelia from other sites (e.g. the tongue).

The signals that are responsible for breakdown of the midline epithelial seam are not yet fully understood. Nevertheless, the breakdown of the basal lamina is likely to be a significant event. The seam is also 'thinned' by growth of the palate and by epithelial cell migration from the region of the seam on to the oral and nasal aspects of the palate. There is also programmed cell death (apoptosis) in the seam. Recent evidence indicates that extracellular matrix molecules may provide the signal and work has been undertaken to assess the role of type IX collagen. At the earliest stages before shelf elevation, the medial edges of the palatal shelves label poorly for type IX collagen compared with floor of the mouth epithelia. Present-day thinking suggests that the control of the synthesis of type IX collagen is influenced by epidermal growth factors.

Once fusion is complete, the hard palate ossifies intramembranously from four centres of ossification, one in each developing maxilla and one in each developing palatine bone:

- The maxillary ossification centre lies above the developing deciduous canine tooth germ and appears in the eighth week of development.
- The palatine centres of ossification are situated in the region forming the future perpendicular plate and appear in the eighth week of development.

Incomplete ossification of the palate from these centres defines the median and transverse palatine sutures. There does not appear to be a separate centre of ossification for the primary palate in humans (in other species there is a separate 'premaxilla').

Development of the jaws

Mandible

The mandible initially develops intramembranously, but its subsequent growth is related to the appearance of secondary cartilages (the condylar cartilage being the most important). The developing mandible is preceded by the appearance of a rod of cartilage belonging to the first pharyngeal (branchial) arch. This is known as Meckel's cartilage and it first appears at about the sixth week of intrauterine life. Meckel's cartilage extends from the cartilaginous otic capsule in the region of the developing ear to a midline symphysis. However, it makes little contribution to the adult mandible, merely providing a framework around which the bone of the mandible forms.

The mandible first appears as a band of dense fibrous tissue on the anterolateral aspect of Meckel's cartilage. During the seventh week of intrauterine life, a centre of ossification appears in this fibrous tissue at a site close to the future mental foramen. From this centre, bone formation spreads rapidly backwards, forwards and upwards, around the inferior alveolar nerve and its terminal branches (the incisive and mental nerves). Further spread of the developing bone in a forwards and backwards direction produces a plate of bone on the lateral side of Meckel's cartilage that corresponds to the future body of the mandible and which extends towards the midline where it comes to lie in close relationship with the bone forming on the opposite side. However, the two plates of bone remain separated by fibrous tissue to form the mandibular symphysis. At a later stage in the development of the body of the mandible, continued bone formation markedly increases the size of the mandible, with development of the alveolar process occurring to surround the developing tooth germs. At an even later stage, Meckel's cartilage resorbs. The neurovascular bundle that initially was located with the developing tooth germs now becomes contained within its own bony canal and there is considerable development of the alveolar process. Although Meckel's cartilage contributes no significant tissue to the developing mandible, nodular remnants of cartilage may be seen in the region of the mandibular symphysis until birth and, in its most dorsal part, Meckel's cartilage ossifies to form ear ossicles (the malleus and incus). Behind the body of the mandible the perichondrium of Meckel's cartilage persists as the sphenomandibular and sphenomalleolar ligaments. The sphenomandibular ligament ossifies at its sites of attachment to form the lingula of the mandible and the spine of the sphenoid bone.

As the developing tooth germs reach the bell stages (see page 114), developing bone becomes closely related to it to form the alveolus. The size of the alveolus is dependent upon the size of the growing tooth germ. Resorption occurs on the inner wall of the alveolus (indicated by Howship's lacunae) while, on the outer wall of the alveolus, bone is deposited (indicated by osteoblasts lining an osteoid seam). The developing teeth therefore come to lie in a trough of bone. Later, the teeth become separated from each other by the development of interdental septa. With the onset of root formation, inter-radicular bone develops in multirooted teeth.

The ramus of the mandible is first mapped out as a condensation of fibrocellular tissue that, although continuous with the developing body of the mandible, is positioned some way laterally from Meckel's cartilage. Further development of the ramus is associated with a backward spread of ossification from the body and by the appearance of secondary cartilages. Between the tenth and fourteenth weeks in utero, three secondary cartilages develop within the growing mandible. The largest, and most important, of these is the condylar cartilage, which, as its name suggests, appears beneath the fibrous articular layer of the future condyle. By proliferation and subsequent ossification, the cartilage is thought by some to serve as an important centre of growth for the mandible, functioning up to about the twentieth year of life. Less important, transitory, secondary cartilages are seen associated with the coronoid process and in the region of the mandibular symphysis.

Postnatally, the ratio of body to ramus is greater at birth than in the adult, indicating a proportional increase with time in the development of the ramus. At birth, there is no distinct chin and the two halves of the mandible are separated by the mandibular symphysis. Ossification of the symphysis is complete during the second year, the two halves of the mandible uniting to form a single bone. The chin becomes most prominent after puberty (especially in the male). There is some evidence that the angle of the mandible decreases from birth to adulthood. Growth of the mandible occurs by the remodelling of bone. In general terms, increase in the height of the body occurs primarily by formation of alveolar bone, although some bone is also deposited along the lower border of the mandible. Increase in the length of the mandible is accomplished by bone deposition on the posterior surface of the ramus with compensatory resorption on its anterior surface, accompanied by deposition of bone on the posterior surface of the coronoid process and resorption on the anterior surface of the condyle. Increase in width of the mandible is produced by deposition of bone on the outer surface of the mandible and resorption on the inner surface. Present evidence suggests that proliferation of the condylar cartilage is a response to growth and not its cause.

Although the mandible is a single bone, it may be thought of as a number of skeletal units, each associated with one or more soft tissue 'functional matrices'. The behaviour of these matrices primarily determines the growth of each skeletal unit. For example, the coronoid process forms a skeletal unit acted upon by the temporalis muscle. Sectioning of the temporalis muscle during early mandibular development may result in atrophy or complete absence of a coronoid process in the adult mandible. Similarly, the alveolar process is influenced by the teeth, the condyle by the lateral pterygoid muscle, the ramus by the medial pterygoid and masseter muscles, and the body by the neurovascular bundle.

Maxilla

As with the mandible, the maxilla develops intramembranously. The centre of ossification appears during the eighth week of intrauterine life, close to the site of the developing deciduous canine tooth. Unlike the mandible, maxillary growth and development is not related to the appearance of secondary cartilages. Because of the maxilla's position in the developing skull, this jaw's growth is influenced by the development of the orbital, nasal and oral cavities. From the region of the developing deciduous canine, ossification spreads throughout the developing maxilla into its growing processes (palatine, zygomatic, frontal and alveolar processes). The ossification of the palatine processes is described on page 102. At one time it was thought that the incisor-bearing part of the maxilla, which develops from the frontonasal process (see page 101), had a separate centre of ossification. It was consequently called the premaxilla. However, it is now clear that ossification spreads from the body of the maxilla into its incisor-bearing component.

Growth of the maxilla occurs by bone remodelling (i.e. surface deposition of bone with associated resorption) and by sutural growth. Among the agents that provide the forces separating the maxilla from the adjacent bones (thus permitting growth at the sutures) are the growing eyeballs, cartilaginous nasal septum and orbital pad of fat. Thus, growth of the maxilla is not an isolated phenomenon but occurs in association with the development of the orbital, nasal and oral cavities. It has been suggested that the growing nasal septum pulls the maxilla forward by means of a septopremaxillary ligament that runs from the anterior border of the nasal septum posteroinferiorly towards the anterior nasal spine and intermaxillary suture. As in the lower jaw, growth in height of the maxilla is related to the development of the alveolar process. The maxillary sinus appears as an out-pocketing of the mucosa of the middle meatus of the nose at the beginning of the fourth month of intrauterine life. Although small at birth, the maxillary sinus is identifiable radiologically. After birth, the maxillary sinus enlarges with the growing maxilla, although it is only fully developed following the eruption of the permanent dentition.

Forward growth of the whole face (including the maxillae) is dependent upon growth of the spheno-occipital synchondrosis at the base of the skull.

Alveolar bone

The mandible and maxillae develop intramembranously. Thus, in a fibrocellular condensation, a centre of ossification appears in which osteoblasts lay down first-formed or woven bone. As the teeth develop, bone extends from the developing mandible and maxillae to surround and protect the teeth, forming the alveolus. The alveolus is separated from the developing enamel organ by the dental follicle. To accommodate the growing tooth germs, the lamellae of the developing alveolar bone undergo resorption, which occurs on the inner wall of the alveolus (indicated by Howship's lacunae) while, on the outer wall of the alveolus, bone is deposited (indicated by osteoblasts lining an osteoid seam). The developing teeth therefore come to lie in a trough of bone. Later, the teeth become separated from each other by the development of interdental septa. With the onset of root formation, inter-radicular bone develops in multirooted teeth. As in other sites, the collagen fibres in the newly formed alveolar bone have a more variable diameter and lack a preferential orientation, giving the bone a matted (basket weave) appearance when viewed in polarized light. This immature bone, termed woven bone, has larger and more numerous osteocytes compared with adult bone. It is formed more rapidly and has a higher turnover rate. Woven bone is subsequently converted to fine-fibred adult lamellar bone. The source of the cells forming alveolar bone is uncertain, although some have suggested that it may be from neural crest cells of the investing layer of the dental follicle (see page 116).

During crown formation, relocation of the tooth germ within the growing jaws may be associated with appropriate patterns of resorption and deposition on the internal surfaces of the alveolar bone. With the onset of tooth eruption, the bone overlying the tooth undergoes resorption to provide a pathway of eruption (see page 118). In addition, as the tooth erupts and the jaws increase in size, bone deposition is prominent in the region of the alveolar crest. The predominant activity in the fundus of the socket is one of bone resorption, except for teeth whose eruptive pathway is greater than the length of the root. On occasions where bone deposition is seen lining the alveolus, it may be related to relocation of the erupting tooth within the growing jaws. Sharpey fibres from the periodontal ligament become attached to the wall of the alveolus during tooth eruption, although the timing is related to whether the tooth is of the deciduous or permanent dentition (see page 210). The bone of the alveolar wall may then be referred to as bundle bone (see page 222).

Development of the tongue

The anterior two-thirds of the tongue develop from three swellings: the two lateral lingual swellings (buds) and the midline median lingual bud (tuberculum impar). Each is formed by proliferation of mesenchyme beneath the endodermal lining of the 1st pharyngeal (branchial) arch. The posterior third of the tongue develops from a single midline swelling, the hypopharyngeal eminence, which is derived mainly from the 3rd pharyngeal arch with a small contribution from the 4th arch. The eminence overgrows the 2nd arch (the copula) to merge with the 1st arch swellings.

The diverse embryological origin of the tongue explains its diverse sensory supply:

- General sensation to the anterior two-thirds of the tongue is supplied by the lingual nerve, a nerve of the 1st pharyngeal arch.
- General sensation and taste to the posterior third of the tongue are supplied by the glossopharyngeal and superior laryngeal nerves, the nerves of the 3rd and 4th arches.
- The perception of taste in the anterior two-thirds of the tongue is associated with the chorda tympani nerve, a branch of the facial nerve, the nerve of the 2nd pharyngeal arch. Since this arch does not contribute tissue to the anterior part of the tongue, in this situation, it is termed a 'pretrematic' nerve.

The muscles of the tongue develop primarily from occipital somites that migrate into the developing tongue carrying their nerve supply, the hypoglossal nerve, with them.

Development of the thyroid gland

This gland develops between the median lingual bud and the hypopharyngeal eminence. On the fully formed tongue, this site is demarcated by the foramen caecum.

Self-assessment: questions

True/false statements

Which of the following statements are true and which are false?

a. The facial processes correspond to centres of growth in the underlying mesenchyme.

b. Ectomesenchyme (neural crest) tissue contributes to the facial processes.

c. Facial processes are separated from each other by epithelial sheets which must be broken down for normal development.

d. The nasal placodes are thickenings of ectoderm from which derive the olfactory hair cells.

e. The frontonasal process is subdivided into medial and lateral nasal processes around the lens placode.

f. An oblique cleft of the lip results from the continuance on the surface of the naso-optic furrow.

g. In the presence of a bilateral cleft lip, the philtrum is innervated by the maxillary nerve.

h. The primary palate is formed by the frontonasal process.

i. The palatal shelves forming the secondary palate are outgrowths of the mandibular processes.

j. Secondary palate formation in humans requires the elevation and then fusion of the palatal shelves in the hard palate but not the soft palate.

k. Palatal shelf elevation occurs because of external forces produced by the developing tongue.

l. During palatal shelf elevation, the amount of the glycosaminoglycan called hyaluronan increases markedly within the shelf.

m. Palatal shelf elevation in humans occurs during the twelfth week of intra-uterine life.

n. Recombination experiments with epithelial and mesenchymal components of the palatal shelves indicate that the epithelium controls mesenchymal behaviour.

o. Type IX collagen, synthesized under the control of epidermal growth factors, may provide a signal for changes occurring at fusion of the palatal shelves.

p. A submucous cleft describes a condition where the palatal mucosa is intact but the underlying bone and musculature are deficient.

q. The hard palate ossifies intramembranously from a centre in the premaxilla.

r. The anterior part of the tongue is derived from the 2nd pharyngeal arch.

s. The developmental division between the anterior and posterior parts of the tongue is shown by the sulcus terminalis.

t. The accessory nerve may innervate the very back part of the tongue, indicating some contribution from the 4th pharyngeal arch.

u. The musculature of the tongue is derived from pre-optic myotomes.

v. The epithelial lining of the tongue is ectodermal in origin.

w. Both the maxilla and the mandible initially develop intramembranously.

x. The centre of ossification for the maxilla appears close to the site of the future deciduous central incisor tooth during the eighth week of intra-uterine life.

y. Unlike the mandible, the maxilla receives no significant contributions from secondary cartilages.

z. Growth of the maxilla is dependent upon forces exerted externally from the growing brain, eye and nasal septum.

aa. Forward growth of the lower jaw is greater than that of the upper jaw.

ab. The maxillary air sinus does not develop until 3 years after birth.

ac. The initial centres of ossification for the mandible lie close to the divisions of the inferior alveolar nerves into incisive and mental branches.

ad. The secondary cartilage within the mandibular condyle is essential for growth of the ramus.

ae. Remodelling of the ramus of the mandible involves resorption of bone on the anterior border and deposition on the posterior border.

af. The mandibular symphysis closes 1 year after birth.

Extended matching questions

Theme: Development of the face, palate and tongue

Lead-in

Select the most appropriate option to answer items 1–5. Each option can be used once, more than once or not at all.

Item list

1. Structure forming the upper lip
2. Epithelial thickening giving rise to inner ear
3. A structure in the developing palate that must degenerate to allow fusion to be completed
4. Structure giving rise to the posterior third of the tongue
5. Site of origin of the thyroid gland

Option list

A. Copula
B. Foramen caecum
C. Frontonasal process
D. Hypopharyngeal eminence
E. Lateral lingual swellings (buds)
F. Lens placode
G. Mandibular process
H. Maxillary process
I. Midline epithelial seam
J. Nasal placode
K. Occipital somites

Self-assessment: questions

L. Otic placode
M. Palatal shelves
N. Tuberculum impar (median lingual bud)

Picture questions

Figure 9.1 (Courtesy of Professor A. G. S. Lumsden)

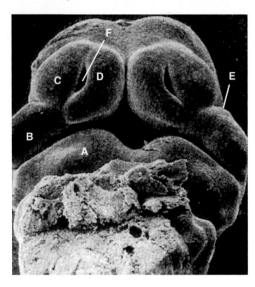

The picture shows the developing face of a fetus during the sixth week of intra-uterine life.
a. Identify the features indicated by the labels A–F.
b. What is the nasal fin and how does it contribute to the development of the upper lip?
c. What is the evidence that vitamin A derivatives are involved in 'pattern formation' during the development of the upper lip?
d. List the main types of facial clefts that can appear.

Figure 9.2

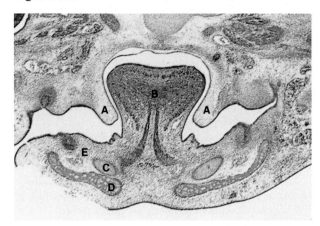

Pictured is a coronal section through the developing head of a fetus during the seventh week of intra-uterine life.
a. Identify the structures indicated by the labels A–E.
b. By which week is the palate elevated and fused?
c. What are the mechanisms responsible for the elevation of the palatal shelves?
d. What are the mechanisms responsible for the fusion of the palatal shelves once they have been elevated?
e. List the main varieties of clefts of the palate.

Self-assessment: questions

Figure 9.3

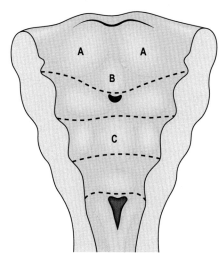

a. In this diagram of the developing tongue, identify regions A–C.

Figure 9.4 (Courtesy of Dr J. Potts)

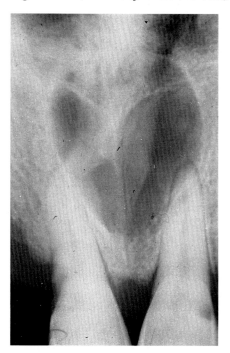

The radiograph shows a large, circular, radiolucent area in the centre of the palate. On surgical examination, a cyst lined with stratified squamous epithelium was discovered and a median palatine cyst of 'developmental' origin was diagnosed.

a. Bearing in mind the mechanism involved during palatogenesis, how would you account for the presence of this cyst?

Figure 9.5 (Courtesy of Dr B. A. W. Brown)

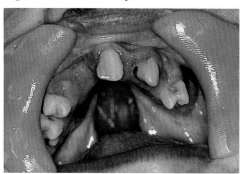

The illustration shows a severe cleft of the palate.
a. What is the incidence of clefts of the palate in human neonates?
b. What is the mode of inheritance for palatal clefts?
c. Is the incidence of cleft palate the same in males and females?
d. From your knowledge of normal palatogenesis, conjecture the mechanisms which may be responsible for palatal clefts.

Self-assessment: questions

Figure 9.6 (Courtesy of Professor J. D. Langdon)

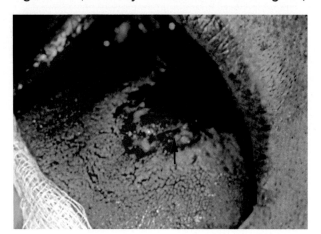

A young man noticed this painless swelling at the back of his tongue in the midline (arrow). Thinking it might be a tumour, he visited his local hospital. The examining doctor believed that the lesion was harmless and had an embryological explanation. To confirm this, the doctor conducted a test which showed that the swelling took up radioactive iodine.

   a. What might the swelling be?

Figure 9.7

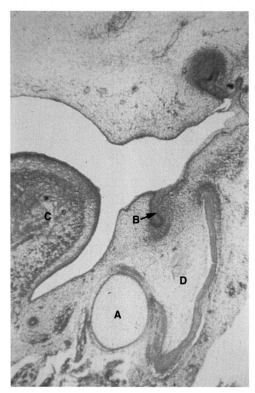

This photomicrograph is a transverse section through the early developing mandible (eighth week of development).

   a. Identify the structures labelled A–D.
   b. What is Meckel's cartilage and to what does it contribute in the adult?
   c. Briefly describe the development of the temporomandibular joint.

Essay questions

1. Review the conflicting views that have been proposed to explain the development of the upper lip and intermaxillary segment.
2. Discuss the various hypotheses that have been proposed to explain palatal shelf elevation.

Self-assessment: answers

True/false answers

a. **True**. The facial processes are also demarcated by grooves which become flattened out by the proliferative and migratory activities of the mesenchymal cells.

b. **True**. The connective tissue cells migrate from the neural crest and muscle cells from the paraxial mesenchyme.

c. **False**. Such sheets were once thought to have a role in the development of facial clefts.

d. **True**. The nasal placodes also 'sink' into the underlying mesenchyme to form the nasal pits (the primitive nasal cavities).

e. **False**. The medial and lateral nasal processes appear around the nasal placodes and pits.

f. **True**. The naso-optic furrow normally would invaginate into the mesenchyme, become a canal and form the nasolacrimal duct.

g. **False**. Although the philtrum of the upper lip is innervated by the maxillary nerve (the nerve of the maxillary process), with a bilateral cleft it is innervated by the ophthalmic nerve (the nerve of the frontonasal process).

h. **True**. Note that it is the primary palate in which the nasal pits lie and that behind the primary palate is a (common) oronasal chamber which becomes separate oral and nasal cavities with the development of the secondary palate.

i. **False**. The palatal shelves are outgrowths of the maxillary processes.

j. **False**. For some mammals, however, formation of the soft palate does not involve palatal shelf elevation.

k. **False**. Present evidence suggests that the force for palatal shelf elevation is produced within the shelves.

l. **True**. Indeed, it has been proposed that it is the hydration of this ground substance component which produces the intrinsic shelf elevation force.

m. **False**. Shelf elevation takes place during the eighth week of intra-uterine life.

n. **False**. The major controlling influence resides with the mesenchymal component.

o. **True**. Immunohistochemical studies indicate the presence of type IX collagen and receptors for epidermal growth factors prior to breakdown of the midline epithelial seam.

p. **True**. Submucous clefts are therefore likely to arise because of failure of the process of fusion of the palatal shelves rather than failure of the process of shelf elevation.

q. **False**. There is no premaxilla in man. All components/processes of the maxillary bone ossify from a single centre that is initially located close to the developing deciduous canine tooth.

r. **False**. It is derived from the 1st pharyngeal arch.

s. **False**. The embryological division probably corresponds with the division of the tongue into different areas of innervation. Consequently, the embryological division would lie just in front of the circumvallate papillae.

t. **False**. The area around the vallecula is innervated by the internal laryngeal nerve (a branch of the vagus).

u. **False**. The musculature of the tongue arises from occipital myotomes (hence the innervation by the hypoglossal nerve).

v. **False**. The epithelial lining is endodermal in origin, the tongue developing from the floor of the pharyngeal arch system.

w. **True**. Most of the facial skeleton develops intramembranously.

x. **False**. The centre of ossification is located close to the developing deciduous canine tooth (there is no premaxilla in humans).

y. **True**. Secondary cartilages have been described in the regions of the zygomatic and alveolar processes, but these rapidly ossify.

z. **True**. There is also considerable surface remodelling.

aa. **True**. This accounts for some of the changing occlusal relationships between the teeth during childhood.

ab. **False**. The maxillary, sphenoidal and ethmoidal sinuses are rudimentary at birth. It is the frontal air sinus which appears much later.

ac. **True**. Thereafter, ossification continues within the condensation of mesenchyme around Meckel's cartilage (the cartilage of the first pharyngeal arch).

ad. **False**. Although important, the role of the secondary cartilage in the mandibular condyle for growth of the ramus is questioned by experiments involving surgical removal of the cartilage.

ae. **True**. The ramus of the mandible also assumes a more vertical relationship to the body of the mandible.

af. **True**. In common with other symphyses, the joint is a secondary cartilaginous joint consisting of a 'sandwich' of bone, cartilage, fibrous tissue, cartilage, bone.

Extended matching answers

Item 1 = Option H. Although it is often reported that the upper lip is formed by the merger of the maxillary processes with the medial nasal processes (from the frontonasal process), evidence from the innervation of the adult upper lip suggests that the upper lip is formed entirely from the maxillary processes that eventually meet in the midline.

Item 2 = Option L. The otic placode is a thickening of the surface ectoderm of the developing face that invaginates and internalizes (by a process not dissimilar to formation of the neural tube) to form the membranous labyrinth of the inner ear.

109

Self-assessment: answers

Item 3 = Option I. Following elevation of the palatal shelves, the shelves fuse but the mesenchyme is initially separated by a 'midline epithelial seam'. This seam breaks down (by apoptosis and/or redifferentiation and migration of the epithelial cells) to provide continuity of the mesenchyme.

Item 4 = Option D. The hypopharyngeal eminence is a swelling on the endodermal surface of the developing pharynx (associated mainly with the 3rd pharyngeal arch). The eminence overgrows the 2nd arch copula (to merge with the lateral lingual buds of the 1st arch) and thus form the posterior third of the tongue.

Item 5 = Option B. The foramen caecum is a small pit on the posterior third of the adult tongue (lying behind the apex of the sulcus terminalis) that demarcated the origin of the thyroid gland between the median lingual bud and hypopharyngeal eminence of the developing tongue. In some situations, a 'lingual thyroid' may be found at this location in an adult patient.

Picture answers

Figure 9.1

a. A = mandibular process. B = maxillary process. C = lateral nasal process. D = medial nasal process. E = naso-optic furrow. F = nasal pit.
b. The nasal fin is a sheet of epithelium located in front of the nasal pit. It was once believed that the nasal fin formed an epithelial partition between the maxillary and medial nasal processes. However, a bridge of mesenchyme known as the maxillary isthmus joins the two processes in front of the nasal fin. The nasal fin is eventually incorporated either into the walls of the nasal pit or into the oronasal membrane. Should the fin become enlarged, it may contribute a line of weakness between the mesenchyme of the maxillary and medial nasal processes, and eventually lead to the formation of a cleft in this region.
c. Pattern formation in some developing organs is controlled by retinoids (vitamin A derivatives), which form morphogenetic gradients within the tissues. Although such gradients have not yet been demonstrated in the face, a similar mechanism seems likely to be present here as the facial primordial are sensitive to exogenous retinoic acid and the mesenchymal cells contain specific retinoic acid receptors.
d. Unilateral cleft lip, bilateral cleft lip, median cleft lip (with nasal defect), oblique facial cleft (with cleft lip), median mandibular cleft, macrostomia. There are also clefts related to the orbit.

Figure 9.2

a. A = palatal shelves. B = developing tongue. C = Meckel's cartilage (cartilage of the 1st branchial arch). D = developing bone of mandible. E = tooth germ.

b. The secondary palate is completed during the twelfth week of development.
c. It now appears that there is a force of elevation intrinsic to the palatal shelves. However, the mechanism responsible is controversial. It has been proposed that the force results from hydration of ground substance components in the shelf mesenchyme and/or from proliferation, migration or contraction of mesenchymal cells.
d. Once elevated, the palatal shelves fuse firstly by adhering together by means of a 'sticky' glycoprotein, then by the epithelial cells developing desmosomes and forming a midline epithelial seam. This seam subsequently thins and breaks down so that there is a merging of the mesenchyme within the palatal shelves. The midline epithelial seam breaks down as a result of programmed cell death and by the migration of the epithelial cells and eventual differentiation into mesenchymal cells.
e. The mildest form of cleft affects the uvula (bifid uvula). Early disturbance of palatal elevation or fusion can result in an extensive cleft of the secondary palate. Should the cleft involve the primary palate, it may extend to one or both sides of the incisive foramen to include the alveolus. A submucous cleft describes a condition where, despite the fact that the palatal mucosa is intact, the bone/musculature of the palate is deficient beneath the mucosa.

Figure 9.3

a. A = lateral lingual swellings/buds (1st pharyngeal arch). B = median lingual bud/tuberculum impar (1st arch). C = hypopharyngeal eminence (mainly from the 3rd arch). Note that the thyroid gland develops between B and C, a site in the adult corresponding with the foramen caecum.

Figure 9.4

a. A median palatine cyst is derived from the epithelium which persists in the fusion line of the two palatal shelves once they have elevated. Normally, the epithelium (the midline epithelial seam) breaks down by a combination of programmed cell death and redifferentiation into mesenchyme or epithelium. However, remnants may become cystic. Because the embryonic epithelium lining the palatal shelves has the potential to differentiate into either respiratory epithelium (pseudostratified, ciliated, columnar epithelium) on the nasal surface or stratified squamous epithelium on the oral surface, the cyst may have an epithelial lining of either type.

Figure 9.5

a. Palatal clefts occur approximately once in every 1000 live births.

Self-assessment: answers

b. Polygenic discontinuous multifactorial mode of inheritance.

c. More common in females (67%).

d. Clefts of the palate may arise because of failure of elevation of the palatal shelves; because of asymmetrical development of the shelves on either side; as a result of deficiency in size of the palatal shelves; because the shelves, although elevated, fail to fuse properly as a result of defective initial contact; because of failure of the midline epithelial seam to form or subsequently break down; or because of deficient migration/proliferation of the mesenchyme across the fused shelves.

Figure 9.6

a. The swelling in the midline of the tongue might appear smooth and could be related to an area related to the embryonic median lingual bud (tuberculum impar). However, the fact that iodine was taken up by the swelling suggests that it is a 'lingual thyroid', the thyroid gland originating embryologically from the region around the foramen caecum. In this case, the gland did not migrate but remained on the tongue as a fully functioning thyroid gland, and should therefore not be removed.

Figure 9.7

a. A = Meckel's cartilage. B = dental lamina. C = developing tongue. D = neurovascular bundle surrounded by developing bone of the mandible.

b. Meckel's cartilage is the cartilage of the 1st pharyngeal (branchial) arch. In the mesenchyme around this cartilage, the body of the mandible is formed (i.e. intramembranously). The cartilage also gives rise to the lingula on the ramus of the mandible, the sphenomandibular ligament, the spine of the sphenoid bone, the malleus and incus ear ossicles, and the sphenomalleolar ligament.

c. The temporomandibular joint develops from mesenchyme lying between the developing mandibular condyle below and the temporal bone above, which themselves develop intramembranously. During the twelfth week of intra-uterine life, two clefts appear in the mesenchyme, producing the upper and lower joint cavities, the remaining intervening mesenchyme becoming the intra-articular disc. The joint capsule develops from a condensation of mesenchyme surrounding the developing joint. At birth, the mandibular fossa is flat and there is no articular eminence, the latter only becoming prominent following the eruption of the deciduous dentition.

Outline essay answers

Question 1

General comments should provide an introduction defining the embryonic upper lip and intermaxillary segment and mentioning that abnormal development in this region leads to the common congenital malformation of clefts of the lip.

A description should follow of the facial processes around the stomodeum and the classical view of fusion of the maxillary processes with the medial nasal processes (part of the frontonasal process) to form the upper lip and the intermaxillary segment.

Three main areas of conflict/controversy should be mentioned:

- The role of the maxillary processes. Knowledge of the innervation of the adult upper lip (i.e. from the infra-orbital branches of the maxillary divisions of the trigeminal nerves) suggests that the upper lip is formed only from the maxillary processes and not the medial nasal processes. In the embryo, the nerve associated with the maxillary process is the maxillary division of the trigeminal nerve, while that associated with a medial nasal process is the ophthalmic division of the trigeminal. The philtrum region of the upper lip is only innervated by the ophthalmic nerve when there is bilateral clefting of the upper lip.

- Epithelial sheets and the nasal fin. It was once believed that the facial processes were bounded by epithelial sheets and that these had to break down before the processes could fuse. It is now known that there are no epithelial sheets and that the facial processes are merely condensations of mesenchyme that proliferate, migrate and eventually fuse. The nasal fin was an epithelial sheet that supposedly separated the maxillary processes from the medial nasal process. While there is indeed a thickening of the epithelial floor of the nasal pits in a region associated with nasal fin, there is not a complete septation between the maxillary and medial nasal processes.

- The premaxilla. While some mammals have a separate region in the upper lip called the premaxilla, which is separate from the remaining maxilla and associated with the developing incisor region, this is not present in humans. Indeed, all of the maxilla and the intermaxillary segment has a single centre of ossification that is located initially close to the developing canine tooth.

Question 2

The introduction should include a description (with diagrams) of the stages of palatogenesis, from the time when there is only a primary palate (behind which is a common oronasal chamber) to the appearance of the palatal shelves (inward extensions of the facial maxillary processes) with

Self-assessment: answers

subsequent elevation/relocation of the shelves from a vertical to a horizontal position. The final stage is of fusion of the palatal shelves and histogenesis. It should be mentioned that palatal shelf elevation is a significant event and that failure of elevation leads to the development of major clefting of the palate. Furthermore, it must be stated that palatal shelf elevation is an event typical of mammalians and that it is very rapid.

The essay should highlight the considerable controversies that have existed concerning the mechanisms responsible for palatal shelf elevation and the fact that a considerable number of hypotheses have been proposed. The hypotheses can be categorized into two groups:

- Those that suggest that there is an extrinsic force pushing or pulling on the shelves
- Those that suggest that there is an intrinsic shelf elevation force generated within the mesenchyme of the palatal shelves.

Examples of extrinsic forces include movements of the tongue, movements of the jaws, and pressure differences above and below the shelves. Early analysis of the events of shelf elevation did not support the notion that there was an extrinsic force, since there appears to be dissociation between the chronologies of events. Furthermore, more recent work involving organ culture of palatal shelves in the absence of tongues and lower jaws shows that palatal shelves still elevate.

Thus, recent research has concentrated on seeking the source of an intrinsic shelf elevation force. Two main hypotheses exist:

- Firstly, it has been proposed that the mesenchymal cells, by their proliferation, migration or contraction, produce the force. Little evidence is available to support this, although a critical number of cells are clearly required for shelf elevation to proceed.

- Secondly, there is the notion that a turgor pressure is generated by hydration of the extracellular matrix, the main candidate molecule being hyaluronan. Early histochemical work showed that hyaluronan was present in abundance just before shelf elevation. Subsequent biochemical research showed that GAG content was significant for shelf elevation to occur (there is less GAG with cleft development) and that there is more hyaluronan present just before elevation than just after elevation of the shelves. Immunohistochemistry has also localized hyaluronan and associated proteoglycans, and shown it to be present in free and bound (to cells) forms. Using organ culture, interference in hyaluronan synthesis (e.g. with hyaluronidase) results in the formation of clefts. However, use of a drug that blocks secretion from the Golgi material, while still allowing hyaluronan production, also prevents shelf elevation. Thus, although there is reasonable evidence that hyaluronan is involved in shelf elevation, there is a further macromolecule 'packaged' through the Golgi (as yet unknown) that makes a significant contribution.

The essay should conclude by mentioning the need for further studies (e.g. for hyaluronan binding sites/receptors) and by suggesting that hyaluronan may exert its effects via the cells and not merely through hydration of the extracellular matrix of the mesenchymal shelf. Finally, it should be highlighted that substances such as retinoids can produce clefts and that the mechanisms by which they exert their effects (and whether or not they affect hyaluronan synthesis or activity) have yet to be elucidated.

Chapter 10

Early tooth development, root development (including cementogenesis) and tooth eruption

Early tooth development 113
Bud stage 114
Cap stage 114
Early bell stage 114
Late bell stage 115
Enamel knot 115
Experimental studies 115
Root development 116
Cementogenesis 116
Tooth eruption 118
Introduction 118
Resorption and shedding
of a deciduous tooth 118
Gubernacular canal 119
Chronology for tooth development 119
Eruptive mechanism 120
Self-assessment: questions 122
Self-assessment: answers 130

Overview

The teeth develop by the mutual cooperation and interaction of an ectodermal tissue (the enamel organ) and mesenchymal tissue (the dental papilla). Root development involves interaction between the enamel organ (specifically an epithelial root sheath) and another mesenchymal tissue (the dental follicle). As tooth development proceeds, there is an increased complexity apparent in terms of histogenesis and morphogenesis (both of these being under the 'control' of the mesenchymal dental papilla). Tooth eruption begins as the root forms and is the process that takes the tooth from its developmental position in the jaw to its functional position in the mouth. Although the mechanisms responsible for the generation of eruptive forces are controversial, evidence suggests that such forces are generated within the dental follicle/periodontal ligament, that they are non-tractional (not involving a 'pulling' force through the fibres of the follicle/periodontal ligament) and that, although multifactorial, they involve, at least in part, the periodontal vasculature/tissue hydrostatic pressure.

The development of the root initially involves the mapping out of the shape of the future root by downgrowths of the cervical loop regions of the enamel organ of the tooth germ to form epithelial root sheaths. This sheath then induces the differentiation of odontoblasts and the secretion of root dentine. As the root sheath extends, it breaks down so that the dental follicle comes to lie adjacent to the root dentine; thence cementogenesis commences, with the eventual incorporation of follicle collagen fibres to form the initial periodontal ligament.

Learning objectives

You should:
- be able to describe the development of the tooth germ from its initial appearance at the dental lamina through to the bell stage of development and up to the point of initiation of dentine and enamel formation, linking the description with events of histogenesis and morphogenesis
- understand the principles underlying ectodermal-mesenchymal interactions during tooth development
- be able to give an account of the development of the root of the tooth
- be able to discuss both the process and mechanisms of tooth eruption (including the resorption and shedding of deciduous teeth).

Early tooth development

The first histological sign of tooth development is the appearance of a condensation of mesenchymal tissue beneath the presumptive dental epithelium of the primitive oral cavity. It is now known that this mesenchymal tissue is of neural crest origin. Subsequently, the oral epithelium thickens and invaginates into the mesenchyme to form a primary epithelial band. The primary epithelial band then divides into two processes: a vestibular lamina and a dental lamina:

- The vestibular lamina contributes to the development of the vestibule of the mouth, delineating the lips and cheeks from the tooth-bearing regions.
- The dental lamina contributes to the development of the teeth and a series of swellings (the tooth germs) develops on the deep surface of the dental lamina.

The tooth germs are classified into bud, cap and bell stages according to the degree of morphodifferentiation and histo-differentiation of their epithelial components (enamel organs).

Bud stage

The enamel organ in the bud stage appears as a simple, spherical, epithelial condensation that is poorly morpho-differentiated and histodifferentiated. It is surrounded by mesenchyme. The epithelial component is separated from the adjacent mesenchyme by a basement membrane.

Cap stage

At the cap stage, and with progressive morphodifferen-tiation, the deeper surface of the enamel organ invaginates to form a cap-shaped structure. There is also histodif-ferentiation with a greater distinction between the more rounded cells in the central portion of the enamel organ and the peripheral cells which are becoming arranged to form the external and internal enamel epithelia. In the late cap stage of tooth development, the central cells of the enamel organ have become separated (though main-taining contact by desmosomes), the intercellular spaces containing significant quantities of glycosaminoglycans. The resulting tissue is termed the stellate reticulum. The cells of the external enamel epithelium remain cuboidal, whereas those of the internal enamel epithelium become more columnar. The part of the mesenchyme lying beneath the internal enamel epithelium is termed the dental papilla, while that surrounding the tooth germ forms the dental follicle.

Early bell stage

Further morphodifferentiation and histodifferentiation of the tooth germ leads to the early bell stage. The configura-tion of the internal enamel epithelium broadly maps out the occlusal pattern of the crown of the tooth. It is during the bell stage that the dental lamina breaks down and the enamel organ loses connection with the oral epithelium. At this stage, the dental follicle has three layers:

- The inner investing layer is a vascular, fibrocellular condensation immediately surrounding the tooth germ. The cells of the inner layer of the dental follicle may be derived from the neural crest.
- The outer layer of the dental follicle is a vascular mesenchymal layer that lines the developing alveolus.
- Between the two layers is loose connective tissue with no marked concentration of blood vessels.

A high degree of histodifferentiation is achieved in the early bell stage. The enamel organ shows four distinct layers: external enamel epithelium, stellate reticulum, stratum intermedium, and internal enamel epithelium.

External enamel epithelium

The external enamel epithelium forms the outer layer of cuboidal cells which limits the enamel organ. It is sepa-rated from the surrounding mesenchymal tissue by a basement membrane. The external enamel epithelial cells contain large, centrally placed nuclei and have relatively small amounts of the intracellular organelles associated with protein synthesis. The cells contact each other via desmosomes and gap junctions. The external enamel epi-thelium is thought to be involved in the maintenance of the shape of the enamel organ and in the exchange of sub-stances between the enamel organ and the environment. The cervical loop, at which there is considerable mitotic activity, lies at the growing margin of the enamel organ where the external enamel epithelium is continuous with the internal enamel epithelium.

Stellate reticulum

The stellate reticulum is most fully developed at the bell stage. The intercellular spaces become fluid-filled, presumably related to osmotic effects arising from the high concentration of glycosaminoglycans. The cells are star-shaped with bodies containing conspicuous nuclei and many branching processes. The mesenchyme-like features of the stellate reticulum include the synthesis of collagens in the tissue. The cells of this layer possess little endoplasmic reticulum and few mitochondria. However, there is a relatively well-developed Golgi com-plex, which, together with the presence of microvilli on the cell surface, has been interpreted as indicating that the cells contribute to the secretion of the extracellular material. Numerous tonofilaments are present within the cytoplasm, and there are desmosomes and gap junctions between the cells.

The main function of the stellate reticulum is 'mechan-ical', protecting the underlying dental tissues against physical disturbance and maintaining tooth shape. It has been suggested that the hydrostatic pressure gener-ated within the stellate reticulum is in equilibrium with that of the dental papilla, allowing the proliferative pat-tern of the intervening internal enamel epithelium to determine crown morphogenesis. The stellate reticulum also produces colony-stimulating factor (CSF-1), trans-forming growth factor beta-1 (TGF-β_1) and parathyroid hormone-related protein (PTHrP). These molecules may be released into the dental follicle and help recruit and activate the osteoclasts necessary to resorb the adja-cent alveolar bone as the developing tooth enlarges and erupts.

Stratum intermedium

The stratum intermedium first appears at the bell stage and consists of two or three layers of flattened cells lying over the internal enamel epithelium (and its derivatives). The cells of the stratum intermedium resemble the cells of the stellate reticulum, although their intercellular spaces are smaller and the cells contain much alkaline phosphatase.

It has been suggested that the stratum intermedium is concerned with:

- the synthesis of proteins
- the transport of materials to and from the enamel-forming cells in the internal enamel epithelium (the ameloblasts)
- the concentration of materials.

Internal enamel epithelium

The cells of the internal enamel epithelium are columnar at the bell stage but, beginning at the regions associated with the future cusp tips (i.e. the sites of initial enamel formation), the cells become elongated. The internal enamel epithelial cells are rich in RNA but, unlike the stratum intermedium and stellate reticulum, do not contain alkaline phosphatase. Desmosomes connect the internal enamel epithelial cells and link this layer to the stratum intermedium. The internal enamel epithelium is separated from the peripheral cells of the dental papilla by a basement membrane and a cell-free zone.

The differentiation of the dental papilla at the early bell stage is less striking than that of the enamel organ. Until the late bell stage, the dental papilla consists of closely packed mesenchymal cells with only a few delicate extracellular fibrils. Histochemically, the dental papilla becomes rich in glycosaminoglycans.

At the early bell stage, downgrowths on the lingual aspect of the enamel organs indicate the early development of the successional (permanent) teeth.

Late bell stage

The late bell stage (appositional stage) of tooth development is associated with the formation of the dental hard tissues. Dentine formation always precedes enamel formation. Detailed accounts of amelogenesis and dentinogenesis are given on pages 144–147 and 165–168. At the late bell stage, enamel and dentine formation commences at the tips of future cusps (or incisal edges). Under the inductive influence of developing ameloblasts (pre-ameloblasts), the adjacent mesenchymal cells of the dental papilla become columnar and differentiate into odontoblasts. The odontoblasts then become involved in the formation of predentine and dentine. The presence of dentine then induces the ameloblasts to secrete enamel.

Enamel knot

During the early stages of tooth development, three transitory structures may be seen: the enamel knot, enamel cord and enamel niche. Of these, the most significant in terms of functional development is the enamel knot. This is a localized mass of cells in the centre of the internal enamel epithelium. Recent studies suggest it may represent an important signalling centre during tooth development (e.g. bone morphogenetic protein (BMP)-2 and BMP-7).

Experimental studies

Tooth development (odontogenesis) is a very complex process involving many growth factors and transcription factors to ensure an ordered, and controlled, development for both individual tooth germs and the whole dentition. Epithelial–mesenchymal interactions are particularly in evidence and require signalling between the two major components of the tooth germ, one derived from the oral epithelium and one from the underlying mesenchyme.

Morphogenesis and histogenesis

Experiments have shown that the epithelium lining the first pharyngeal (branchial) arch has 'odontogenic potential'. This potential only exists in the very early stages of odontogenesis because, after initiation, the 'control' of tooth development passes to the mesenchyme. At the cap stage of tooth development, the principal organizer is the dental papilla, in terms of both morphogenesis and histogenesis. The result of culturing dental papilla mesenchyme with epithelium from the developing foot pad is normal tooth development, illustrating the importance of the dental papilla. On the other hand, if the enamel organ of a tooth is cultured with mesenchyme from the developing foot pad, tooth development does not occur. Furthermore, should an incisor enamel organ be combined with a molar papilla, the resulting tooth is molariform and, if a molar enamel organ is combined with an incisor papilla, the resulting tooth is incisiform.

Presumptive incisor and molar regions

It has been established that the presumptive incisor and molar regions contain some difference in their homeobox gene arrays (in the incisor region Msx-1 (but not Barx-1) is expressed; in the molar region Barx-1 (but not Msx-1) is expressed). The odontogenic homeobox code can be considered in the light of a 'field model hypothesis', where each tooth germ starts the same but different concentrations of morphogens (e.g. growth factors) in the local environment are responsible for producing different tooth types. In contrast to the 'field model hypothesis', a 'clonal model hypothesis' has been forwarded to explain tooth form. Accordingly, the tooth type is prespecified and is not dependent on the environment within the jaws. Consequently, if a molar tooth germ is cultured in a site well away from the jaws the complete series of molars can form by budding off from this single precursor.

Bioactive signalling molecules

During tooth development, 'messages' pass between the epithelium and mesenchyme to produce changes of increasing complexity (i.e. differentiation) within the cell layers. It has been clearly shown that bioactive signalling molecules in the form of small proteins pass between the epithelium and mesenchyme, and usually have important interactions with the receptors on the cell membrane.

Ten

Experimental evidence suggests that induction is due to the presence of the initial extracellular matrix, a thin layer situated between the epithelium and mesenchyme and comprising the basal lamina and adjacent region.

Root development

Root development proceeds after the crown has formed and involves interactions between the dental follicle, the dental papilla, and a structure derived from the cervical loop region of the enamel organ called the epithelial root sheath (of Hertwig). At the late bell stage of tooth development, when amelogenesis and dentinogenesis are well advanced, the external and internal enamel epithelia at the cervical loop of the enamel organ form a double-layered epithelial root sheath, which proliferates apically to map out the shape of the future root. The primary apical foramen at the growing end of the epithelial root sheath may subdivide into a number of secondary apical foramina by the ingrowth of epithelial shelves from the margins of the root sheath, which subsequently fuse near the centre of the root. The number and location of these epithelial shelves correspond to the number and location of the definitive roots of the tooth, and may be under the inductive control of the dental papilla. When a permanent tooth first erupts, only about two-thirds of the length of the root is complete. A wide, 'open' root apex is present in these situations, surrounded by a thin, regular knife-edge of dentine. It takes about 3 more years for root completion to occur.

During root development, growth of the epithelial root sheath occurs to enclose the dental papilla, except for an opening at the base (the primary apical foramen). Beneath the dental papilla the epithelial sheath usually appears angled to form the root diaphragm. Note that, between the two epithelial layers, there is no stellate reticulum or stratum intermedium. The dental follicle lies external to the root sheath and forms cementum, periodontal ligament and alveolar bone. In the region of the root diaphragm, the epithelial root sheath is seen as a continuous sheet of tissue sandwiched between the undifferentiated mesenchyme of the dental papilla and the dental follicle. Above the root diaphragm, towards the developing crown, the cells of the internal layer of the epithelial sheath induce the peripheral cells of the dental papilla to differentiate into odontoblasts. Following the onset of dentinogenesis in the root, the epithelial cells of the root sheath lose their continuity, becoming separated from the surface of the developing root dentine to form epithelial rests in the periodontal ligament (see page 206). The mesenchymal cells of the dental follicle adjacent to the root dentine now differentiate into cementoblasts, and cementogenesis commences.

Cementogenesis

The tissues of the dental follicle in the developing root are comprised of three layers:

- Adjacent to the epithelial root sheath is the inner investing layer of the dental follicle, which is said to be derived from the neural crest.
- Adjacent to the developing alveolar bone is the outer layer of the dental follicle.
- The outer layer is separated from the inner layer by an intermediate layer.

The outer and intermediate layers are mesodermal in origin. Cells of the inner layer of the dental follicle differentiate into the cementoblasts. Once cementogenesis has begun, cells of the remaining dental follicle become obliquely oriented along the root surface and become the fibroblasts of the periodontal ligament.

Cementogenesis is here considered in terms of the formation of primary (acellular) cementum and then of secondary (cellular) cementum. As for the crown, the hard tissues that comprise the root (i.e. cementum and dentine) develop under the control of epithelial/mesenchymal interactions. Unlike the crown, the epithelial component involved in root formation retains a simpler morphology, rapidly loses its continuity with adjacent cells, and is not evident as a conspicuous layer during initial cementum formation.

Primary (acellular) cementum

Once the crown has fully formed, the internal and external enamel epithelia proliferate downwards as a double-layered sheet of somewhat flattened epithelial cells, the epithelial root sheath (of Hertwig) that maps out the shape of the root(s). The process of cementogenesis is initiated at the cervical margin and extends apically as the root grows downwards. The epithelial root sheath is separated by a basal lamina on both of its surfaces from the adjacent connective tissues of the dental follicle and dental papilla. The epithelial root sheath induces the adjacent cells of the dental papilla to differentiate into odontoblasts. As these odontoblasts initially retreat inwards, they synthesize and secrete the organic matrix of the first-formed root predentine. As the odontoblasts do not leave behind an odontoblast process in this initial few microns of tissue, its structureless (and later glass-like) appearance is responsible for the term hyaline layer that is given to this (approximately 10 μm) layer once it is mineralized. The epithelial root sheath is in contact with the initial predentine layer for only a short distance before the continuity of its cells is lost (i.e. the sheath 'fenestrates'). There is evidence that the epithelial root sheath cells secrete enamel-related protein(s) into the collagenous matrix of the hyaline layer at the cement–dentine boundary. Thus, the hyaline layer is formed by contributions from both the odontoblast and epithelial root sheath layers. The enamel-related protein(s) has been identified as amelogenin, although there is some dispute as to whether another enamel-related protein, ameloblastin, is also present. The function of such enamel-related proteins is unclear but may concern epithelial/mesenchymal interactions involving the induction of odontoblasts and cementoblasts, and/or the process of mineralization. During the subsequent mineralization of cementum and the hyaline layer, the enamel-related protein(s) is lost, although remnants may be retained in the granular layer of the root dentine. Mineralization of the first-formed dentine does not initially occur at the outermost surface of the hyaline layer, but a few microns within it. From this initial centre, mineralization spreads both inwards towards the pulp and outwards towards the periodontal ligament (centrifugally). Thus, the outermost part of the hyaline layer undergoes delayed mineralization.

The cause of 'fenestration' of the epithelial root sheath is not known, but may be due to programmed cell death (apoptosis). Fibroblast-like cells of the adjacent dental follicle pass through the fenestrations and come to lie close to the surface of the hyaline layer. These cells become cementoblasts associated with the formation of primary cementum but they do not form a conspicuous layer on the forming root surface and may retreat and mingle with adjacent fibroblasts of the periodontal ligament. The precise origin of the fibroblast-like cells is not clear. They might appear to be derived from the cells of the investing layer of the dental follicle. However, there is also evidence suggesting that they may be derived from epithelial root sheath cells as a result of epithelial/mesenchymal transformation. Whatever their origin, these cells are responsible for producing a 'fibrous fringe' on the surface of the dentine. During the next phase of development in the formation of acellular cementum, the delayed mineralization front in the hyaline layer gradually spreads outwards (centripetally) until this layer is fully mineralized and then continues on into the first few microns of the 'fibrous fringe'. In this manner, the first few microns of primary cementum are firmly attached to the root dentine. At this stage, the collagen fibres in the adjacent periodontal ligament are oriented to be more parallel to the root surface and have not yet gained an attachment to the 'fibrous fringe'.

As with bone, the early stage of acellular cementum formation results in the secretion by the associated cementoblasts of various non-collagenous proteins (e.g. osteopontin, cementum-attachment protein, bone sialoprotein), cytokines and growth hormones. The precise roles of such molecules await clarification but it has been suggested that they may play a role in bonding the cementum to the outer surface of the root dentine. The subsequent development of acellular cementum involves:

- its slow increase in thickness
- the establishment of continuity between the principal collagen fibres of the periodontal ligament with those of the 'fibrous fringe' at the surface of the root dentine
- continued slow mineralization of the collagen.

It is only with the establishment of continuity between periodontal ligament fibres and those of the initial 'fibrous fringe' that the tooth can be properly supported within the socket. Once periodontal ligament fibres become attached to the surface of the cementum layer, the cementum may be classified as acellular extrinsic fibre cementum (see page 195). It increases slowly and evenly in thickness throughout life at a rate of about 2 μm per year. Although the cementoblasts may not form a distinctive and recognizable layer of cells that can be distinguished from adjacent cells

of the periodontal ligament, some cells lying between the perpendicularly oriented periodontal fibre bundles may become more cuboidal and contain small amounts of the intracellular organelles associated with protein synthesis and secretion. Such secretion is polarized at the surface of the cells adjacent to the cementum surface and, together with the slow rate of formation, ensures that the cells are not entombed by their own secretion.

Mineralization of the cementum matrix does not appear to be controlled by its cells and initiation of mineralization probably occurs from the dentine. Indeed, when mineralization of initial root dentine is interfered with, there is inhibition of cementogenesis. The adjacent periodontal ligament fibroblasts are rich in alkaline phosphatase and may also play a role in mineralization. Mineralization proceeds very slowly in a linear fashion. Owing to the slow progress of mineralization, there is usually no evidence of a layer of precementum associated with acellular cementum.

Cementogenesis occurs rhythmically, periods of activity alternating with periods of quiescence. Structural lines may be visible within the tissue, indicating the incremental nature of its formation. The periods of decreased activity are associated with these incremental lines, which are believed to have a higher content of ground substance and mineral and a lower content of collagen than the adjacent cementum. These lines may also reflect changes in crystallite orientation. The periodicity of the incremental lines might be annual and can be used to age individuals. As acellular cementum is formed very slowly, the incremental lines are closer together than corresponding lines seen in cellular cementum that is deposited more rapidly.

Secondary (cellular) cementum

Following the formation of primary cementum in the cervical portion of the root, secondary cementum appears in the apical region of the root at about the time the tooth erupts. Secondary cementum is also formed in the furcation area of the cheek teeth. This type of cementum is associated with an increase in the rate of formation of the tissue. The early inductive changes associated with the development of odontoblasts and dentine appear to be similar to those described for primary cementum. However, following the loss of continuity of the epithelial root sheath, large basophilic cells are seen to differentiate from the adjacent cells of the dental follicle against the surface of the root dentine. These cells form a more distinct cuboidal layer of cementoblasts adjacent to the root surface. They generally possess more cytoplasm and more cytoplasmic processes than the cells associated with the formation of acellular cementum. The basophilia at the light microscope level corresponds to roughened endoplasmic reticulum at the ultrastructural level and indicates that the cementoblasts secrete the collagen (together with ground substance) that forms the intrinsic fibres of the secondary, cellular cementum. These fibres are oriented parallel to the root surface and do not extend into the periodontal ligament. Associated with the increased rate of formation, a thin unmineralized precementum layer (about 5 μm thick) will be present on the surface of cellular cementum. Mineralization in the deeper layer of the precementum occurs in a linear manner but, overall, this type of cementum is less mineralized than primary cementum. As in bone, the multipolar mode of matrix secretion by the cementoblasts and its increased rate of formation result in cells becoming incorporated into the forming matrix, and these are converted into cementocytes. Thus, this is a cellular cementum and, since it usually presents as the intrinsic fibre type, this type of cementum does not act in a supportive role, there being no Sharpey fibres from the periodontal ligament inserted into it. Incremental lines will be present in secondary (cellular) cementum but, due to the increased rate of formation, are more widely spaced than in acellular cementum.

As the chemical composition of primary and secondary cementum differs, it is assumed that this reflects differences in the secretory activity of the cells involved. Thus, dentine sialoprotein, fibronectin and tenascin, as well as a number of proteoglycans (e.g. versican, decorin and biglycan), are present in cellular cementum but not in acellular cementum. This may be related to the presence of cementocytes, as many of the proteoglycans are located at the periphery of the lacunae and canaliculi. The precise origin of the cells in the dental follicle associated with the formation of cellular cementum awaits clarification. The possibility exists that different cell populations are responsible for the formation of primary (acellular) and secondary (cellular) cementum. Due to the similarity between osteoblasts and cementoblasts, it has been suggested that stem/progenitor cells primarily associated with alveolar bone could migrate into the periodontal ligament and provide a source of new cementoblasts.

The development of the periodontal ligament is described on page 210.

Tooth eruption

Introduction

Tooth eruption is the process whereby a tooth moves from its developmental position in the jaw into its functional position in the mouth. However, there is no evidence to suggest that eruption entirely ceases once a tooth meets its antagonist in the mouth. Prior to the formation of the root of the tooth, there is concentric growth of the tooth within its follicle without any active bodily movement in a direction indicating eruption towards the oral cavity. Once the root starts to form, the active phase of eruption commences.

As a tooth approaches the oral cavity, the overlying bone is resorbed and there are marked changes in the overlying soft tissues. The enamel surface is covered by the reduced enamel epithelium, which is a vestige of the enamel organ. As the tooth erupts, the outer cells of the reduced enamel epithelium proliferate into the connective tissue between the cusp tip and the oral epithelium. It has been suggested that these proliferating epithelial cells secrete enzymes that degrade collagen. Reduced enamel epithelial cells may also remove breakdown

products resulting from resorption of connective tissue. Depolymerization of the non-fibrous components of the extracellular matrix has been detected in the connective tissue overlying erupting teeth. Although a relationship between the degeneration of the connective tissue and the pressure exerted by the underlying erupting tooth has not been established, ischaemia is thought to be a contributory factor. Many of the fibroblasts in the connective tissue overlying an erupting tooth cease fibrillogenesis, actively take up extracellular material (as evidenced by intracellular collagen profiles) and synthesize acid hydrolases. Eventually, the cells degenerate.

The development of the dentogingival junction occurs as the tooth emerges into the oral cavity. As the tooth approaches the oral epithelium, the cells of the outer layer of the reduced enamel epithelium and the basal layer of the oral epithelium actively proliferate and eventually unite. The epithelium covering the tip of the tooth then degenerates at its centre, enabling the crown to emerge through an epithelial-lined pathway into the oral cavity. Further emergence of the tooth results from active eruptive movements and passive separation of the oral epithelium from the crown surface. When the tooth first erupts into the mouth, the reduced enamel epithelium is attached to the unerupted part of the crown, thus forming an epithelial seal — the junctional epithelium. It is generally believed that the reduced epithelial component of the junctional epithelium is eventually replaced by oral epithelium. With continued eruption, as more of the crown is exposed, a gingival crevice is formed.

Resorption and shedding of a deciduous tooth

Resorption and shedding of a deciduous tooth occurs to enable eruption of a permanent tooth (excluding the permanent molars). Initially, each deciduous tooth and its developing permanent successor share a common alveolar crypt, the permanent tooth germ being situated lingually to the developing deciduous tooth. With continued growth, the permanent tooth comes to lie near the root apex of the deciduous tooth within its own bony crypt. During the early eruptive stages of the permanent tooth, the bone separating it from its deciduous predecessor is resorbed. Following this, resorption of the hard tissues of the deciduous tooth takes place by the activity of multinucleated, osteoclast-like cells termed odontoclasts. The odontoclasts lie within resorption lacunae (Howship's lacunae). Odontoclasts, like osteoclasts, differentiate from circulating monocyte-like cells. They are vacuolated and have long cytoplasmic processes, forming a brush border with the tooth surface. The odontoclasts have an abundance of ribosomes and a large number of mitochondria. The Howship's lacunae in resorbing teeth tend to be larger and more spherical than lacunae in bone. The vascular, resorbing tissue is termed the resorbing organ of Tomes.

For a deciduous incisor or canine, root resorption initially occurs on the lingual surface adjacent to the developing permanent tooth. With subsequent movement and relocation of the teeth in the growing jaws, the developing permanent tooth comes to lie directly beneath the deciduous tooth and further resorption occurs from the apex. For a deciduous molar, root resorption often commences on the inner surfaces where the permanent premolars initially develop. The premolars later come to lie beneath the roots of the deciduous molar and further resorption occurs from the root apices. The shift in position of the deciduous tooth relative to the permanent successor may account for the intermittent nature of root resorption. The initiation of root resorption may be an inherent developmental process or it may be related to pressure from the permanent successor against the overlying bone or tooth. To assess which of these explanations is correct, permanent tooth germs have been surgically removed, when it was seen that resorption of the deciduous predecessors still occurred, although this was delayed. These findings are also consistent with the clinical observation that shedding of a deciduous tooth still occurs but is retarded where the successor is congenitally absent or occupies an abnormal position within the jaw. It has also been suggested that increased masticatory loads affect the pattern and rate of deciduous tooth resorption.

Resorption of deciduous teeth is not a continuous process. During rest periods, reparative tissue may be formed, leading to a reattachment of the periodontal ligament. The tissue of repair is cementum-like and the cells responsible for its formation are similar in appearance to cementoblasts. If the repair process prevails over resorption, the tooth may become ankylosed to the surrounding bone, with loss of the periodontal ligament. Ankylosis may also be caused by trauma or infection of a tooth. Where a deciduous tooth becomes ankylosed and cannot move, its position within the jaw remains constant so that, as the height of the alveolar bone increases, the tooth appears to sink gradually below the level of the adjacent teeth. Such ankylosed teeth are referred to as 'submerged' teeth. The submergence may continue to such an extent that the teeth become completely buried within bone.

Gubernacular canal

A specialized feature associated with the erupting permanent tooth is the presence of a gubernacular canal. This canal occurs where the roof of the alveolar crypt of the permanent tooth is not complete. The canal enables the dental follicle of the tooth germ to communicate with, and be attached to, the overlying oral mucosa. The gubernacular canal contains the gubernacular cord, composed of a central strand of epithelium (derived from the dental lamina) surrounded by connective tissue. The connective tissue is organized into inner and outer layers. Collagen fibres of the inner layer show greater organization and run mainly parallel to the long axis of the epithelium. In the outer layer, the collagen fibres are fewer and less organized. Differences between the layers can also be discerned with

respect to the vasculature, the vessels in the outer layer being larger. During eruption, the gubernacular cords decrease in length but increase in thickness and become less dense. Surgical removal of the cord does not prevent eruption of the permanent tooth.

Chronology for tooth development

Eruption rates of teeth are greatest at the time of crown emergence:

- Permanent maxillary central incisors are reported to erupt at about 1 mm/month.
- The rates for mandibular second premolars have been determined to be about 4.5 mm in 14 weeks.
- For permanent third molars, where space is available, eruption rates of 1 mm in 3 months have been recorded.

As teeth emerge into the oral cavity, there is initially a period of slow eruption when the crown is carried towards the oral mucosa. For permanent teeth, this period may last 2 to 4 years. A tooth erupts most rapidly as it enters the oral cavity, at which time the length of its root is about two-thirds complete. Eruption then slows as the tooth approaches the occlusal plane. Once the tooth has emerged into the oral cavity it may take 1 to 2 years to reach the occlusal plane. The emergence of the crown is partly due to axial movement of the tooth (active eruption) and partly due to retraction of the adjacent soft tissues (passive eruption).

Because no individuals are exactly alike, the chronology for tooth development shown in Tables 10.1 and 10.2 is approximate. Variations of 6 months either way are not unusual, but the tendency is for teeth to erupt late rather than early. Generally, the development of the permanent

Table 10.1 Chronology of the deciduous dentition and the order of eruption

Tooth	First evidence of calcification (months in utero)	Crown completed (months)	Eruption (months)	Root completed (years)
Maxillary				
A	3–4	4	7	1½–2
B	4½	5	8	1½–2
C	5	9	16–20	2½–3
D	5	6	12–16	2–2½
E	6–7	10–12	21–30	3
Mandibular				
A	4½	4	6½	1½–2
B	4½	4	7	1½–2
C	5	9	16–20	2½–3
D	5	6	12–16	2–2½
E	6	10–12	21–30	3

Unless otherwise indicated, all dates are postpartum. The teeth are identified according to the Palmer–Zsigmondy system.

Table 10.2 Chronology of the development of the permanent dentition and time of eruption

Tooth	First evidence of calcification	Crown completed (years)	Eruption (years)	Root completed (years)
Maxillary				
1	3–4 months	4–5	7–8	10
2	10–12 months	4–5	8–9	11
3	4–5 months	6–7	11–12	13–15
4	1½–1¾ years	5–6	10–11	12–13
5	2–2½ years	6–7	10–12	12–14
6	Birth	2½–3	6–7	9–10
7	2½–3 years	7–8	12–13	14–16
8	7–9 years	12–16	17–21	18–25
Mandibular				
1	3–4 months	4–5	6–7	9
2	3–4 months	4–5	7–8	10
3	4–5 months	6–7	9–10	12–14
4	1¾–2 years	5–6	10–12	12–13
5	1¼–2½ years	6–7	11–12	13–14
6	Birth	2½–3	6–7	9–10
7	2½–3 years	7–8	12–13	14–15
8	8–10 years	12–16	17–21	18–25

All dates are postpartum. The teeth are identified according to the Palmer–Zsigmondy system.

dentition is more advanced in girls; there does not appear to be any sex difference in the development of the deciduous dentition.

Eruptive mechanism

At present, little is known about the nature, source and magnitude of the eruptive forces. The theories advanced to explain the mechanism of tooth eruption can be divided into two main groups. One view suggests that the tooth is pushed out as a result of forces generated beneath and around it, by alveolar bone growth, root growth, blood pressure/tissue fluid pressure or cell proliferation. Alternatively, the tooth may be pulled out as a result of tension within the connective tissue of the periodontal ligament. Present experimental evidence shows that the eruptive mechanism:

- is a property of the periodontal ligament (or its precursor, the dental follicle)
- does not require a tractional force pulling the tooth towards the mouth
- is probably multifactorial, in that more than one agent has important contributions to the overall eruptive force
- could involve a combination of fibroblast activity (although the evidence to date remains poor) and vascular and/or tissue hydrostatic pressures.

Experiments involving root resection or root transection of the continuously growing incisors of rodents (or rabbits) indicate that the periodontal ligament is the probable source for the generation of the forces responsible for eruption. Root resection involves the surgical removal of the proliferative odontogenic tissues at the base of the continuously growing incisor; root transection involves cutting the incisor into proximal and distal portions. Both surgical procedures result in a situation where the tooth (or the distal segment following transection) remains merely as a fragment attached to the jaw by a periodontal ligament, but without the possibility of root growth and with degeneration of the pulp. Furthermore, there can be no contribution to eruption from bone growth as none occurs at the base (fundus) of the socket. The resected and transected incisors continue to erupt to the point where they are exfoliated from the socket. Although the periodontal ligament is implicated in the generation of the eruptive force, experiments show that, for teeth of limited growth, this property can be undertaken by its precursor, the dental follicle. When a developing unerupted premolar tooth is surgically removed and replaced with a metal replica, the replica will 'erupt', provided that the dental follicle is retained.

Investigation into the eruptive behaviour of the continuously growing, lathyritic incisor confirms that the eruptive force is unlikely to involve a tractional element that pulls the tooth towards the oral cavity. Lathyrogens are drugs that specifically inhibit the formation of collagen cross-links, thereby disrupting the fibre network in the periodontal ligament. Compared with controls, eruption rates of lathyritic rodent incisors are unaffected, provided that occlusal forces (which could traumatize the already weakened ligament) are reduced by regular trimming of the tooth to the gingival level. Further evidence against a tractional eruptive force comes from a study showing that teeth can erupt in the absence of well-developed periodontal fibres. Furthermore, experiments on teeth of limited growth show that, provided there is a dental follicle, teeth will erupt without roots and therefore without attachment of the follicle fibres into the tooth.

That eruption is multifactorial is indicated by the fact that there are at least two factors involved in the eruptive mechanism — a cortisone-sensitive factor and a cortisone-insensitive factor — and two major systems have been implicated in the generation of the eruptive force. One view holds that the force is produced by the activity of periodontal fibroblasts through their contractility and/or motility; the other that vascular and/or tissue hydrostatic pressures in and around the tooth are responsible for eruption.

Role of the periodontal ligament fibroblasts in eruption

A role for the periodontal ligament fibroblasts in eruption is based upon the notion that these cells can exert a tractional force onto the tooth through the collagen network or through cell-to-cell contacts. However, there is considerable evidence against the requirement for a tractional eruptive force acting through the periodontal collagen network. Furthermore, there is nothing to indicate that the fibroblasts can exert a force under physiological conditions sufficient to move a tooth in a direction favouring eruption. Neither has it been possible to devise procedures to affect selectively periodontal fibroblast activity in vivo to assess whether the experimental procedures have predictable effects on eruption. It has been shown that the drug colchicine, by its known disturbance of intracellular microtubules, reduces cell motility and this might explain the drug's significant retardatory effect on eruption. However, colchicine influences more than just cell migration (for example, it also affects connective tissue turnover). To date, the evidence relating to the fibroblast activity hypothesis relies almost entirely upon consideration of the morphology of the fibroblasts and upon the possible characteristics of the system, which would sustain the eruptive forces over long periods of time. When periodontal fibroblasts are cultured on plastic they assume the appearance and behaviour of migratory cells, but when cultured in a collagen gel they generate tension by their contractility and assume the appearance of myofibroblast-like cells (i.e. fibroblasts with some of the properties of smooth muscle cells). In vivo, however, periodontal fibroblasts show features of neither migratory cells nor myofibroblasts. Instead, they show all the characteristics of a cell actively synthesizing and secreting protein rather than those of a motile/contractile cell. Nevertheless, there is evidence of sustained migration of periodontal fibroblasts in vivo. Studies indicate that periodontal fibroblasts move occlusally at a rate equal to that of eruption. Furthermore, if the eruption rate is increased there is a concomitant increase in the rate of migration. Although providing some evidence of a shift in the position of periodontal fibroblasts, such work does not in itself indicate whether the cells are moving actively to generate the force of eruption or whether they are merely being transported passively within the ligament, the eruptive force being generated by another mechanism.

Role of the periodontal vasculature in the generation of eruptive forces

A role for the periodontal vasculature in the generation of eruptive forces can be derived either directly through blood pressure or indirectly by influencing periodontal tissue (hydrostatic) pressures. Whether acting directly or indirectly, the periodontal vascular hypotheses clearly do not require a tractional mode of activity within the periodontal tissues. That vascular pressures can alter the position of a tooth in its socket is shown by the fact that a tooth moves in synchrony with the arterial pulse. Furthermore, spontaneous changes in blood pressure have been shown to influence eruptive behaviour. In addition, experimental alterations to the periodontal vasculature following the administration of vasoactive drugs or interference with the sympathetic vasomotor nerve supply also result in predictable changes in eruption-like behaviour. To sustain eruptive movements according to the vascular hypotheses, it is necessary to postulate that periodontal tissue pressures are high, that there are pressure differentials along the periodontal ligament, and that changes in such pressures change eruptive behaviour. Indeed, there is evidence to support all three postulates. To assess whether the biochemical composition of the periodontal ligament is consistent with the production of an eruptive force by 'vascular' means, analysis of the periodontal ground substance at different stages of tooth development has shown that a proteoglycan, with possibly significant osmotic influences on the tissue, increases in quantity during the active phase of eruption. Finally, it has been shown that, for both the degree of vasculature and the numbers of fenestrations on the capillaries within the periodontal ligament, marked changes occur with different phases of eruption (e.g. the number of fenestrations is three times greater during eruption than after eruption). Thus, the sum of the evidence suggests that the periodontal vasculature could provide one factor in the multifactorial mechanism of eruption.

Ten

Self-assessment: questions

True/false statements

Which of the following statements are true and which are false?

a. The vestibular lamina lies lingual to the dental lamina.

b. The enamel organ is derived from ectomesenchyme (neural crest) cells.

c. Tooth germs at the early bell stage of development can be seen by the eighth week of intra-uterine life.

d. The stratum intermedium is a single layer of cells lying between the internal enamel epithelium and the stellate reticulum.

e. The stellate reticulum is rich in RNA.

f. Stellate reticulum cells show tonofilaments.

g. The enamel cord is a transient group of cells extending from the stratum intermedium into the stellate reticulum.

h. The enamel knot, an important signalling centre during tooth development, is found in the centre of the stellate reticulum of the tooth germ.

i. The cementum and the periodontal ligament originate from the dental follicle.

j. Continued differentiation of the tooth germ does not occur when an enamel organ and dental papilla are cultured on either side of a millipore filter with a pore size of 1 μm.

k. At the cap stage of development, combination in culture of an incisor enamel organ and a molar dental papilla gives rise to an incisor-shaped tooth when allowed to develop further.

l. Root development commences immediately after crown formation.

m. The epithelial root sheath comprises the internal and external enamel epithelia, separated by stratum intermedium but no stellate reticulum.

n. As with the crown, the internal enamel epithelial cells of the root sheath enlarge during their inductive stage.

o. Cells of the epithelial root sheath give rise to cementoblasts.

p. The pulp-limiting membrane is attached at its margins to alveolar bone.

q. In multirooted teeth, ingrowth of the epithelial shelves from the root sheath takes place along paths of high vascularity.

r. Principal fibres of the periodontal ligament are poorly organized at the time of eruption in succedaneous teeth.

s. As for dentine, calcospherites can be observed during the mineralization of cementum.

t. As in the formation of bone, a layer of unmineralized cementum matrix a few microns thick is seen during cementogenesis.

u. Coronal cementum can be deposited on enamel following degeneration of the reduced enamel epithelium.

v. When viewing an orthopantomogram of a child aged 9 years, the following permanent teeth would be expected to have erupted: all incisors and canines, and the first and second molars.

w. At birth, the 20 gum pads corresponding to the unerupted deciduous teeth are often brought into a functional occlusion.

x. At 5 years of age, the deciduous incisors show considerable wear and often occlude edge to edge.

y. Between the ages of 6 and 13 years, the human dentition is described as a 'mixed' dentition.

z. Spacing of the deciduous dentition is uncommon.

aa. The first permanent molars often erupt with a cusp-to-cusp relationship.

ab. Postpubertal loss of space anteriorly may result from forces exerted by the permanent third molar teeth.

ac. Prior to their emergence into the mouth, each deciduous tooth is overlain by a gubernacular canal.

ad. The cells responsible for the resorption and shedding of deciduous teeth are distinct in origin and form from osteoclasts responsible for bone resorption.

ae. As a tooth erupts through the oral mucosa, its reduced enamel epithelium becomes the initial junctional epithelium.

af. Following the loss of an antagonist tooth in the opposite jaw, a tooth often 'over-erupts'.

ag. The main phase of axial tooth eruption begins prior to root formation.

ah. Experiments involving root resection of the rodent incisor indicate that the eruptive force(s) is generated within the dental pulp.

ai. Hypotensive agents acting on the dental vasculature are associated with decreased eruption-like movements.

aj. In vitro studies suggest that the periodontal fibroblasts may have contractile or migratory properties which might explain tooth eruption.

Extended matching questions

Theme: Early tooth development

Lead-in

Select the most appropriate option to answer items 1–5. Each option can be used once, more than once or not at all.

Item list

1. The name given to the thickening of the presumptive oral epithelium that first marks the site of dental development

2. The name given to the tooth germ when dentine and enamel are first formed

3. The tissue of the enamel organ histochemically rich in alkaline phosphatase

4. The tissue that gives rise to ameloblasts

5. The tissue that controls both histogenesis and morphogenesis of the tooth germ

Self-assessment: questions

Option list

A. Bell stage
B. Bud stage
C. Cap stage
D. Cervical loop
E. Dental follicle
F. Dental lamina
G. Dental papilla
H. Enamel knot
I. Epithelial root sheath (of Hertwig)
J. External enamel epithelium
K. Internal enamel epithelium
L. Primary epithelial band
M. Stellate reticulum
N. Stratum intermedium

Theme: Chronology of tooth development

Lead-in

Select the most appropriate option to answer items 1–5. Each option can be used once, more than once or not at all.

Item list

1. Time of onset of calcification of deciduous maxillary first incisors
2. Time of completion of crowns of permanent mandibular first molars
3. Time of eruption of permanent maxillary first incisors
4. Time of eruption of permanent mandibular first premolars
5. Time of completion of roots of permanent maxillary second premolars

Option list

A. 4 months in utero
B. 6 months in utero
C. 8 months in utero
D. Birth
E. 2 years
F. 3 years
G. 6 years
H. 8 years
I. 9 years
J. 10 years
K. 11 years
L. 13 years
M. 16 years
N. 18 years

Picture questions

Figure 10.1

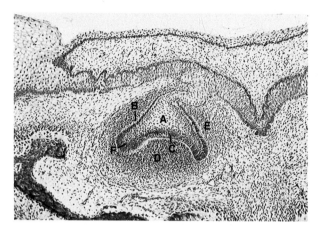

a. Which stage of tooth development is illustrated here and when is it first reached?
b. Identify the structures labelled A–E.
c. What biochemical substance characterizes A?
d. What is the name of region F?

Figure 10.2

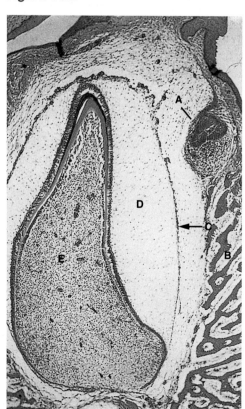

Self-assessment: questions

a. What stage of development is illustrated here?
b. Identify the structures labelled A–E. What is the possible function of D?
c. Is the lingual side situated to the right or left of this micrograph?

Figure 10.3 (Courtesy of Dr P. Smith)

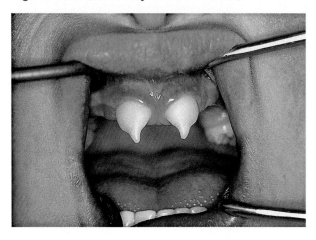

This illustration is of an 8-year-old child suffering from the disorder known as ectodermal dysplasia.
a. What do you deduce are the main dental signs of this disorder?

Figure 10.4 (Figure A courtesy of Professor J. D. Langdon, Figure B courtesy of Professor D. A. Luke)

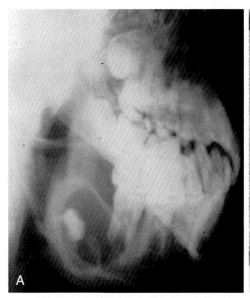
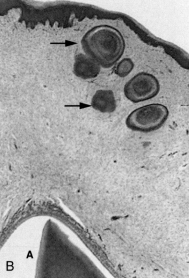

a. What is the connection between the pathological condition seen on the lateral radiograph in Figure 10.4A and the micrograph in Figure 10.4B?

Self-assessment: questions

Figure 10.5

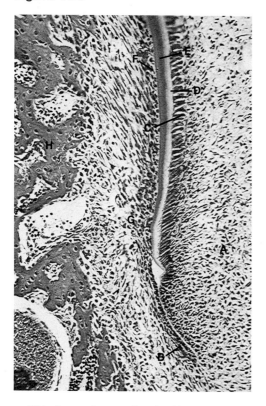

This figure shows a developing root.
a. Identify the structures labelled A–H.
b. To which adult structures does B give rise?

Figure 10.6 (Courtesy of Dr P. D. A Owens)

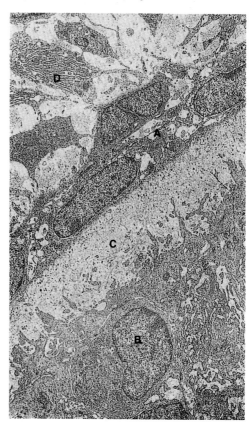

The picture is an electron micrograph of a developing root.
a. Identify the structures labelled A–D.
b. List three possible functions for B.
c. What is the fate of B?
d. What is the principal protein component of C?

Self-assessment: questions

Figure 10.7

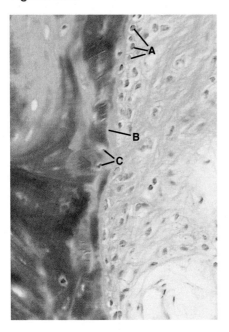

In this section of a developing root surface:
a. Identify the structures labelled A–C.
b. What is the origin of the cells labelled 'A'?

Figure 10.8 (Courtesy of Professor C. Franklyn)

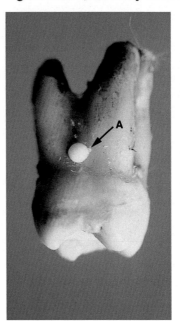

a. Identify structure A.
b. Account for its formation.

Self-assessment: questions

Figure 10.9 (Figure A courtesy of Dr M. E. Atkinson, Figure B courtesy of Dr J. Sauyave)

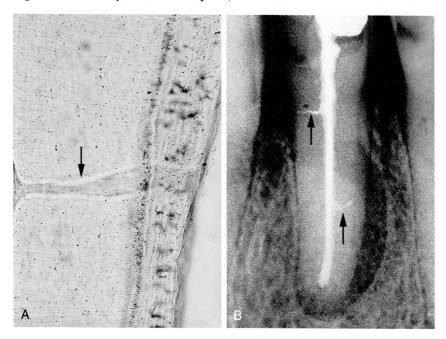

a. Identify the structure arrowed in the ground section (10.9A) and in the radiograph (10.9B).
b. How does it originate?
c. What is its clinical significance?

Figure 10.10

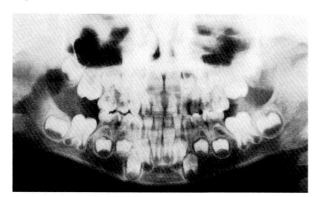

a. From this orthopantomogram, give the patient's dental age.

Figure 10.11

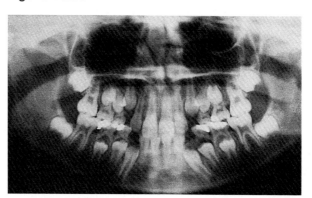

a. From this orthopantomogram, give the patient's dental age.

Self-assessment: questions

Figure 10.12 (Courtesy of Royal College of Surgeons of England)

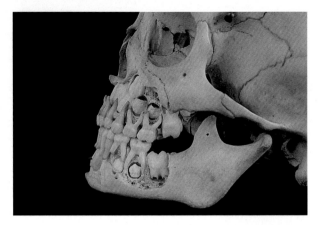

a. Age this skull, briefly giving reasons for your answer.

Figure 10.13

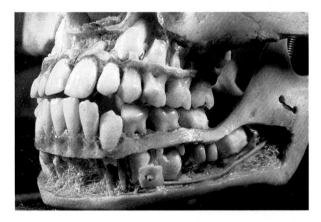

a. Age this skull, briefly giving reasons for your answer.

Figure 10.14 (Courtesy of Dr P. Smith)

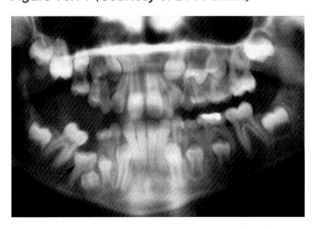

a. What abnormality is evident on this orthopantomogram?
b. How would you attempt to explain the cause of the abnormality?

Figure 10.15

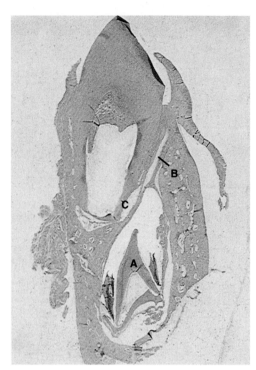

This light micrograph shows a deciduous tooth being replaced by a permanent tooth.
a. Identify the structures labelled A–C.
b. What is the pattern of resorption of a deciduous mandibular canine tooth? How would you distinguish the root of a tooth which has been resorbed from one which has been fractured, and also from a root which shows incomplete development?
c. What are the changes that take place in the soft tissues overlying the crown of an erupting deciduous tooth?
d. What is the evidence indicating that the force(s) of eruption is generated by pressure within the periodontal ligament and not by a tractional force through its collagen network?

Self-assessment: questions

Figure 10.16

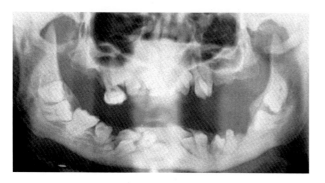

a. What unusual features are evident in this orthopan-tomogram of a 25-year-old patient?
b. What structures may present barriers to an erupting tooth and thereby delay its appearance in the mouth?
c. What are the various stages passed though to achieve a 'normal' (anatomical) occlusion of the permanent dentition from the deciduous dentition?

Essay questions

1. Describe the interactions between ectoderm and mesenchyme during tooth development, illustrating your answer with some of the experimental research conducted to investigate ectodermal–mesenchymal interactions.
2. Discuss the statement that 'tooth eruption is too complex to provide a simple explanation for a single tissue component (prime mover) responsible for the generation of eruptive forces'.

Self-assessment: answers

True/false answers

a. **False**. The vestibular lamina lies buccal to the dental lamina.

b. **False**. The dental papilla and dental follicle contain ectomesenchymal cells.

c. **False**. The early bell stage is reached at about the fourteenth week of development.

d. **False**. The stratum intermedium consists of a few layers of cells.

e. **False**. The stellate reticulum is rich in glycogen and glycosaminoglycans. It is the ameloblast cell layer that is rich in RNA. The stratum intermedium is rich in alkaline phosphatase.

f. **True**. The cells also have many cell contacts and possess a relatively well differentiated Golgi complex.

g. **True**. Where the enamel cord meets the external enamel epithelium, a small invagination termed the enamel navel may be seen.

h. **False**. The enamel knot is an important signalling centre during tooth development (e.g. for BMPs) but it is located in the centre of the internal enamel epithelium and not the stellate reticulum.

i. **True**. Some of the alveolar bone may also arise from the dental follicle.

j. **True**. Differentiation will occur only with a pore size greater than 2 μm.

k. **False**. The combination would result in a molar tooth.

l. **False**. Root development commences some time after crown formation is complete (perhaps a period of some months).

m. **False**. The epithelial root sheath comprises only the external and internal enamel epithelia.

n. **False**. The internal enamel epithelial cells do not increase in size during induction of root dentinogenesis.

o. **False**. Cementoblasts arise from cells of the investing layer of the dental follicle. However, there is some evidence that the first-formed cementoblasts might arise from the epithelial root sheath.

p. **False**. It merges with the fibres of the developing periodontal ligament.

q. **False**. Its growth occurs along paths of low vascularity.

r. **True**. This differs from the situation in deciduous teeth and is relevant to theories of tooth eruption which implicate collagen fibre involvement.

s. **False**. Mineralization is linear.

t. **True**. This layer of precementum is found in cellular (secondary) cementum but not in acellular cementum.

u. **True**. Coronal cementum is found particularly in the cheek teeth of herbivorous mammals and in some teeth of continuous growth.

v. **False**. Although all the permanent incisors, the permanent first molars and possibly the mandibular canines have erupted by the age of 9 years, the permanent maxillary canines and second molars would be unerupted.

w. **False**. The maxillary and mandibular gum pads rarely come into occlusion, the space between them being occupied by the tongue.

x. **True**. The edge-to-edge bite results from greater forward growth of the mandible compared with the maxilla.

y. **True**. A 'mixed' dentition describes the situation where there are both deciduous and permanent teeth in the mouth at the same time.

z. **False**. At the time when the permanent teeth are beginning to erupt (6 years), the deciduous teeth appear spaced because of growth of the jaws.

aa. **True**. The first molars take up their 'normal' adult relationship once the deciduous second molars are shed.

ab. **True**. However, mesial drift has been ascribed to other factors (e.g. contraction through the transseptal fibre system).

ac. **False**. The permanent teeth show gubernacular canals.

ad. **False**. The cementoclasts/dentinoclasts/odontoclasts are, like the osteoclasts, derived from circulating blood cells of the monocyte/macrophage lineage, and all have the same basic ultrastructural features.

ae. **True**. Although, with time, the junctional epithelium may be replaced by the oral epithelium and thereby loses its association with the reduced enamel epithelium.

af. **True**. It is thus possible that the forces responsible for the eruptive mechanism remain even when the tooth has reached its functional position.

ag. **False**. The main phase of eruption begins with the development of the root. However, both clinical and experimental studies indicate that rootless teeth can erupt and that a tractional force acting through the periodontal ligament (collagen fibres) is not responsible for eruption.

ah. **False**. Root resection experiments suggest that the eruptive force is generated within the periodontal ligament (but see (ag) above).

ai. **False**. The periodontal vasculature, consisting mainly of capillaries, shows increased vascular pressures with hypotensive agents and therefore there are associated increased eruption-like movements.

aj. **True**. However, the features of periodontal fibroblasts in culture are remarkably different from the fibroblasts in vivo.

Extended matching answers

Theme: Early tooth development

Item 1 = Option F (L). The primary epithelial band gives rise to a vestibular lamina (that clefts to differentiate the developing lip from the tooth-bearing region) and a dental lamina upon which tooth germs will eventually appear.

Self-assessment: answers

Item 2 = Option A. The late bell stage is also termed the 'appositional' stage and is characterized firstly by the synthesis and secretion of some dentine (beginning at the cuspal/incisal region), and subsequently by the synthesis and secretion of enamel.

Item 3 = Option N. The alkaline phosphatise-rich stratum intermedium (of the enamel organ) lies immediately above the internal enamel epithelial cells. Alkaline phosphatase is an important enzyme involved in the process of mineralization of biological tissues.

Item 4 = Option J. The internal enamel epithelial cells are responsible for forming the ameloblasts that synthesize and secrete enamel matrix.

Item 5 = Option G. Experiments involving recombination of enamel organs and dental papillae in various combinations show that, although oral epithelium is responsible for initiating tooth development, the dental papilla is responsible for controlling both histogenesis and morphogenesis. So, for example, a molar enamel organ combined with an incisor papilla will result in the development of an incisor tooth.

Theme: Chronology of tooth development

Item 1 = Option A. The crown of a deciduous maxillary first incisor commences calcification at about 3–4 months in utero.

Item 2 = Option F. The crown of the permanent mandibular first molar commences calcification at birth but is completed between 2.5 and 3 years.

Item 3 = Option H. The permanent maxillary first incisor erupts between 7 and 8 years.

Item 4 = Option K . The permanent mandibular first premolar erupts between 10 and 12 years.

Item 5 = Option L. Root completion occurs 2 to 3 years after eruption. The permanent maxillary second premolar erupts between 10 and 12 years and the root is completed between 12 and 14 years.

Picture answers

Figure 10.1

a. Late cap stage. This is reached by about 12 weeks of development.
b. A = stellate reticulum. B = external enamel epithelium. C = internal enamel epithelium. D = dental papilla. E = dental follicle (investing layer).
c. Glycosaminoglycans.
d. F = Cervical loop (a region of high mitotic activity).

Figure 10.2

a. Late bell (appositional) stage.
b. A = successional tooth germ. B = developing alveolus. C = external enamel epithelium. D = stellate reticulum. Its function is probably a mechanical one, protecting the underlying dental tissues against physical disturbance and thereby maintaining tooth shape. E = dental papilla.
c. The lingual side is to the right, the side on which the permanent tooth develops in relation to its deciduous predecessor.

Figure 10.3

a. Hereditary ectodermal dysplasia affects ectodermally derived structures. As is evident from the photographs, a variable number of teeth, both deciduous and permanent, fail to develop. Indeed, virtually all of the teeth may be absent. In addition, the teeth may have a conical or fang-shaped appearance. This especially applies to the maxillary incisors which may also be enlarged. Other epidermal appendages may be affected, and the patient may lack hair and sweat glands.

Figure 10.4

a. The structures arrowed in Figure 10.4B are known as epithelial pearls (of Serres), and represent remnants of the dental lamina. In Figure 10.4A, the mandibular third molar has failed to erupt. Note that the roots are fully formed. The cause of this condition is related to the presence of the overlying radiolucent area, which probably represents a dentigerous (eruption) cyst caused by proliferation and cyst formation from remnants of the dental lamina.

Figure 10.5

a. A = epithelial root sheath. B = predentine. C = odontoblast layer in root. D = dental papilla. E = dentine. F = developing cementum. G = developing periodontal ligament. H = developing alveolar bone.
b. Structure B, the epithelial root sheath, gives rise to the epithelial cell rests seen in the adult periodontal ligament. These structures, whose function is not understood, can give rise to cysts.

Figure 10.6

a. A = cell of epithelial root sheath. B = odontoblast. C = predentine. D = cell of dental follicle.
b. The epithelial root sheath helps map out the shape of the root, induces root dentine formation, and may secrete components into the first-formed cementum material.
c. Cells of the epithelial root sheath form the epithelial rests present in the periodontal ligament. Under certain conditions, these 'rests' may become cystic.
d. The predominant protein in predentine is type I collagen.

Self-assessment: answers

Figure 10.7

a. A = cementoblast layer. B = precementum. C = cementocytes being incorporated into matrix.
b. Cementoblasts arise from stem cells in the periodontal ligament. These cells may lie in the vicinity of blood vessels. It is not clear whether there is a common stem cell for cementoblasts, fibroblasts and osteoblasts in the periodontal ligament, or whether each cell line has its own separate stem cell.

Figure 10.8

a. Epithelial pearl. This comprises a localized mass of enamel, with a core of dentine, found on the root.
b. It is thought that, in the region affected, stellate reticulum and stratum intermedium develop between the internal and external epithelial of the root sheath. This provides the ability to form some enamel locally.

Figure 10.9

a. Lateral root canal in ground section and in root-filled tooth.
b. Although the aetiology is not known for certain, it is likely that the epithelial root sheath grows around an aberrant blood vessel, leaving a lateral channel which forms a lateral root canal.
c. As lateral root canals may occur in the inter-radicular regions, gingival recession may lead to their exposure in the oral cavity with the possibility of pain and pulpal inflammation resulting.

Figure 10.10

a. The dental age is 5 years.

Figure 10.11

a. The dental age is 9 years.

Figure 10.12

a. The deciduous dentition is fully erupted and the roots fully developed, giving a minimum age of 3 years. The crowns of the mandibular permanent premolars are well on the way to completion. The first permanent molars are unerupted but their roots are about one-third formed, giving a dental age of about 5–5½ years.

Figure 10.13

a. The permanent incisors and first permanent molars have erupted. Root development on the first molars is almost complete, giving a minimum age of 9 years.

The crown of the mandibular second permanent molar is complete and root development is just commencing. The mandibular permanent canine is just erupting. These factors suggest the dental age of the skull is about 9 years.

Figure 10.14

a. The mandibular right first permanent molar is buried within the jaw and the space it normally occupies within the dental arch has been reduced by tilting of the adjacent teeth. The maxillary right first permanent molar is similarly, but less, affected.
b. During their development, either before or soon after they had erupted into the mouth, the affected first molar teeth probably became ankylosed to the bone of the socket. They were then unable to erupt any further and, with subsequent growth of the jaws and alveolar processes, they gradually became submerged and incorporated into the bone of the jaws. They may then be referred to as 'submerged teeth'. The mandibular tooth probably became ankylosed earlier than the maxillary tooth, as the second molar has erupted more mesially. The reason for the original ankylosis is not understood. The tooth commonly affected is the second deciduous molar.

Figure 10.15

a. A = erupting permanent tooth. B = gubernacular canal. C = resorbing root of deciduous tooth.
b. The permanent mandibular canine tooth would initially develop below, and on the lingual aspect of, the deciduous mandibular canine. As the permanent tooth starts to erupt, it is associated with resorption of the deciduous canine on the lingual surface of its root. With subsequent movement and relocation of the teeth in the growing jaws, the permanent tooth comes to lie directly beneath the deciduous tooth and resorption occurs from the apex. An isolated tooth which shows evidence of resorption can be readily distinguished from roots showing fractures or incomplete development. For incomplete root development, the apical root canal is relatively large (open) and its margin has a smooth knife-edge. For a resorbing root, the surface is rough and irregular. For a fractured root, the surface is smooth and the pulp opening is usually narrow.
c. As the tooth erupts, the outer cells of the reduced enamel epithelium (the vestige of the enamel organ which forms a thin layer over the crown of the erupting tooth) proliferate into the connective tissue between the tooth and the oral epithelium. These proliferating epithelial cells may secrete enzymes which degrade the collagen. In addition,

Self-assessment: answers

the fibroblasts in the connective tissue overlying the erupting tooth cease fibrillogenesis and, as judged by the abundance of intracellular collagen profiles, they actively take up extracellular material. Eventually, the fibroblasts themselves degenerate (the nuclei becoming pyknotic). The reduced enamel epithelium cells may also aid eruption by removing the breakdown products resulting from the resorption of the overlying connective tissue. Experiments have shown that the dental follicle has some role to play in the production of an eruptive pathway in the tissues above the erupting tooth.

As the tooth approaches the oral epithelium, the cells of the outer layer of the reduced enamel epithelium and the basal cells of the oral epithelium unite. The epithelium covering the tip of the tooth then degenerates at its centre, enabling the crown to emerge through an epithelial-lined pathway into the oral cavity. Further emergence of the tooth results from active eruptive movements and passive separation of the oral epithelium from the crown surface. With continued eruption, the reduced enamel epithelium becomes the initial junctional epithelium, forming a seal between the oral environment above and the periodontal connective tissues below.

d. That the periodontal ligament and its precursor, the dental follicle, is the source of the force(s) of eruption is well documented. However, the force(s) does not need to be tractional, acting through the periodontal collagen by way of their attachments into the root of the tooth. There have been several clinical observations that rootless teeth erupt. Furthermore, production of rootless teeth by irradiation or surgery does not prevent eruption. Some permanent teeth also erupt into the mouth in the absence of a well-organized, fibrous network in the periodontal ligament, and experiments with lathyrogens (which disrupt the collagen by specifically affecting the formation of collagen cross-links) are also without effect on eruption (provided the tooth is maintained free of the bite to avoid the influence of trauma on the weakened periodontal ligament).

Figure 10.16

a. Although the teeth are present and the roots fully formed, the teeth have all failed to erupt (and are also malaligned). This is characteristic of a rare genetic abnormality known as cleidocranial dysostosis. The reason for the lack of eruption is not known, although the biochemistry of the connective tissue is affected in this disorder.

b. Delayed eruption of teeth may be caused by many factors, although most are local rather than systemic. Amongst the various structures/local conditions which could prevent eruption are: adjacent unerupted teeth, or teeth with unusual angulations; crowded dentitions; unresorbed deciduous teeth or retained tooth fragments; supernumerary teeth; malpositioning of the erupting tooth itself (including abnormal location for its initial development); presence of dental pathologies (e.g. eruption cysts); resistance provided by overlying soft tissues (which might involve failure to resorb the overlying tissues to produce an eruptive pathway); early loss of a deciduous tooth with drifting of adjacent teeth to block the eruptive pathway.

c. Between the ages of 6 and 13 years, the dentition is said to be 'mixed', comprising both deciduous and permanent teeth. The first molars are the first of the permanent teeth to erupt. Initially, they have a cusp-to-cusp relationship (the flush terminal plane), which is governed by the position of the deciduous second molars. The first permanent molars take up their 'normal' adult relationship once the deciduous second molars are shed. The permanent incisors erupt between the ages of 6 and 9 years. Since the permanent incisors are much larger than their deciduous predecessors, they are accommodated into the dental arches, not just by the utilization of the space left by the deciduous incisors, but also by lateral growth of the alveolar arches and the greater proclination of the permanent incisors. Frequently, when the permanent incisors erupt, they fan out (incline distally) so that there may be a significant diastema between the central incisors. This appearance has been termed the 'ugly duckling' stage, the diastema usually closing following eruption of the permanent canines. The canines and premolars, which usually erupt between the ages of 9 and 12 years, are readily accommodated into the dental arches, since the combined mesio-distal dimensions of the deciduous predecessors are usually greater than the permanent canines and premolars. Once all the deciduous teeth are shed, the occlusion appears similar to that in the adult and space for the permanent molar teeth is provided by continued growth of the mandible and maxilla.

Outline essay answers
Question 1

The introduction to the essay should describe in general terms the development of a tooth germ from an ectodermal (perhaps endodermal) enamel organ and a mesenchymal dental papilla. The description should cover the range of tooth germs from the bud to the bell stage. Brief mention should be made of the neural crest origin of the dental mesenchyme.

Information should be provided as to why the tooth germ has served as a 'model' for investigating ectodermal–mesenchymal interactions. Of particular importance is the

Self-assessment: answers

fact that the tooth germ is experimentally 'manipulable' since one can trypsinize the tooth germ to separate it into its ectodermal and mesenchymal components and subsequently recombine them in tissue culture.

Experiments to show the importance of ectoderm in the initiation of tooth development should be described. Other experiments should be mentioned that show how, subsequent to initiation, the dental papilla controls both morphogenesis and histogenesis in tooth development.

Experiments using micropore films placed between an enamel organ and a dental papilla should be described in order to highlight the nature of the inductive signals passing between the enamel organ and the dental papilla, and to show the importance of the basement membrane.

Finally, the role of growth factors and homeobox genes in ectodermal–mesenchymal interactions should be outlined. The temporal sequence and site in which these appear should be briefly described. Then, for example, one can describe the experiment where the transcription factor Barx-1, normally found in the mesenchyme of molars, was extended forwards to occupy the dental mesenchyme in the incisor region (that normally exhibits Msx-1 and 2). Subsequent tissue culture of this incisor region produced a molariform tooth.

Question 2

The introduction to the essay should define tooth eruption and indicate that the mechanism of tooth eruption that is responsible for generating eruptive forces not only is present during the main stage of emergence of the tooth into the mouth, but is also maintained after the tooth has reached its functional position (N.B. over-eruption). There should then follow a brief history of the theory for a 'prime mover' (a single biological component responsible for generating eruptive forces) and the variety of hypotheses that have been proposed. Briefly, evidence should be provided that the periodontal ligament/dental follicle is involved, although these tissues will not provide a tractional force through their fibrous networks.

The possible mechanisms in the periodontal ligament/follicle responsible for eruption should be elucidated and, in particular there should be a brief description of the possible roles of the periodontal fibroblasts and/or of periodontal vascular/tissue hydrostatic pressures.

Comment should be made on the fact that the mechanism of eruption is likely to be multifactorial and how there is experimental evidence for this; it is not just a 'cry of despair' because of the inability to agree upon a prime mover.

The final paragraph of the essay should indicate that eruption is also multifactorial in terms of the process of eruption. In addition to the requirement to generate eruptive forces, there is the production of an eruptive pathway to facilitate movement of the tooth towards the mouth. Furthermore, the tissues must remodel to sustain eruptive movements and, importantly, the amount (and rate) of eruption is dependent upon the forces of eruption exceeding forces resisting eruption.

Mechanisms of mineralization

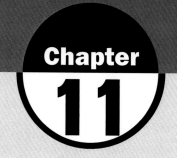

Matrix vesicle-mediated mineralization   **135**
Heterogenous nucleation   **136**
Mineralization of circumpulpal dentine   **136**
Initial mineralization of root dentine   **136**
Mineralization of bone   **136**
Mineralization of enamel   **137**
Mineralization of cementum   **137**
   Self-assessment: questions   **139**
   Self-assessment: answers   **140**

Overview

Mineralization of biological tissue is both strictly regulated and unique to each mineralized tissue. For each tissue, the mineral crystal in question is hydroxyapatite. The mechanisms of mineralization of bone and dentine share close similarities whereby an unmineralized matrix, osteoid or predentine, is calcified by a combination of matrix vesicle-mediated mineralization and heterogenous mineralization. Enamel is mineralized purely by heterogenous mineralization. However, for all three tissues, a number of tissue-specific proteins and proteoglycans tightly regulate mineralization by inhibiting mineralization processes or by guiding mineral deposition. Such proteins, and the cells that synthesize them, are therefore crucial in controlling the rate of mineralization, allowing ordered growth of the mineral crystals and preventing premature crystal fusion.

Learning objectives

You should:
- know the mechanisms relating to matrix vesicle-mediated mineralization and understand the concept of heterogenous nucleation (epitaxy) as related to mineralization of bone and dentine organic matrix
- understand the similarities with and differences from the mineralization of enamel
- understand the role of bone- and dentine-specific proteins in inhibiting or promoting mineralization.

When considering the basic concepts of mineralization of bone and dentine it becomes clear that mineralization is a controversial subject. Very close similarities exist in the mineralization of bone and dentine, whereas the mineralization of enamel is unique. To understand mineralization we have to answer several important questions:

- What initiates mineralization?
- Where does the mineral come from?
- What controls the rate of mineralization?
- Where are mineral crystals deposited?

Although the area is still subject to much debate, it is clear that the matrix-producing cells (the osteoblasts, odontoblasts and ameloblasts) are essential and key elements in initiating and regulating mineralization of the various hard tissues. They:

- produce the organic matrix that becomes mineralized
- control the transport of calcium ions into the matrix
- determine the presence and distribution of specific matrix components (proteoglycans and glycoproteins) that regulate the process.

The basic mechanisms for mineralization are matrix vesicle-mediated mineralization and heterogenous mineralization or epitaxy.

Matrix vesicle-mediated mineralization

Hydroxyapatite cannot be precipitated directly, as it is too complex and requires a high degree of saturation of calcium and phosphate. To obtain hydroxyapatite, we must first precipitate a less stable, simpler calcium phosphate called brushite and then transform this into hydroxyapatite. However, there is not enough calcium or phosphate in serum to precipitate brushite so that, to form hydroxyapatite mineral where none existed before, there is a need for a mechanism to raise calcium and phosphate concentrations within a localized environment. This first mineral in mantle dentine, early bone and calcified cartilage is provided by matrix vesicles. These vesicles provide a controlled micro-environment to concentrate calcium and phosphate, in the presence of a variety of enzymes (including alkaline phosphatase). Mineral crystals develop within the vesicles and eventually burst out and become associated with the organic collagenous matrix of predentine or osteoid. These vesicles 'bud off' from the odontoblast process membrane in dentine formation, forming membrane-bound organelles of approximately 30–200 nm in size. As matrix vesicles are the only crystalline structures present in the first-formed dentine (mantle dentine) and bone, they have been credited with having an initiating role in mineralization.

Mineral crystal formation involves two stages:

- Firstly, nucleation or the formation of small embryo crystals
- Secondly, crystal growth, which is characterized by the deposition of calcium and phosphate onto the crystal surface.

Heterogenous nucleation

In heterogenous nucleation, crystal growth is induced by the provision of a second, solid phase on which a crystal lattice may be formed. Crystal growth is better promoted on crystalline material having similar lattice spacings, a concept known as epitaxy. In the context of mineralizing tissues, the prime candidate is the organic matrix. This method requires the 'seeding' of small quantities of hydroxyapatite crystals into the matrix and allowing it to grow at the expense of the calcium and phosphate surrounding it.

Mineralization of circumpulpal dentine

Investigations into the mineralization of circumpulpal dentine have suggested that odontoblasts actively transport calcium ions to the mineralization site via active transport through the cell. This intracellular route actively controls the level of calcium in the mineralizing area and maintains calcium concentrations that are not in equilibrium with other body fluids. Deposition of calcium occurs on to a template formed by type I collagen, and mineral crystal deposition occurs at the gap zone within the collagen fibrils. A pool of chondroitin sulphate (CS), decorin and biglycan is secreted at the mineralization front and is transported intracellularly along the odontoblast process. Although general levels of proteoglycans at the mineralization site and in mineralized dentine are lower than those found in predentine, the CS-rich proteoglycans are distributed in mineralized connective tissues interfibrally and associated with the gap zones of the collagen fibrils. It is this CS proteoglycan pool that is associated with guiding mineral deposition, as the CS may be involved in transport of calcium and phosphate to gap zones in the collagen.

Another important glycoprotein in directing mineralization is dentine phosphoprotein (DPP). This dentine-specific protein is secreted at the mineralizing front and is highly phosphorylated and highly acidic, thus having a high affinity for calcium and hydroxyapatite surfaces. Changes in the conformation of the protein allow it to bind increasing numbers of calcium ions. In high concentrations, it inhibits crystal formation and so, by controlling the release and level of DPP, the odontoblast controls the initiation of mineralization and rate of deposition.

Several other proteins have been shown *in vitro* to be associated with mineralization. The classical bone-associated glycoproteins are also found within the dentine.

Osteopontin is a phosphorylated protein capable of promoting mineralization, and osteonectin has been shown to inhibit growth of hydroxyapatite crystals whilst promoting the binding of calcium and phosphate to collagen.

Other factors may also play a role in limiting or controlling mineralization. Collagen is found in many other soft connective tissues that are not mineralized. Although specific glycoproteins and proteoglycans have been shown to have differing roles in promoting and inhibiting mineralization and crystal growth (including the presence of dermatan sulphate proteoglycans in predentine), other factors are also important in regulating mineralization. Pyrophosphate is found in soft tissues and body fluids and actively inhibits mineralization. In hard tissues, pyrophosphatase can be identified and degrades any pyrophosphate present, allowing mineralization to occur.

Why two mechanisms?

Matrix vesicles are required for the mineralization of mantle dentine, not only as there is the need to produce mineral where none existed before, but also because the matrix formed is secreted from newly differentiating odontoblasts, with some contribution from the adjacent dental papilla cells. Not all the matrix components are present and some nucleation sites are not expressed. There is also the need to form mineral that can be seeded onto the matrix. After mantle dentine has been synthesized and secreted, and odontoblast differentiation is complete, the odontoblasts express the matrix components required for nucleation sites and the initial hydroxyapatite crystal seeds grow at the expense of calcium and phosphate that pass into the matrix through the cell.

Initial mineralization of root dentine

It is worth noting two features where there are differences between the mineralization of coronal dentine and that of root dentine. These concern the first-formed root dentine, which is called the hyaline layer:

- The first concerns the secretion into this layer from the adjacent epithelial root sheath cells of the enamel-related protein ameloblastin. Whether this protein is associated with differentiation of cells or with mineralization awaits clarification.
- The second feature is that mineralization does not commence in the outermost surface of the hyaline layer but a few microns inside. The subsequent extension of mineralization outwards is thought to allow for better bonding of the cementum and dentine (see page 137).

Mineralization of bone

Mineralization of bone has strong similarities with that of dentine in that the initial process is governed by matrix vesicle-mediated mineralization, with matrix vesicles budding off from the plasma membrane of the osteoblast, followed by heterogenous nucleation. Calcium and phosphate ions required for mineralization are derived from the plasma. As with the mineralization of predentine, mineralization of osteoid requires remodelling of the original tissue matrix to remove inhibitory proteoglycans. Osteoid contains a collagenous matrix rich in dermatan sulphate, proteoglycans (DS-decorin and DS-biglycan) and versican. These proteoglycans inhibit mineralization. However, as the osteoid is remodelled, these proteoglycans are enzymatically degraded (probably through the action of certain matrix metalloproteinase (MMP) species). At the mineralization site, fresh pools of CS proteoglycans are synthesized, secreted and distributed in the bone matrix interfibrally, where they are associated with the gap zones of the type I collagen fibres. As with dentine mineralization, it is this CS proteoglycan pool that is associated with guiding mineral deposition, as the CS may be involved in transport of calcium and phosphate to the gap zones in the collagen. Mineral crystals themselves become associated with the gap zone of the collagen. The presence of other tissue-specific proteins such as osteopontin, osteocalcin and bone sialoprotein further influences the mineralization in a similar manner to that seen in dentine mineralization. In the case of bone, it is these proteins that are important in regulating mineralization.

Mineralization of enamel

The mechanism of mineralization of enamel differs from that seen in the mesenchymally derived hard tissues bone and dentine. No matrix vesicles are present, so the sole mechanism is heterogenous nucleation/epitaxy and the seeding of a mineral crystal on the organic matrix. The organic matrix in enamel is unique in that it contains no collagen. However, the presence of enamel-specific proteins, amelogenins and non-amelogenins (e.g. enamelins) has an important role in nucleation and regulation of mineralization:

- Non-amelogenins act as seeds/epitactic sites for initial crystal deposition.
- Amelogenins provide regulation by inhibiting crystal growth. During enamel maturation, amelogenins are broken down, allowing crystal growth and hard tissue formation.

Amelogenins

Calcium reaches the matrix through the enamel organ by active transport systems, using carrier proteins in cell membranes. Calcium may also flow through concentration gradients from blood plasma to the developing enamel matrix, about 90% of which is formed by amelogenins, the remaining 10% being non-amelogenin protein. The first-formed enamel contains random crystal sizes and morphology, and these initial crystals grow by fusion of nucleation sites. However, once prismatic enamel starts to form, growth or maturation of the hydroxyapatite

crystallites occurs by increasing the length of the crystals, not the width, and this is controlled by the amelogenin. The amelogenin self-assembles into spherical structures, 15–20 nm in diameter. These spherical structures are known as amelogenin nanospheres. These nanospheres can interact with other components and may form an organizing structure. For example, they bind tightly to enamel crystals through the C terminal part of the molecule, which is cleaved off soon after secretion. This is the key to understanding how the amelogenin nanospheres regulate hydroxyapatite crystal growth.

The amelogenin nanospheres control growth by acting as spacers between the crystals, providing space for new crystal deposition and inhibiting uncontrolled mineralization. They achieve this by promoting growth in the C axis (length of the crystal) and prevent premature crystal–crystal fusion. It is this mechanism that explains the unusually long initial enamel crystal appearance. Biomineralization continues as proteinase activity, through the action of enamelysin and enamel matrix serine proteinase 1 (EMSP1), degrading the amelogenin that inhibits mineral deposition. In the maturation phase of amelogenesis, the matrix proteins have a reduced role to play, as most organic material has been degraded and lost, and the matrix proteins are removed long before crystal growth ends.

Non-amelogenin proteins

Concerning the non-amelogenin proteins, enamelin is thought to act as a nucleation site, as it has been suggested that it may interact with the crystallites. However, evidence for this is limited. The role in mineralization of the other non-amelogenin proteins, tuftelin and ameloblastin, is still open for debate, although ameloblastin may be involved due to its localization to the prism boundary region.

Mineralization of cementum

Mineralization of cementum follows similar processes to that seen in dentine and bone, which is not unsurprising considering that the biochemical composition of both tissues is closely related. However, the initiation of mineralization differs, as matrix vesicles have not been described in the first-formed cementum. Whether underlying dentine crystallites form the seeding mechanism or whether this is entirely regulated by the organic matrix of cementum awaits clarification.

Acellular extrinsic fibre cementum

In the case of acellular extrinsic fibre cementum (AEFC) during root development, the fibroblast-like cells (periodontal fibroblasts?) at the surface of the unmineralized dentine surface secrete collagen into the dentine matrix so that the dentine fibres intermingle with those from the cementum. Mineralization of the dentine starts internally and eventually spreads across into the cementum, presumably regulated by non-collagenous proteins (see page 136). Initial AEFC consists of a mineralized layer with a short fringe of collagen fibres structured perpendicular to the root surface. The fibroblast-like cells at the surface migrate away from the tissue while still secreting collagen so there develop alternating bands of more and less mineral content arranged in parallel to the root surface. AEFC lacks a recognizable layer of precementum (cementoid) and mineralization proceeds very slowly.

Cellular intrinsic fibre cementum

Cellular intrinsic fibre cementum (CIFC) is deposited on the dentine surface towards the root apex of cheek teeth.

Unlike AEFC, the cementoblasts of CIFC form a more recognizable cuboidal layer and deposit collagen fibres, which intermingle with those from the dentine. The cementoblasts also secrete non-collagenous proteins which are deposited between the collagen fibres, regulating mineral deposition. A layer of unmineralized matrix, termed cementoid, can be seen to be present at the surface of the mineralized cementum, as the formation rate is faster than that occurring in AEFC and, as with dentine, there is a mineralization front between the two tissues. Although this cementoid is now generally perceived to exist, it is less regular and apparent than predentine or osteoid.

Self-assessment: questions

True/false statements

Which of the following statements are true and which are false?

a. The first deposits of mineral in the mantle dentine are seen within matrix vesicles.

b. A globular pattern of mineralization is seen at the mineralization front of dentine.

c. After mantle dentine formation, mineralization occurs in association with the dentine extracellular matrix.

d. Hydroxyapatite crystal growth is controlled by enamelins.

e. Chondroitin sulphate-rich proteoglycans inhibit mineralization.

f. Amelogenin nanospheres control crystal growth by promoting growth in the width of the crystal.

g. Enamelins act as epitactic sites for initial crystal deposition.

h. Enamelysin is involved in the maturation of the enamel matrix.

i. The initiation of mineralization of cementum and dentine is similar.

j. The first-formed layer in coronal and radicular dentine shows identical patterns of mineralization.

k. Like dentine, the surface of cementum possesses a distinct unmineralized layer of precementum (cementoid).

Extended matching questions

Theme: Mechanisms of mineralization

Lead-in

Select the most appropriate option to answer items 1–6. Each option can be used once, more than once or not at all.

Item list

1. Osteoid contains a collagenous matrix rich in
2. Promotion of crystal growth on a crystalline material having similar lattice spacings
3. Bind tightly to hydroxyapatite crystals through the C terminal part of the molecule which is cleaved off soon after secretion
4. Is secreted at mineralizing front and is highly phosphorylated and highly acidic, with a high affinity for calcium and hydroxyapatite surfaces
5. Pre-dentine contains a collagenous matrix rich in
6. Helps remove the inhibition of mineral deposition in the maturation phase of amelogenesis

Option list

A. Heterogenous nucleation
B. Osteoid
C. Matrix vesicle
D. Dermatan sulphate proteoglycans
E. Chondroitin sulphate proteoglycans
F. Enamel matrix serine proteinase 1 (EMSP-1)
G. Tuftelin
H. Dentine phosphoprotein
I. Pyrophosphatase
J. Amelogenin
K. Enamelin
L. Epitaxy

Essay questions

1. Discuss the mechanisms involved in dentine mineralization, including the formation of mantle dentine and how the process may be regulated.

Self-assessment: answers

True/false answers

a. **True**. Matrix vesicles bud off from the odontoblast process and mediate the mineralization process for mantle dentine.

b. **True**. Calcospherites fuse together to give rise to a globular pattern of mineralization.

c. **True**. Hydroxyapatite crystals are 'seeded' onto the collagen matrix as mineralization proceeds by heterogenous nucleation or epitaxy.

d. **False**. Crystal growth is controlled by the amelogenin nanospheres acting as spacers between the crystals, providing space for new crystal deposition, inhibiting crystal and inhibiting uncontrolled mineralization.

e. **False**. Chondroitin sulphate proteoglycans are secreted at the mineralization front and may guide and direct mineralization. Dermatan sulphate proteoglycans inhibit mineralization.

f. **False**. Amelogenin nanospheres promote growth in the C axis or length of the crystal, preventing premature crystal–crystal fusion.

g. **True**. Enamelin is thought to act as a nucleation site, as it has been suggested that it may interact with the crystallites, but this is still not fully understood.

h. **True**. Enamelysin or MMP-20 proteolytically degrades the organic matrix of enamel during the maturation phase of amelogenesis.

i. **False**. The initiation of the first-formed dentine, mantle dentine, is via matrix vesicles. However, matrix vesicles are not present during the mineralization of cementum.

j. **False**. Whereas mineralization of mantle dentine in the crown occurs at the surface and moves inwards (centripetally), that of the hyaline layer in the root commences a few microns deep to the surface layer and gradually spreads outwards (centrifugally) as well as inwards. The outward spread aids in bonding the cementum to the dentine.

k. **False**. While this statement is true for cellular cementum, it does not apply to acellular cementum which, due to its slow rate of formation, lacks a distinct layer of precementum.

Extended matching answers

Item 1 = Option D. Dermatan sulphate proteoglycans inhibit mineralization and osteoid is an unmineralized organic matrix. These proteoglycan species are removed when osteoid is remodelled for mineralization.

Item 2 = Option L. Epitaxy is the concept of the promotion of crystal growth on a material with similar lattice spacings. In the case of dentine and bone this is the collagen matrix.

Item 3 = Option J. Amelogenins bind tightly to enamel hydroxyapatite crystals through the C terminal part of the molecule, and this interaction is key to how the self-assembled amelogenin nanospheres regulate hydroxyapatite crystal growth.

Item 4 = Option H. Dentine phosphoprotein is secreted at the mineralization front of dentine. It is highly phosphorylated and is thus highly acidic. Changes in the conformation of the protein allow it to bind increasing numbers of calcium ions and it regulates mineralization during dentinogenesis.

Item 5 = Option D. Dermatan sulphate proteoglycans inhibit mineralization and predentine is an unmineralized organic matrix. These proteoglycan species are synthesized and secreted by the odontoblasts and removed by proteolytic enzymes when predentine is remodelled prior to mineralization.

Item 6 = Option F. EMSP-1 degrades the amelogenin that inhibits mineral deposition, and this occurs in the maturation phase of amelogenesis, when most of the matrix proteins are degraded and lost.

Outline essay answers

Question 1

Homogenous nucleation is the spontaneous precipitation of hydroxyapatite and occurs during the mineralization of mantle dentine. However, hydroxyapatite cannot precipitate within the organic matrix, as there is some difficulty in forming stable embryo crystal to allow for crystal growth, and other calcium phosphate salts form in preference to hydroxyapatite. Matrix vesicles, containing the crystalline material in a small micro-environment, bud off from the plasma membrane of the odontoblast process and these are responsible for the initial mineralization of dentine. These vesicles are rich in phosphatase activity (used to concentrate Ca and PO_4 and form hydroxyapatite) and are required, as hydroxyapatite cannot form by homogenous nucleation directly because there is insufficient Ca and PO_4 in the plasma.

Circumpulpal dentine is mineralized by heterogenous nucleation. Heterogenous nucleation is also known as epitaxy and is the ability of nucleating sites to attract Ca and PO_4 ions and induce aggregation of ions to form mineral. The mechanism needs substrate with a similar lattice structure to mineral and having similar lattice spacings. Collagen acts at the epitactic sites and deposition of crystals occurs in the gap zone of collagen type I. Subsequent seeding occurs on deposited hydroxyapatite crystals. Proteoglycans rich in dermatan sulphate side-chains, such as DS-decorin and DS-biglycan, inhibit the formation of mineral; as predentine is remodelled, these species are replaced by chondroitin sulphate-rich proteoglycans, which facilitate mineral deposition. Chondroitin sulphate proteoglycans are distributed in mineralized connective

Self-assessment: answers

tissues interfibrally; they are associated with the gap zones of the collagen fibres and appear to be involved in the transport of calcium and phosphate to this gap zone. Dentine phosphoprotein (DPP) also promotes mineralization and is a very acidic glycoprotein present only within dentine and not within predentine. It has a high affinity for calcium and hydroxyapatite surfaces and may induce hydroxyapatite nucleation and control crystal growth. The acidic nature of the glycoproteins present in dentine appears to be important in regulating hydroxyapatite crystal nucleation and growth. DPP in high concentrations can also inhibit crystal formation, so by controlling the release and levels of DPP in the tissue environment, the odontoblast regulates mineralization.

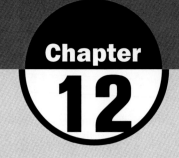

Dental tissues. I
Enamel: structure, composition and development

Chapter 12

Enamel structure	**142**
Physical properties	142
Composition	142
Enamel prisms	143
Incremental lines	143
Surface enamel	144
Enamel–dentine junction	144
Enamel formation	**144**
Presecretory stage	144
Secretory stage	145
Transition stage	145
Maturation stage	146
Post-maturation stage	147
Self-assessment: questions (Enamel structure)	148
Self-assessment: answers (Enamel structure)	151
Self-assessment: questions (Enamel formation)	155
Self-assessment: answers (Enamel formation)	157

Enamel structure

Overview

Enamel is the hardest of the mineralized tissues and covers the crown of the tooth. It differs significantly from other mineralized tissues in the nature of its organic content as a result of its epithelial origin. It is non-vital and non-sensitive, and cannot be repaired once lost. It has an underlying prismatic structure. Enamel may be lost through various processes such as dental caries, attrition, erosion and abrasion, and can be built up by numerous restorative procedures.

Learning objectives

You should:
• know the composition and structural features of enamel
• appreciate the nature of surface enamel and the changes that take place with age
• have a detailed knowledge of how structural features in enamel relate to clinical practice.

Physical properties

Enamel covers the crown of the tooth. It is thickest over cusps and incisal edges (about 2.5 mm) and thinnest at the cervical margin. Enamel is the hardest of biological tissues and is very resistant to wear. It has little tendency to deform, has a low tensile strength and is brittle. However, any tendency to fracture is avoided by the more flexible support of the underlying dentine. Surface enamel is harder, denser and less porous than subsurface enamel. Enamel is the least porous of the dental hard tissues, its porosity representing about 5% of the volume.

Composition

Concerning the composition of enamel, 96% by weight (and 88–90% by volume) is comprised of mineral in the form of crystallites of hydroxyapatite, $Ca_{10}(PO_4)_6(OH)_2$, but in a form that contains impurities. The remaining non-mineral component of enamel is comprised of about 3% water and 1% organic material.

Calcium hydroxyapatite

Calcium hydroxyapatite is present as large crystals approximately 70 nm in width and 25 nm thick, which may extend across the whole width of the tissue. They are regular hexagonal structures when viewed in cross-section and the core may be more soluble than the periphery. Solubility of enamel decreases as development proceeds. Each unit cell of the crystallite consists of a hydroxyl group surrounded by three calcium ions. These ions are surrounded by three phosphate ions. Six calcium ions in a hexagon enclose the phosphate ions.

Crystal formation is a slow process, usually involving several different intermediates, meaning that the structural arrangement and stoichiometry of ions in the initial formed solid is different to that in the final formed crystal. Numerous different forms of calcium phosphate mineral can be found in enamel. Octacalcium phosphate crystals are thought to be precursors of the final formed hydroxyapatite.

Ionic substitution

Ionic substitution regularly takes place within the enamel surface. The hydroxyapatite crystal is highly uniform, regular and organized; however, some substitutions and variations can occur. Other ions may replace the 'normal' ones. In this case, carbonate may substitute for a phosphate or hydroxyl (most occurs at the phosphate site) and has a destabilizing effect. This depends upon local pCO_2 concentration and occurs exclusively during development (2% at the surface and 5% towards the dentine–enamel junction); it is one reason for the much higher solubility product of enamel compared to pure hydroxyapatite. Magnesium may also replace calcium ions and this has a destabilizing effect on the hydroxyapatite crystal lattice, but is a very limited substitution.

Of clinical importance, fluoride may substitute for hydroxyl ions, making the lattice more stable and therefore increasing resistance to acidic dissolution. Fluoride levels are greater at the outer enamel surface but fall dramatically through the tissue towards the dentine; this is probably due to it being acquired during enamel maturation.

Water

Water accounts for about 3% by weight of enamel (approximately 5–10% by volume). Water is related to the porosity of tissue. Some lies between the crystals and surrounds the organic material; however, some may become trapped within crystal defects and the remainder can form a hydration layer coating the crystals.

Organic matrix

The organic matrix in mature enamel mainly comprises two unique groups of proteins. About 90% are grouped as non-amelogenins (such as enamel and tuftelin), with small traces or fragments of amelogenins. In developing enamel, these ratios are reversed. The organic matrix of enamel is considered in more detail on pages 146–147.

Enamel prisms

The basic structural unit of enamel is the enamel prism (rod), running from the enamel–dentine junction to the surface. In a cross-section of human enamel, the prisms may be seen to be keyhole-shaped and alternate, so that the tail of a prism lies between the heads of two prisms in the row below (i.e. pattern 3 enamel). The prisms are 5–6 μm in diameter. Adjacent prisms are delineated by the prism boundary, an optical feature produced by sudden changes in crystallite orientation at that site. No such sudden changes are present in the prism core.

Although in the outer third of enamel prisms run parallel to each other when viewed in a longitudinal section of the crown, in the inner two-thirds adjacent bands of enamel approximately 50 μm wide (and containing groups of about 10–20 prisms) show prisms running in different directions as they spiral outwards; some groups of prisms are cut more

transversely, others more longitudinally. When viewed in polarized or reflected light, this produces the optical phenomenon known as Hunter–Schreger bands. This complex pattern of prisms may limit crack propagation.

The surface layer of enamel in newly erupted permanent teeth is non-prismatic. Here, the enamel crystallites are all aligned at right angles to the surface and parallel to each other. Non-prismatic enamel occurs as a result of the absence of Tomes processes from the ameloblasts in the final stages of enamel deposition.

Incremental lines

During development, enamel is formed rhythmically, periods of activity alternating with periods of rest. This is associated with slight changes in the enamel resulting in the appearance of incremental lines. There are two main types of incremental line: short period (cross-striations) and long period (enamel striae).

Cross-striations

The cross-striations are diurnal, being formed every 24 hours. Cross-striations appear as lines that cross enamel prisms at right angles to their long axes, being approximately 4 μm apart.

Enamel striae

Enamel striae represent approximately weekly incremental lines and are seen in longitudinal sections of the crown as prominent lines that run obliquely across the enamel prisms to the surface. In horizontal sections they form concentric rings. They represent the successive positions of the enamel-forming front and for this reason do not reach the surface in the initial layers of enamel deposited over the tip of cusps or incisal margins. The periodic nature of this feature may be assessed by counting the number of cross-striations between successive enamel striae, the average being 7 days (range 6–10). Enamel striae in the middle portion of enamel are about 25–35 μm apart. In cervical enamel, where enamel is formed more slowly and cross-striations may be only about 2 μm apart, the striae are closer together.

Perikymata grooves and ridges

Over the whole of the lateral enamel, enamel striae reach the surface in a series of fine grooves running circumferentially around the crown. These grooves are known as the perikymata grooves and are separated by ridges, the perikymata ridges. In deciduous teeth, enamel striae and perikymata are only ever clearly seen in the cervical enamel of deciduous second molars.

Neonatal line

Enamel striae are less pronounced or absent from enamel formed before birth. A particularly marked stria is formed at birth – this is the neonatal line and reflects the metabolic changes at birth. Prisms appear to change both direction and thickness at the time of this event.

Surface enamel

The surface of enamel is, perhaps, its most clinically significant region as it is here that dental caries is initiated, restorations are attached and bleaches and fluoride remineralization preparations applied. Compared with subsurface enamel, surface enamel is harder, less porous, less soluble and more radio-opaque. It is richer in some trace elements (especially fluoride) but contains less carbonate. The enamel surface presents a variable appearance, exhibiting features such as aprismatic enamel, perikymata, prism-end markings, cracks, pits and elevations.

Enamel–dentine junction

The boundary between enamel and dentine is known as the enamel–dentine junction. It is scalloped and this feature is particularly evident beneath cusps and incisal edges. The convexities of the scallops project from the enamel into the dentine. Features seen at the enamel–dentine junction include enamel spindles, enamel tufts and enamel lamellae.

Enamel spindles

These are narrow, club-shaped structures extending up to 25 μm into the enamel; they may represent odontoblast processes that, during the early stages of enamel development, insinuate themselves between the ameloblasts. Enamel spindles are most commonly seen beneath cusps and, due to their alignment, are best viewed in longitudinal sections of enamel.

Enamel tufts

These are more extensive than enamel spindles and are seen in the inner third of the enamel. Resembling tufts of grass, they appear to travel in the same direction as the prisms. The prism boundaries in the tufts are hypomineralized and contain more enamel protein. They recur at approximately 100 μm intervals along the enamel–dentine junction and, owing to their alignment, are best visualized in transverse sections of enamel.

Enamel lamellae

These are thin, sheet-like faults that run through the entire thickness of the enamel. Like the enamel tufts, they are hypomineralized and best visualized in transverse sections of enamel. Enamel lamellae may arise:

- developmentally, in which case they would be filled with enamel proteins
- after eruption as cracks produced during loading of enamel, in which case they would be filled with saliva and oral debris.

Enamel formation

Overview

Being epithelial in origin, enamel formation differs in many respects from that associated with the other mineralized dental tissues. When initially formed, young enamel is only lightly mineralized (about 20–30%) and contains a high proportion of unique enamel proteins. However, it subsequently undergoes a process of maturation whereby its very high level of mineral content (96%) is attained and excess enamel proteins and water are removed. The more complicated pattern of development of enamel is reflected in the changing morphology of the ameloblast during development.

Learning objectives

You should:
- know the different stages that occur during enamel formation and be able to relate the changing structure of the ameloblast with its changing functions
- appreciate the composition of the organic matrix and how this changes during enamel formation
- understand how the structural features observed in the adult tissues are related to the development of the tissue
- be capable of comparing and contrasting enamel and dentine formation.

Enamel formation (amelogenesis) commences at the late bell stage of tooth formation, the earlier changes having been described in Chapter 10. During the early bell stage, the enamel organ comprises four distinct layers:

- External enamel epithelium
- Stellate reticulum
- Stratum intermedium
- Internal enamel epithelium.

Prior to the formation of dentine and enamel, the shape of the tooth has already been outlined following epithelial/mesenchymal interactions during tooth morphogenesis. The peripheral cells of the dental papilla adjacent to the internal enamel epithelium are undifferentiated, while the internal enamel epithelial cells have assumed a columnar appearance. The two groups of cells are separated by a basement membrane.

During the formation of enamel, the internal enamel epithelial cell undergoes a number of changes in its morphology, each being related to different functions. These can be considered for convenience in five stages: presecretory, secretory, transitional, maturation and post-maturation.

Presecretory stage

In the stage leading up to the secretion of the enamel matrix, the presecretory stage, initial signs of differentiation occur at the cusp-tip or incisal edge and gradually spread down the sides of the crown. The internal enamel epithelial cell becomes more columnar and there is a 'reversal of polarity', with the nucleus moving towards the stratum intermedium end of the cell. There is a build-up of intracellular organelles associated with protein synthesis (e.g. endoplasmic reticulum and Golgi material) at the opposite distal end of the cell adjacent to the dental papilla. The internal enamel epithelial cells at this more advanced stage can be termed 'pre-ameloblasts' and they induce the adjacent cells of the dental papilla to become odontoblasts, which then secrete the first-formed dentine of the crown (mantle dentine). Although no extracellular enamel matrix is present at this stage, small amounts of enamel proteins are synthesized and may be involved in epithelial/mesenchymal interactions.

With the initial formation of dentine, there is breakdown of the basement membrane separating the pre-ameloblasts from the adjacent dental papilla, probably resulting from the release of enzymes from the pre-ameloblast, which may also phagocytose the breakdown products.

Secretory stage

The secretory stage is characterized by the synthesis and secretion of the enamel matrix and its initial light mineralization. At the ultrastructural level, there is an increase in endoplasmic reticulum as well as vesicles containing material representing the organic matrix of enamel. The contents of the vesicles (secretory granules) are discharged into the extracellular space at the distal end of the cell against the surface of the first-formed dentine. Almost as soon as the enamel matrix is released extracellularly, the initial calcium hydroxyapatite crystallites appear within it as thin, needle-like crystallites. The cells can now be termed ameloblasts. As the ameloblasts migrate outwards (centrifugally), small processes from the odontoblasts may get caught up between them. When the early enamel starts to mineralize around them, these processes will become entrapped as enamel spindles.

Prismatic structure of enamel

The first few microns of enamel at the site of the enamel–dentine junction are aprismatic (prismless/non-prismatic), as the distal end of the ameloblast is flat and the initial crystallites do not show sudden changes in orientation. As the ameloblasts continue to move away from the dentine surface, a cone-shaped process (Tomes process) soon forms at the distal, secretory end of the ameloblasts. As the forming enamel crystallites align at right angles to the surface of the ameloblasts, it is the Tomes process that is responsible for producing sudden changes in crystallite orientation and the resulting prismatic structure of enamel. When this is considered in three dimensions, it can be seen that four ameloblasts contribute to each enamel prism and that each ameloblast contributes to four prisms. Numerous cell contacts are present between adjacent ameloblasts. At the ends of the ameloblast, these form the terminal bar apparatus. Additional cell contacts are present between ameloblasts and cells of the stratum intermedium. The boundary of the prism is formed ahead of the central prism core, giving the forming enamel surface a 'picket-fence' arrangement. Increments of enamel are deposited on each other and enamel formation extends from the cusp-tips down the sides of the tooth. Just before the enamel reaches its final thickness, the Tomes process disappears and the distal surface of the ameloblast becomes flattened, so that the final 20–100 μm at the surface is prismless. The composition of 'young' immature enamel at this stage comprises up to about 30% organic matrix and about 20–30% mineral in the form of thin crystallites of hydroxyapatite, the remaining 40–50% comprising water.

The complex paths traced out by the ameloblasts as they move outwards are responsible for generating the Hunter–Schreger bands, with groups of prisms in adjacent layers of enamel moving in different directions. However, towards the surface they move in similar directions so that Hunter–Schreger bands are not evident in the outer third of the crown.

The secretory phase ends once the full thickness of enamel matrix has been laid down.

Incremental markings

Periodic changes in the nature or orientation of the enamel crystallites or enamel matrix or enamel prisms produce short-period or long-period incremental markings. A diurnal rhythm produces a daily cross-striation across each prism approximately 4 μm apart, while approximately every 7 days (range 6–10), an enamel stria (of Retzius) is produced outlining the mineralizing front and running obliquely to the surface. These striae end on the surface of the enamel as perikymata, except for the first-formed striae overlying the cusps of the tooth. In teeth mineralizing before birth, an exaggerated stria, the neonatal line, is present representing the enamel formed during the general disturbance in metabolism occurring over the few days following birth.

Transition stage

The young enamel that is deposited initially is high in water and protein content, low in mineral content, and porous. The process that converts it to fully mineralized enamel is termed maturation. Enamel maturation is carried out by the same ameloblast cells that secreted the primary matrix, but in a very changed form. The period during which the ameloblasts change from a secretory to a maturation form is the transition stage. During this phase, enamel secretion stops and some of the matrix is removed. A reduction in height of the ameloblasts signals the onset of the transition. The number of ameloblasts is reduced by as much as 50% by apoptosis (programmed cell death). In those ameloblasts that remain, the organelles associated with protein synthesis (e.g. the rough endoplasmic reticulum and the Golgi apparatus) are reduced by autophagocytosis. The amount of stellate reticulum is reduced so that blood vessels invaginating the external enamel epithelium come to lie close to the proximal end (base) of the ameloblasts.

Maturation stage

Once the entire thickness of the enamel has formed, it is structurally complete and possesses the morphological features seen in mature enamel. Newly formed enamel consists of about 65% water, 20% organic material and 15% calcium hydroxyapatite crystallites by weight. The stage during which enamel changes from its lightly calcified and organic-rich state into its final highly mineralized and organic poor state is termed the maturation stage. In addition to a quantitative loss of organic matrix from 30% to 1%, there is also a qualitative change; young enamel protein is comprised of approximately 90% amelogenins and 10% non-amelogenins, whereas in adult enamel 90% of the protein is comprised of non-amelogenins and 10% of amelogenin proteins. During maturation, enamel crystallites increase in width and thickness at the expense of water and organic matrix. Calcium and phosphate ions move through the ameloblasts and into the maturing enamel, while water and degraded enamel proteins pass in the opposite direction. During this process, the average thickness of the crystallites increases from about 1.5 nm to about 25 nm. The degradation of the enamel matrix, probably by serine proteases released from the enamel organ, seems to precede mineral gain. Indeed, at the initial stage of maturation, the space caused by matrix loss is occupied by water, with the enamel becoming more porous.

To reflect the change in function from the secretory stage to the maturation stage, the ameloblasts undergo morphological changes. Having a reduced height and a great reduction in the amount of organelles associated with protein synthesis, the distal end of the cell shows numerous infoldings, forming a striated border. The ameloblast in this form is described as ruffle-ended. This morphology alternates with that of the smooth-ended ameloblast, in which the striated border is absent. Modulation between the two forms appears to occur between five and seven times during maturation. This modulation may indicate alternation between resorptive phases, during which water and organic components are removed, and secretory phases, when mineral ions are added to the maturing enamel. Maturation takes a considerable period of time and, like enamel formation, proceeds from the tips of the cusps down towards the cervical margins (and fissures).

Not all areas within enamel will achieve full mineralization. Near the enamel–dentine junction, hypomineralized regions with a prismatic appearance are found as enamel tufts. Other faults give rise to enamel lamellae.

Enamel matrix

At this point, it is necessary to consider the composition and functions of the developing enamel matrix in more detail.

Amelogenin

Approximately 20% of young, developing enamel is almost all proteinaceous. The majority of the developing enamel organic matrix are amelogenins, secreted by the ameloblasts.

This protein is rich in proline and glutamine, and is 178 amino acids in length with a hydrophobic core and protein–protein interaction domain. Within the enamel matrix, it self-assembles into spherical nanospheres that lie between the hydroxyapatite crystals, acting as spacers that allow the crystals to grow as enamel matures. It has a hydrophilic, mineral-binding domain, binding tightly to the enamel crystals through the C-terminal, which is cleaved shortly after secretion. This is the key to regulating crystal growth, as these nanospheres promote growth of the hydroxyapatite crystals, preventing premature crystal–crystal fusion. Amelogenin is degraded by proteolytic enzymes as enamel matures.

Non-amelogenins

The remaining proteins forming a small (10%) component of the organic matrix are grouped together as non-amelogenins. These include enamelin, tuftelin and ameloblastin:

- Enamelin is the largest enamel protein and is an acidic glycoprotein. This means that it has a high affinity for binding hydroxyapatite. It is rapidly processed after secretion and may interact with enamel crystals and be involved with nucleation, although evidence of this is limited.
- Tuft protein is highly anionic and can be found within the enamel tufts at the dentine–enamel junction.
- Ameloblastin is a tooth-specific protein expressed by cells of the inner enamel epithelium, in ameloblasts and transiently in odontoblasts during tooth development. Ameloblastin cleavage products lacking the C-terminus have been found to accumulate at the prism boundary throughout the enamel layer. Its localization suggests a possible role in regulating mineralization.

Proteinases

Proteinases are also expressed within the developing enamel matrix. Enamel matrix contains metalloproteinases during early enamel development and serine proteinases during the late stages of enamel formation. Their roles are involved with proteolytic processing of the enamel proteins and, as such, drive enamel maturation by degrading those proteins which inhibit mineral deposition. Such proteinases include enamelysin (MMP-20) and enamel matrix serine proteinase-1 (EMSP-1):

- Enamelysin is secreted primarily during the secretory and transition stages of enamel development. It is secreted from the secretory face of the Tomes process directly into the enamel matrix. The 45 kDa active MMP cleaves amelogenin at the majority of sites observed in vivo.
- EMSP-1 is a trypsin-like serine proteinase and is expressed in the pulp tissue as well as enamel. Activity of this enzyme is markedly increased during the transition stage of enamel development and remains at a

high level throughout maturation. Its optimal activity is at pH 5.7, which is the pH present within the enamel matrix during maturation.

Nucleation

Nucleation is the mechanism whereby a hydroxyapatite crystal is seeded onto the organic matrix, allowing it to grow at the expense of calcium and phosphate surrounding it. In enamel, the process of heterogeneous nucleation, also known as epitactic nucleation (epitaxis), occurs. This is defined as the growth of one crystalline substance on a different solid surface having similar lattice spacings, the organic matrix.

Biomineralization of enamel

Biomineralization of enamel takes place in a tissue-specific micro-environment. The size, morphology and stability of the formed crystals are determined by the degree of super-saturation of calcium and phosphate in the fluid phase, and are influenced by the presence of a large number of regulators (matrix proteins). Calcium reaches the matrix through the enamel organ by intercellular and transcellular pathways. Active transport systems, using carrier proteins in cell membranes, may be involved, and calcium may also flow through concentration gradients from blood plasma to enamel matrix. First-formed enamel is poorly organized, with random crystal sizes and morphology. Initial crystals grow by fusion of nucleation sites but, once a prismatic structure takes shape, growth is by increased length, not width, and controlled by amelogenin nanospheres.

Nanospheres control growth by acting as spacers between the crystals, providing space for new crystal deposition and inhibiting crystal fusion. There is good correlation between the size of the nanospheres and spacing of the enamel crystallites, suggesting that the width of the nanospheres controls the final thickness of the enamel crystals. In the maturation phase, the matrix proteins have a reduced role to play, as most organic material has been degraded and lost. Matrix proteins are removed long before crystal growth ends. Such degraded matrix proteins may accumulate in the extracellular space around the ameloblast cells where they may inhibit cell activity and so control or limit the thickness of enamel deposition.

Post-maturation stage

Once maturation of the enamel is complete, the ameloblasts undergo further changes in morphology associated with changes in function, which can be considered as the post-maturation stage. The cells become flattened and a thin, amorphous layer of protein, the primary enamel cuticle, separates the cells from the surface enamel. This cuticle can be considered as a basal lamina and the distal, flattened end of the ameloblast are linked to it by hemidesmosomes. Together with the shrunken remnants of the enamel organ, the ameloblast layer forms the reduced enamel epithelium. During eruption, this reduced enamel epithelium protects the enamel surface from the possible addition of a surface layer of cementum as it erupts through the adjacent connective tissue. The primary enamel cuticle, together with the remnants of the enamel organ (reduced enamel epithelium), form Nasmyth's membrane. Once the tooth has erupted into the oral cavity, the surface layer shows a further slight increase in mineralization through interaction with saliva.

On eruption, the reduced enamel epithelium undergoes yet another transformation as it is converted into the junctional epithelium (see page 144).

Twelve

Self-assessment: questions (Enamel structure)

True/false statements

Which of the following statements are true and which are false?

a. Enamel contains 4% by weight of organic matrix.
b. Hydroxyapatite crystals in enamel are flattened hexagonal rods with an average thickness of about 30 nm.
c. In pattern 3 enamel, the heads of the prisms point occlusally and the tails cervically.
d. The prismatic structure of enamel is not evident in carefully demineralized sections.
e. Enamel prisms run a straight course from the enamel–dentine junction to the surface enamel.
f. Fluorapatite dissolves more slowly in acid than hydroxyapatite.
g. Enamel matrix is evenly distributed throughout the tissue.
h. The diameters of enamel prisms are three times as large at the surface than at the enamel–dentine junction.
i. Enamel spindles are present in greatest numbers beneath the cusps or incisal margins.
j. Deciduous enamel appears whiter than permanent enamel due to its being more opaque.
k. Pattern 1 enamel is the most widely distributed type of human enamel.
l. Enamel over the cusps of permanent teeth can reach a maximum thickness of 1 mm.
m. Polarized light highlights prism boundaries because it can demonstrate changes in crystallite orientation.
n. Hunter–Schreger bands are prominent in the outer third of enamel.
o. Enamel matrix in adult enamel consists primarily of enamelins (non-amelogenins).
p. Enamel spindles project inwards between 10 and 40 μm from the enamel surface.
q. Throughout its life, the crown of a tooth is covered by an organic integument.

Extended matching questions

Theme: Enamel structure

Lead-in

Select the most appropriate option to answer items 1–6. Each option can be used once, more than once or not at all.

Item list

1. An incremental line reflecting a diurnal rhythm of enamel secretion during development
2. Grooves and ridges resulting from incremental lines reaching the surface of enamel
3. Long-period incremental lines
4. Thought to be extensions of dentinal tubule/odontoblast processes through the enamel–dentine junction
5. Very thin structural faults running through the entire thickness of the enamel
6. Regions where there are sudden changes in crystallite orientation

Option list

A. Cross-striations
B. Enamel broch
C. Enamel lamellae
D. Enamel pearl
E. Enamel spindles
F. Enamel striae
G. Enamel tufts
H. Gnarled enamel
I. Hunter–Schreger bands
J. Neonatal line
K. Perikymata
L. Prism boundaries

Theme: Enamel organic matrix

Select the most appropriate option to answer items 1–6. Each option can be used once, more than once or not at all.

Item list

1. Substitutes for hydroxyl ions in the hydroxyapatite crystal lattice
2. Process enamel proteins and enamel maturation
3. Self-assemble into specific structures acting as spacers between the developing enamel mineral crystals
4. Stabilizes the hydroxyapatite crystal lattice
5. Contributes 30–35% of early enamel matrix
6. Is the largest enamel protein

Option list

A. Epitaxis
B. Amelogenins
C. Enamelin
D. Collagen type I
E. Collagen type III
F. Hydroxyapatite
G. Ameloblastin
H. Enamelysin
I. Magnesium
J. Tuftelin
K. Fluoride
L. Organic matrix

Self-assessment: questions (Enamel structure)

Picture questions

Figure 12.1 (Courtesy of Dr D. F. G. Poole)

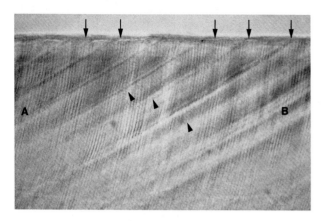

a. Identify the oblique lines indicated by arrow heads.
b. Is this a longitudinal or transverse section of enamel?
c. Which of the borders (A or B) is more cervical?
d. What is the approximate time gap between two adjacent oblique lines?
e. Are the oblique lines spaced regularly apart throughout enamel?
f. What structural features are represented by the arrows, and are such structures found all over the enamel surface?

Figure 12.2 (Courtesy of Dr R. Sprinz)

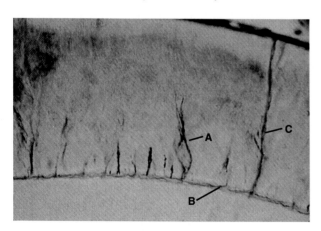

a. Identify the structures labelled A–C.
b. Has this ground section been cut longitudinally or transversely?
c. How could you determine whether C was a definite structure or an artefact?
d. Would structure A be retained following demineralization?

Figure 12.3 (Courtesy of Dr D. F. G. Poole)

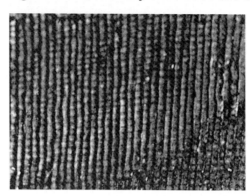

In this ground longitudinal section of enamel viewed in polarized light:
a. Identify the vertical lines, giving their distance apart.
b. What produces the appearance of these lines?
c. What is the thickness of these lines in the light microscope and in the transmission electron microscope?
d. Identify the horizontal lines.
e. Are the structures identified in part (e) visible with the transmission electron microscope and are they evenly spaced?

Figure 12.4 (Courtesy of Professor D. K. Whittaker)

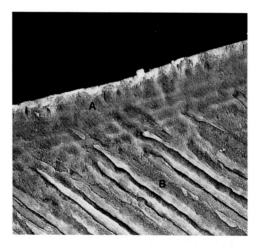

In this scanning electron micrograph of enamel:
a. Identify zone A.
b. Account for its appearance compared with the zone B.
c. With regard to zone A, are there any differences between deciduous and permanent teeth?
d. Are there any physicochemical differences between zones A and B?
e. Why is a knowledge of etching patterns in zone A important?

Self-assessment: questions (Enamel structure)

Figure 12.5 (Courtesy of Dr D. F. G. Poole)

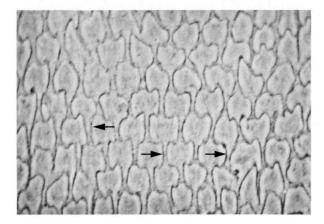

This is a ground section of enamel.
a. Are the basic structural units illustrated here cut transversely or longitudinally?
b. Classify this pattern of enamel.
c. What is the average diameter of the basic structural unit?
d. What is the main explanation given to account for the appearance of the boundaries (arrowed)?
e. Is the occlusal surface of the tooth directed towards the top of the micrograph or towards the bottom?

Figure 12.6 (Courtesy of Drs R. J. Hillier and G. T. Craig)

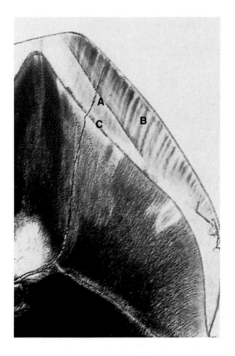

a. Identify structure A in this longitudinal ground section of a deciduous canine.
b. Which region of enamel is the oldest, that in zone B or that in zone C?
c. Do all teeth exhibit structure A?
d. Is the degree of occlusal wear present typical for such teeth?

Figure 12.7

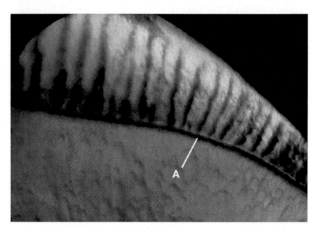

In this longitudinal ground section of a crown viewed in polarized light:
a. Name the principal feature seen in the upper half of this micrograph.
b. Account for the banded appearance.
c. Do the bands normally traverse the whole thickness of the tissue?
d. Identify the dark line A.

Essay questions
1. What structural features of enamel have clinical significance?
2. What are the main age changes that occur in enamel?
3. Describe the hydroxyapatite structure found within enamel and explain how ionic substitutions can strengthen the crystal lattice.
4. Compare and contrast the composition and structure of enamel and dentine.

Self-assessment: answers (Enamel structure)

True/false answers

a. **False**. Enamel contains about 1% by weight of organic matrix, with 3% water.

b. **True**. The width is about 70 nm and the length is indeterminate.

c. **True**. In a cross-section of pattern 3 enamel, the tail of a prism is seen to lie between the heads of two prisms in the row below.

d. **False**. The presence of prisms in carefully demineralized sections may indicate regional variations in the organic matrix.

e. **False**. The variation in prism direction is responsible for the Hunter–Schreger bands.

f. **True**. The lower solubility of fluorapatite is the reason for giving fluoride tablets to children.

g. **False**. Enamel matrix is heterogeneous, much being present as tuft protein at the enamel–dentine junction.

h. **False**. There is little variation in prism diameters throughout enamel.

i. **True**. Because of their orientation, they are most readily seen in longitudinal sections of enamel.

j. **True**. Therefore in deciduous enamel less of the underlying yellow dentine shows through the enamel.

k. **False**. Pattern 1 enamel displays circular prisms, and is most often located close to the enamel–dentine junction.

l. **False**. In permanent teeth, the average thickness of enamel is 2.5 mm.

m. **True**. Enamel shows both intrinsic and form birefringence.

n. **False**. They are present in the inner two-thirds of enamel where groups of prisms decussate.

o. **True**. In developing enamel, the enamel matrix consists mainly of amelogenins.

p. **False**. Enamel spindles project from the enamel–dentine junction.

q. **True**. Before eruption, it is covered by Nasmyth's membrane; after eruption, by the acquired pellicle.

Extended matching answers

Theme: Enamel structure

Item 1 = Option A. These cross-striations are about 4 μm apart and run across the long axis of prisms. They may represent areas where the enamel prisms narrow.

Item 2 = Option K. Counting the number of perikymata along the surface of a tooth will give an indication of how long the crown took to form. Perikymata may be lost following abrasion. Perikymata are rare on the surface of deciduous teeth.

Item 3 = Option F. The distance between adjacent enamel striae represents an interval of approximately 1 week and are roughly 30–40 μm apart. The striae formed over the cusp or incisal edge of a tooth do not reach the surface, but represent about 6 months' development of enamel.

Item 4 = Option E. Enamel spindles are most common over the cusp or incisal edge of a tooth and are best visualized in a longitudinal section of the crown.

Item 5 = Option C. Enamel lamellae developing during tooth development will be filled with remnants of enamel matrix. Those developing as cracks once a tooth has erupted will be filled with salivary deposits. They are best visualized in horizontal sections of the crown.

Item 6 = Option L. The sudden changes of crystallite orientation at prism boundaries are related to the presence of Tomes processes during amelogenesis. The sudden change in crystallite orientation is also evident in polarized light.

Theme: Enamel organic matrix

Item 1 = Option K. Fluoride is the most common ionic substitution in the hydroxyapatite crystal lattice and replaces the hydroxyl ions within it.

Item 2 = Option H. Enamelysin or MMP-20 is involved with proteolytic processing of the enamel proteins and as such drives enamel maturation by degrading those proteins which inhibit mineral deposition.

Item 3 = Option B. Amelogenins self-assemble into nanospheres which sit in association with the developing hydroxyapatite crystals, providing space for new crystal deposition, inhibiting crystal fusion and controlling final thickness of the enamel crystals.

Item 4 = Option K. The fluoride/OH exchange strengthens the lattice crystal and makes it more resistant to acid dissolution.

Item 5 = Option L. The early enamel matrix is up to 30% organic matrix, containing amelogenins, enamelins and other proteins. These are proteolytically degraded and removed as the enamel matures.

Item 6 = Option C. Although its exact role is still unclear, enamelin is the largest enamel protein and is an acidic glycoprotein. This means that it has a high affinity for binding hydroxyapatite.

Picture answers

Figure 12.1

a. A = Enamel striae (of Retzius).

b. Longitudinal section, due to the oblique orientation of the enamel striae (in a cross-section they would be arranged circularly).

c. A, as the enamel striae pass downwards and inwards from the enamel surface.

d. The enamel striae are thought to represent an approximately 7-day incremental feature.

Self-assessment: answers (Enamel structure)

e. No. They lie closer together near the enamel–dentine junction and at the enamel surface where the daily increments of enamel are smaller.

f. Perikymata occur where enamel striae reach the surface. However, enamel striae do not reach the surface over the cusps and incisal margins.

Figure 12.2

a. A = enamel tuft. B = enamel–dentine junction. C = enamel lamella.

b. Transversely, as enamel tufts and lamellae are mainly seen in this plane of section.

c. If C were an artefact (i.e. a crack), it would disappear if the section were demineralized. In a demineralized section, the true enamel lamella would show its organic nature.

d. Yes, as enamel tufts are hypomineralized areas of enamel.

Figure 12.3

a. The lines indicated are those of the prism boundaries. The distance between prism boundaries is 5 µm.

b. Prism boundaries are seen because of sudden changes in crystallite orientation.

c. At the light microscope level, prism boundaries are about 1 µm thick while, with the electron microscope, their thickness is barely measurable, being measured in terms of a few nanometres.

d. Cross-striations.

e. Cross-striations are not visible using the electron microscope. Their distance apart varies from about 2.5 µm (near the enamel–dentine junction and the surface enamel) to about 4 µm in the main body of enamel.

Figure 12.4

a. A = aprismatic surface zone of enamel.

b. Its lack of a prismatic structure as in the subsurface zone (B) relates to the absence of a Tomes process during its development.

c. The aprismatic zone in deciduous teeth is said to be wider.

d. Surface enamel is harder, less porous and less soluble than subsurface enamel. There are also chemical differences (e.g. surface enamel has more fluoride and less carbonate than subsurface enamel).

e. Knowledge of etching patterns may help us understand the process of dental caries and clinical procedures such as the application of bonding materials and fissure sealants.

Figure 12.5

a. The enamel prisms have been sectioned transversely.

b. The keyhole type of arrangement of the enamel prisms in staggered rows is pattern 3.

c. The average diameter of the enamel prism is of the order of about 5 µm.

d. Prism boundaries are seen as the result of an optical effect caused by sudden changes in crystallite orientation at these regions.

e. As the tails of prisms are directed cervically, the occlusal surface lies beyond the top of the micrograph.

Figure 12.6

a. A = neonatal line.

b. Zone C (below the neonatal line) represents the first-formed enamel and is therefore the oldest.

c. No. Apart from all the deciduous teeth, only the first permanent molars possess a neonatal line, indicating mineralization commencing before birth.

d. Yes, as deciduous enamel is softer than permanent enamel.

Figure 12.7

a. The banded appearance in the enamel is termed the Hunter–Schreger bands.

b. The appearance is the consequence of alternating groups of prisms being cut in different planes, some being sectioned more transversely and others more longitudinally. This reflects the different paths taken by adjacent groups of ameloblasts as they travel away from the amelodentinal junction towards the surface.

c. No. In the outer portion of enamel the enamel prisms all run in the same direction and are therefore sectioned in the same plane.

d. This represents mantle dentine.

Outline essay answers

Question 1

Surface enamel, being at the interface between the tooth and the environment, has considerable clinical significance. It is the site at which dental caries first attacks enamel. In a carious lesion, loss of mineral is seen in the subsurface tissues, the surface layer seemingly remaining unaffected. This is due to remineralization of ions at the surface as they pass out from subsurface regions. In the body of the lesion, the enamel striae are exaggerated. From an understanding of the development of a carious lesion, methods of remineralizing the early lesion can be developed.

Self-assessment: answers (Enamel structure)

Surface enamel is harder than subsurface enamel. It is not fully mineralized until 1 or 2 years after it erupts into the mouth, the final maturation being the result of interactions with saliva. If fluoride is incorporated into the diet (or drinking water) during development, fluorapatite crystals may form in preference to hydroxyapatite, and are more resistant to demineralization as a result of acid produced by plaque bacteria.

Different acids at different concentrations can produce a variety of patterns of partial prism dissolution to provide a roughened surface suitable for adherence of restorative materials (acid conditioning), including fissure sealants. This reduces or eliminates the need for mechanical retention cut into sound tissue. For agents mechanically binding to enamel, it is necessary to produce microporosities in the surface by acid-etch techniques. Thus, when bonding agents are applied to such a surface, microscopic tags can be seen invaginating into the roughened surface. Where a prismless layer of enamel is encountered, a more prolonged etching time needs to be applied to penetrate into the underlying prismatic layer. In early carious lesions, the decalcification of enamel produced by bacteria within plaque appears to proceed preferentially along the enamel striae, whilst leaving the surface relatively intact. Thus, knowledge of enamel structure and its reactions to acid has important clinical ramifications.

When cavities are prepared, a knowledge of the microanatomy of enamel, particularly in terms of prism orientation, is essential to conserve as much as possible of the original strength of the tissue. Cutting cavities into enamel with rotary instruments will inevitably lead to subsurface cracking. Fortunately, some adhesive materials are capable of reinforcing this weakened substrate.

Micropores in surface enamel may accumulate chromogenic material from the diet that may bind to the organic matrix. Such material may be degraded and removed by the application of tooth whitening agents such as hydrogen peroxide. Enamel pearls and projections on the root may predispose to plaque accumulation and gingivitis and should be removed.

Question 2

A small amount of post-eruptive maturation occurs in surface enamel following eruption of a tooth into the oral cavity as a result of interchange of ions with the saliva. With age, there is loss of enamel by three different mechanisms:

- Attrition loss involving tooth-to-tooth contact. This occurs both occlusally and interproximally. The potential space to be expected during interproximal wear is generally closed up by mesial drift. Thus, although initial tooth contact areas are small, these become broader with age.

- Abrasion loss involving friction between the tooth and external material. A common cause is toothbrush abrasion seen on the labial and buccal surfaces of teeth.
- Erosion loss involving contact with acidic agents. Erosion may be extrinsic (e.g. soft drinks) or intrinsic (gastric acids following chronic regurgitation). In cases of bulimia, the erosion characteristically affects the palatal surfaces of the upper anterior teeth.

This loss of enamel will also lead to the disappearance of perikymata on the surface in affected areas.

The natural colour of enamel may darken with age. This may be due to the loss of enamel, allowing the underlying dentine to show more prominently through the semitranslucent enamel. Also, organic coverings such as plaque may discolour the tooth and such material may fill any cracks that appear in the enamel. If the plaque mineralizes, supragingival calculus may become attached to the enamel.

There will be changes in the chemical composition of enamel, particularly as a result of ion interchange at the surface with saliva. The most important of these will be an increase in fluoride content with age.

Question 3

Hydroxyapatite is represented by the stoichiometric formula $Ca_{10}(PO_4)_6(OH)_2$. It consists of a regular hexagonal structure with a hydroxyl group surrounded by three calcium ions. These are surrounded by three phosphate ions. Six calcium ions in a hexagon enclose the phosphate ions.

Ionic substitutions can significantly strengthen the crystal lattice or destabilize it, depending on which ions are substituted. Fluoride substitutes for hydroxyl ions and has a stabilizing effect on the crystal lattice, strengthening it. Fluoride is concentrated at the enamel surface and falls dramatically towards the underlying dentine. Such ionic substitution is the principle behind fluoride in dentifrices, as the strengthened crystal lattice is less soluble and more resistant to caries.

Question 4

Composition

Both are composed of an inorganic component of hydroxyapatite crystals, an organic component and water. However, by weight enamel is 96% mineral, 3% water and 1% organic, whereas by weight dentine is 70% mineral, 20% organic and 10% water. Enamel is therefore harder and less resistant to wear than dentine.

Regarding the organic component, whereas the organic matrix of dentine is principally collagen, that of enamel is principally amelogenin and non-amelogenin proteins. The

Self-assessment: answers (Enamel structure)

collagen in dentine provides a more flexible support than the proteins in enamel, which is brittle.

Dentine contains a non-collagenous ground substance of many proteins (e.g. dentine phosphoprotein, osteopontin, dentine sialoprotein) not present in enamel. This reflects the different origin of the two tissues: enamel by oral epithelial cells, dentine by neural crest (ectomesenchyme) cells.

Regarding the mineral component, the hydroxyapatite crystals of enamel are larger than those of dentine.

Structure

Both enamel and dentine are composed of repeat units (prisms and tubules).

Both are deposited incrementally with both short-term lines (cross-striations in enamel and von Ebner lines in dentine) and long-term lines (striae in enamel, Andresen lines in dentine).

Both show heterogeneity in structure, enamel having prismatic and non-prismatic areas, and dentine having zones, such as mantle dentine, a granular layer, a hyaline layer.

Both possess hypomineralized areas. In enamel these are the enamel spindles, tufts and lamellae; in dentine these are interglobular areas.

The orientation of the prisms and tubules both show variability. In enamel, the changing direction of prisms gives rise to the Hunter–Schreger bands in the inner two-thirds. The variability of the tubules gives rise to the primary (and secondary) curvatures.

Unlike enamel, dentine is permeated by the dentinal tubules containing odontoblast processes and nerve fibres. This accounts for dentine being more permeable, sensitive and responsive.

As the enamel-forming cells are lost on eruption, enamel cannot react to stimuli or attrition, apart from simple physicochemical interchanges with ions in saliva. The dentine-forming cells (odontoblasts) are present at the periphery of the pulp throughout life so that dentine forms continuously, accounting for the presence of a predentine layer, physiological secondary dentine and tertiary dentine. Within dentine tubules, peritubular dentine is formed, narrowing the tubules and often completely obliterating them (translucent dentine). The peritubular dentine also has a different composition to intertubular dentine, being more mineralized, lacking collagen and having additional forms of calcium phosphates.

Dentine is capable of resorption by odontoclasts, as seen in the resorption of the roots of deciduous teeth and in examples of internal and external resorption of permanent teeth. Enamel does not resorb.

Self-assessment: questions (Enamel formation)

True/false statements

Which of the following statements are true and which are false?

a. Secretory ameloblasts are approximately 5 μm wide and 10 μm long.
b. During reversal of polarity within the ameloblast, the Golgi material migrates to the distal end of the cell.
c. In young immature enamel, the ratio of amelogenins to non-amelogenins is about 19:1.
d. The daily rate of enamel formation is greater at the enamel surface than in the central region.
e. As for dentine, the initiation of enamel mineralization occurs by means of matrix vesicles.
f. Ameloblasts are hexagonal in cross-section.
g. Aprismatic (prismless) enamel can be correlated with the size of the Tomes process.
h. Nasmyth's membrane comprises the reduced enamel epithelium and the primary enamel cuticle.
i. A thin, unmineralized layer, about 2 μm thick, exists at the formative enamel surface.
j. Compared with amelogenins, non-amelogenins have a lower molecular weight and are rich in proline.
k. The Hunter–Schreger bands are incremental lines reflecting the diurnal rhythm of enamel formation.

Extended matching questions

Theme: Enamel formation

Lead-in

Select the most appropriate option to answer items 1–6. Each option can be used once, more than once or not at all.

Item list

1. That part of the ameloblast responsible for prism formation
2. Reflects the daily incremental nature of enamel formation
3. Non-prismatic enamel
4. Associated with ameloblasts during their maturation phase
5. Enamel tufts
6. Approximate percentage of mineral in young enamel

Option list

A. Found at the surface of enamel
B. Hunter–Schreger bands
C. Perikymata
D. Cross-striations
E. Tomes process
F. Hyaline layer
G. Occupies full thickness of enamel
H. Striated border/microvilli
I. Hypomineralized enamel
J. 20%
K. 60–70%

Picture questions

Figure 12.8

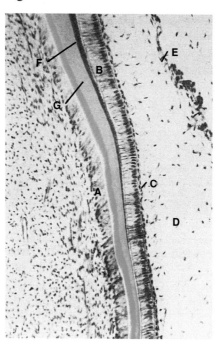

a. Identify the structures labelled A–G.
b. What are the principal organic components of F and G?
c. Has reversal of polarity occurred in the cells in layer B at the bottom of the micrograph?

Figure 12.9 (Courtesy of Professor A. Boyde)

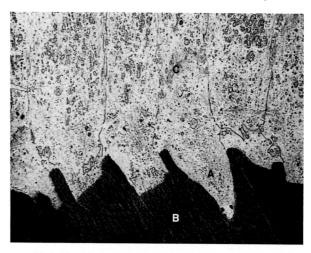

a. Identify the structures labelled A–C.
b. What structural feature 'separates' A and C?
c. What is the relationship of A to the basic structure of enamel?

Self-assessment: questions (Enamel formation)

Figure 12.10

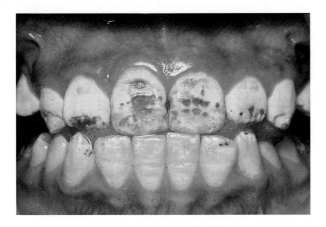

a. What may be responsible for the appearance of the enamel in this 14-year-old patient?

Essay questions

1. How do the structures seen in a longitudinal section of enamel reflect the development of the tissue?
2. How does the changing morphology of the ameloblast reflect the changing functions of the cell during its life cycle?
3. What are the principal constituents of the enamel organic matrix?

Self-assessment: answers (Enamel formation)

True/false answers

a. **False**. The cells are highly columnar and, depending on species, can be up to 50 μm long.

b. **True**. In addition, the nucleus migrates to the opposite (basal or proximal) and non-secretory end of the cell adjacent to the stratum intermedium.

c. **True**. The bulk of the amelogenins are removed during enamel maturation so this ratio is reversed in mature enamel.

d. **False**. The slower daily rate towards the end of enamel formation explains why the cross-striations are closer together at the enamel surface.

e. **False**. Matrix vesicles are not present in enamel, and mineralization probably extends from the adjacent and already mineralized dentine or is effected by the enamel proteins.

f. **True**. Each ameloblast contributes to the formation of more than one enamel prism; each prism receives contributions from four ameloblasts.

g. **False**. Aprismatic enamel is formed in the absence of a Tomes process.

h. **True**. Nasmyth's membrane merges with the overlying oral epithelium to provide an epithelial lined pathway for the erupting tooth.

i. **False**. Enamel matrix is mineralized almost as soon as it is secreted. Hence there is no equivalent layer to predentine.

j. **False**. Non-amelogenins have a higher molecular weight (about 55 000) and are richer in glycine.

k. **False**. Hunter–Schreger bands reflect the path of migration of ameloblasts. It is the cross-striation that reflects the diurnal rhythm of enamel.

Extended matching answers

Item 1 = Option E. As enamel crystallites are oriented parallel to the surface of a cell, the morphology of the Tomes process accounts for the sudden change in crystallite orientation at the prism boundary.

Item 2 = Option D. The short-period cross-striations represent the daily incremental lines traversing the long axis of enamel prisms. Approximately seven cross-striations are found between adjacent enamel striae, confirming the weekly time-course of the long-period striae.

Item 3 = Option A. The absence of prisms at the enamel surface can be correlated with the loss of the Tomes processes at this site. This prismless layer is slightly thicker in the weekly enamel of deciduous teeth than in that of permanent teeth.

Item 4 = Option H. The presence of a striated/microvilli border (alternating with a smooth border) has been associated with the withdrawal of water and organic matrix from enamel and its replacement with mineral during the maturation phase of the ameloblast.

Item 5 = Option I. The enamel tufts, representing hypomineralized regions of enamel, are regions that also contain more enamel matrix. They are best visualized in horizontal sections of the crown.

Item 6 = Option J. The mineral content of about 20% of young enamel is converted to adult enamel containing about 96% mineral.

Picture answers

Figure 12.8

a. A = odontoblast layer. B = ameloblast layer. C = stratum intermedium. D = stellate reticulum. E = external enamel epithelium. F = enamel matrix. G = dentine matrix.

b. The principal organic components of young enamel matrix (F) are the amelogenins, while that of dentine (G) is collagen.

c. Yes. It occurs in presecretory ameloblasts (i.e. pre-ameloblasts).

Figure 12.9

a. A = Tomes process. B = developing enamel. C = ameloblast.

b. Terminal bar apparatus related to cell complexes.

c. The presence of a Tomes process is responsible for the prismatic appearance of enamel, resulting in the sudden changes in crystallite orientation at prism boundaries. The absence of a Tomes process during the formation of surface enamel has been associated with prismless enamel in this region.

Figure 12.10

a. This 14-year-old patient is from a region where there are high levels of fluoride in the drinking water. This has resulted in toxic effects during the period of enamel formation of many of the teeth. The mottled appearance of the enamel is known as fluorosis and can occur when fluoride levels in the drinking water are in excess of 1 part per million. The enamel affected by fluorosis is hypocalcified but it is also acid-resistant. Fluorosis has to be distinguished from other defects in the enamel such as amelogenesis imperfecta.

Outline essay answers

Question 1

The basic unit of enamel seen in a ground longitudinal section of the crown will be the enamel prism. The prism boundaries are seen as lines about 5 μm apart running obliquely to the surface along the sides of the tooth, but more horizontally towards the cervical margins. The prism boundaries reflect sudden changes in crystallite orientation

Self-assessment: answers (Enamel formation)

and are related to the presence of Tomes processes in ameloblasts during the secretory phase. The disappearance of these processes at the end of the secretory phase accounts for the presence of non-prismatic (prismless) enamel in the surface layer.

As enamel formation is an intermittent rather than a continuous process, incremental markings are produced where the structure/composition of enamel is slightly different. Although the precise cause is not known, it may be the result of slight differences in:

- the quality of the enamel (either inorganic or organic)
- crystallite orientation
- prism dimensions.

Two types of incremental lines are seen: short-period and long-period lines. The short-period lines reflect a diurnal periodicity and are seen running transversely across the prisms at about 4 μm distances (cross-striations). Towards the cervical margin, where enamel is deposited more slowly, the cross-striations may be only 2 μm apart. The long-period markings reflect an approximately weekly rhythm, producing a change at the mineralizing front, and run oblique to the main direction of the prisms. These form the enamel striae. As enamel commences its deposition at the tip of cusps (or incisal edges) and is deposited centrifugally, the layers are laid down on top of each other, gradually lengthening and extending down the crown towards the cervical margin. The initial striae over the cusps therefore do not reach the surface. The striae on average are about 30–40 μm apart, but are closer together towards the cervical margin where enamel is formed more slowly. The ameloblasts do not all stop secreting at the same time at the surface. Those that stop first result in grooves at the surface (perikymata grooves), while on either side a slight continuation in formation is seen as ridges (perikymata ridges).

In deciduous teeth (and the mesiobuccal cusp of the first permanent molar), an exaggerated stria forms the neonatal line, representing the enamel formed during the nutritional disturbance accompanying the first few days after birth. The enamel contained within the neonatal line represents prenatal enamel, and that formed external to the line represents postnatal enamel. The enamel of deciduous teeth differs in some respects from that of permanent teeth. The incremental lines are far less conspicuous. The prismless layer at the surface is slightly thicker. The ameloblasts seem to mature at the surface at the same time, so that perikymata are rarely evident.

In moving outwards towards the surface, adjacent groups of ameloblasts in the inner two-thirds of enamel take slightly different paths. When this enamel is viewed in longitudinal ground section, groups of prisms will be sectioned in different planes, some being cut more longitudinally and others being cut more transversely. Each will react differently when viewed in transmitted (or polarized)

light. The effect is to produce alternating black-and-white bands known as the Hunter–Schreger bands. In the outer part of the enamel, all the ameloblasts move in the same direction so that Hunter–Schreger bands are not usually present.

As the ameloblasts initially move away from the odontoblasts, cell processes from the latter cells may be pulled along by the ameloblasts. When the initial layer of enamel mineralizes around these processes, they form the enamel spindles seen mainly over the cusps (and incisal edges).

If the question dealt with transverse rather than longitudinal sections, additional features that would be seen are the enamel tufts (representing hypomineralized groups of prisms extending into the inner enamel from the enamel–dentine junction) and enamel lamella (representing hypomineralized fault lines extending across the whole thickness of enamel). In addition, the enamel striae would be arranged circumferentially like the rings of a tree.

Question 2

At the early stage of tooth development, the internal enamel epithelial cell is a relatively undifferentiated low columnar cell with little evidence of polarization of its organelles. In this form it is free to divide and, interacting with the underlying cells of the dental papilla, maps out the shape of the crown of the tooth (morphogenetic stage). Prior to this, at an even earlier stage, the precursor of the internal enamel epithelial cell has already acted in an instructive capacity to specify the neural crest tissue migrating into the 1st arch to become odontogenic.

The first significant change in internal enamel epithelial cells at the early bell stage is seen at the tip of the future cusps when the cells elongate to become more columnar, this requiring a build-up of the cytoskeletal elements within the cell, such as microtubules. In addition, the cell undergoes a reversal of polarity, the nuclei coming to lie at the proximal part of the cell adjacent to the stratum intermedium and the Golgi material moving to the distal (secretory) end of the cell, where there is also a build-up of other organelles related to future production and secretion of the organic matrix. The cells may now be termed pre-ameloblasts and the change in their morphology is associated with the induction of the adjacent peripheral cells of the dental papilla to become odontoblasts; secretory organelles within the pre-ameloblasts may release signalling molecules to influence this process. This increased differentiation of the pre-ameloblasts is also correlated with the cells losing their ability to undergo cell division.

Once the odontoblasts have commenced laying down dentine, the cell membrane at the distal end of the pre-ameloblasts becomes irregular with many projections and pits, and vesicles and vacuoles appear in the cytoplasm. These

Self-assessment: answers (Enamel formation)

changes may, in part, be associated with the removal of the basal lamina. The pre-ameloblasts are then converted into ameloblasts that begin to deposit enamel matrix (secretory phase). This function is reflected in continued elongation of the cell and a further build-up of its intracellular organelles, with the appearance of secretory vesicles containing components of the organic matrix of enamel that will be exocytosed on to the dentine surface. Numerous cell contacts are present between neighbouring ameloblasts, forming terminal webs at both the proximal and distal ends of the cells. The distal, secretory end of the ameloblast during the formation of the initial few microns is flat, giving rise to a zone of non-prismatic enamel. However, soon afterwards, this surface develops a cone-shaped projection called a Tomes process. It is the presence of the Tomes process that is responsible for producing the sudden changes in crystallite orientation that result in the presence of the prismatic structure in enamel. The organic matrix synthesized in ameloblasts is carried in secretory vesicles to be exocytosed at the distal surface of the cell, where very thin enamel crystallites appear almost simultaneously. The different surfaces of the Tomes process may show slight differences in structure, indicating different functions.

When the full thickness of the enamel matrix has been reached, the Tomes process disappears, so that the last few microns of enamel at the surface will be non-prismatic.

At this stage, the enamel comprises about 30% mineral, 20–30% organic and about 40–50% water, and can be referred to as young, immature enamel. As no more enamel protein will be required, the ameloblast will undergo a further change in its morphology. It will shorten and show a great decrease in its intracellular organelles, such as roughened endoplasmic reticulum and Golgi material. Many ameloblasts will die and show evidence of apoptosis. The process whereby immature enamel is converted into its adult form, comprising about 96% mineral, is called maturation and involves the withdrawal of virtually all the organic matrix and water and its replacement with calcium and phosphate ions. This function, which is undertaken by the ameloblast, is reflected in a further change in its morphology. Vesicles and mitochondria build up in the distal part of the cell, whose distal surface modulates between two forms. It may possess numerous microvilli, forming a striated border (ruffle-ended form), or it may be smooth-ended. The many vesicles are thought to be associated with the removal and degradation of organic matrix from maturing enamel. In the ruffle-ended ameloblast, the distal cell contacts are 'leaky' and it is thought that enamel matrix can be removed via an intercellular route between ameloblasts. In the smooth-ended state, where it is thought the distal cell contacts are close, calcium and phosphate ions pass across the ameloblast to boost mineral levels in the maturing enamel. Because these high levels of calcium ions would normally be toxic to the cells, special mechanisms must be present to ensure that the calcium is conveyed through (or between) the cells without damaging it, utilizing, for example, calcium-binding mechanisms and calcium channels.

Once maturation of the enamel is complete, the ameloblasts become flattened and retain few intracellular organelles. They are separated from the enamel surface by a basal lamina termed the primary enamel cuticle; the cells themselves contain hemidesmosomes at this interface. The primary enamel cuticle, together with the remnants of the enamel organ (reduced enamel epithelium), form Nasmyth's membrane (see page 147); during eruption, this protects the enamel surface.

As the tooth erupts into the oral cavity, the reduced enamel epithelium undergoes a final, radical rearrangement of its layers, proliferating and merging with the overlying oral epithelium to provide an epithelial-lined pathway of eruption and then initially forming the junctional epithelium.

Question 3

The organic matrix is unique to enamel and accounts for 1–2% of total mature enamel composition, but approximately 25–30% of developing enamel matrix; the matrix is almost entirely composed of protein material. The major organic components of the developing enamel organic matrix are the amelogenins. This group of proteins accounts for 80–90% of the total secreted protein within developing enamel, the remaining 10% being the non-amelogenins.

Study of the functions of the enamel proteins is made difficult by the large number of amelogenin and amelogenin-related proteins. This is due to a combination of three features:

- Following their initial secretion, enamel proteins undergo a series of complex degradative changes carried out by various proteolytic enzymes that result in the accumulation of many smaller enamel proteins and peptides.
- The presence of alternative RNA splicing of the mRNA transcript. Thus, the same amino acid sequence is present at either end, but with deficiencies occurring in the middle.
- The presence of the amelogenin gene(s) on both the X and Y sex chromosomes, producing slightly different proteins; the amelogenin gene on the X chromosome has 106 base pairs while that on the Y chromosome has 112 base pairs. However, the male-specific proteins represent only a minor proportion of the total enamel protein. The functional significance of this sexual dimorphism is not known. This has forensic implications, as the sex of an individual could be determined from viable nuclear material by detecting the nature of the amelogenin gene.

Self-assessment: answers (Enamel formation)

The nascent amelogenin is rich in proline and glutamine, and is 178 amino acids in length, with a hydrophobic core and protein–protein interaction domain. This protein can self-assemble into spherical nanospheres that lie between the hydroxyapatite crystals, acting as spacers that allow the hydroxyapatite crystals to grow as enamel matures. It has a hydrophilic, mineral-binding domain, binding tightly to the enamel crystals through the C-terminal, which is cleaved shortly after secretion. Amelogenin is degraded by proteolytic enzymes as enamel matures. The other proteins are grouped together as non-amelogenins and include enamelin, tuftelin and ameloblastin. Enamelin is the largest enamel protein and is an acidic glycoprotein, with high binding affinity for hydroxyapatite. It is rapidly processed after secretion and may interact with crystals and be involved with nucleation. Tuft protein is highly anionic and can be found within the enamel tufts at the dentine–enamel junction. Ameloblastin is a tooth-specific protein and cleavage products have been identified in the prism boundary region throughout the enamel layer. Its localization suggests a possible role in regulating mineralization. Enamel matrix also contains metalloproteinases during early enamel development and serine proteinases during the late stages of enamel formation. Their roles are involved with proteolytic processing of the enamel proteins and, as such, drive enamel maturation by degrading those proteins which inhibit mineral deposition. Such proteinases include enamelysin (MMP-20), which is secreted primarily during the secretory and transition stages of enamel development. The active MMP cleaves amelogenin at the majority of sites observed in vivo. Enamel matrix serine proteinase-1 (EMSP-1) is a trypsin-like serine proteinase whose activity is dramatically increased during the transition stage of enamel development and remains at a high level throughout maturation. The pH for optimal activity of the enzyme is 5.7, which is the same as that within the enamel matrix during maturation.

Dental tissues. II
Dentine/pulp complex: structure, composition, development and oral pain

Structure and composition of dentine	**161**
Physical properties	161
Chemical composition	162
Dentinal tubule	162
Regional variations in dentine structure and composition	163
Incremental lines	164
Age-related and posteruptive changes	164
Dentine sensitivity	165
Dentine development (dentinogenesis)	**165**
Differentiation of odontoblasts	165
Organic matrix	166
Mineralization of mantle dentine	166
Dentinogenesis in the root	167
Secondary dentine	167
Tertiary dentine	168
Development of the pulp	168
Dental pulp	**169**
Organization and composition of the dental pulp	169
Blood supply	170
Lymphatic vessels	170
Nerve supply	170
Pain	171
Age-related changes	173
Self-assessment: questions (Structure and composition of dentine)	174
Self-assessment: answers (Structure and composition of dentine)	177
Self-assessment: questions (Dentine development)	181
Self-assessment: answers (Dentine development)	183
Self-assessment: questions (Dental pulp)	186
Self-assessment: answers (Dental pulp)	187

Structure and composition of dentine

Overview

Dentine is the mineralized connective tissue that forms the bulk of the tooth. It surrounds and protects the dental pulp. In the crown it is covered by enamel, in the root by cementum. Unlike enamel, dentine is sensitive and is formed throughout life, giving rise to secondary dentine. Though the odontoblasts that form the tissue have processes that lie in tubules within the dentine, the cell bodies lie at the periphery of the pulp, constituting a dentine/pulp complex. Being a living tissue, dentine can react to trauma by forming tertiary dentine.

Learning objectives

You should:
- know the composition and main structural features of dentine and be able to contrast these with enamel
- appreciate the different zones in dentine and understand the changes that take place in its structure with age. As with other dental tissues, you should be able to relate structure to function
- know the basis of dentine sensitivity
- understand how dentine reacts to trauma and how it bonds to restorative materials, as such knowledge has clinical relevance.

Dentine is the mineralized connective tissue that forms the bulk of the tooth. In the crown it is covered by enamel, in the root by cementum. It surrounds and protects the dental pulp. Unlike enamel, dentine is formed throughout life and is sensitive so that it is able to react to stimuli.

Physical properties

Dentine is pale yellow in colour. As enamel is semitranslucent, it is the underlying dentine that imparts the slight yellowish colour on the crown. Dentine is softer than enamel but harder than cementum. The combination of its organic matrix and mineral composition gives it both strength and a degree of flexibility. Dentine is traversed by a system of very narrow tubules that render it permeable. However, this permeability is reduced by the development of peritubular dentine.

Chemical composition

The chemical composition of dentine by weight is approximately 70% inorganic, 20% organic and 10% water. The inorganic component is in the form of (impure) calcium hydroxyapatite crystallites that give it its hardness. The crystallites are smaller than enamel, having a width of about 35 nm and a thickness of about 10 nm. The organic component of dentine consists of collagen fibrils embedded in an amorphous ground substance.

Collagen

Collagen gives dentine its strength. The fibrils comprise over 90% of the organic matrix and are mainly type I collagen (with very small traces of type III and type V); they have a mean diameter of approximately-100 nm.

Concerning its structure and formation, type I collagen has:

- a triple helix of two α-1 and one α-2 chains
- intracellular formation of procollagen (triple helix formation/secretion)
- propeptides removed in processing of procollagen to tropocollagen
- fibril formation with alignment of tropocollagen molecules, guided by non-collagenous proteins, e.g. decorin
- pyridinoline cross-link formation between lysine and hydroxylysine residues; this increases as predentine is modified, allowing for mineralization of dentine.

The collagen fibril orientation, along with the presence of proteoglycans, can be said to be the scaffold on which mineral can be deposited, and collagen itself is a good nucleator of hydroxyapatite. Hydroxyapatite crystal deposition occurs at the gap zone within collagen fibrils of dentine.

Non-collagenous proteins

Comprising only about 10% of the organic matrix, there are a large number of non-collagenous proteins in dentine. Although their functions are poorly understood, they are concerned with collagen formation and mineralization, and with odontoblast cell function and adhesion. The non-collagenous proteins include the proteoglycans decorin and biglycan, with the glycosaminoglycan side-chains of chondroitin-4-sulphate and chondroitin-6-sulphate. Also contained within this non-collagenous matrix are specific dentine phosphoproteins, acidic proteins, including Gla-protein, osteopontin, osteonectin, dentine and bone sialo-proteins, and numerous growth factors such as TGF-β1, BMP-2, BMP-4, BMP-6, BMP-7, insulin-like growth factor (IGF) and vascular endothelial growth factor (VEGF).

Acidic proteins

Acidic proteins such as γ-carboxyglutamate-containing proteins (Gla-proteins) are found in dentine in low amounts. It is not known what their function is, but their acidic nature allows them to bind strongly to hydroxyapatite crystallites, and therefore they may play some role in directing or guiding mineral deposition as predentine matures through to dentine. The other acidic proteins, osteopontin and osteonectin, may also be important in directing mineralization, and these are classically associated with bone. Dentine matrix protein is another acidic phosphorylated protein found in dentine and bone, and may also be involved in regulating nucleation of mineral crystals.

Dentine phosphoproteins

The two dentine phosphoproteins, dentine sialoprotein (DSP) and dentine phosphoprotein (DPP) are post-transcriptionally cleaved from the same gene product from the dentine sialophosphoprotein (DSPP) gene. The two proteins may have similar, but slightly different roles:

- DPP is secreted at the mineralizing front and is not present in predentine. It is highly phosphorylated (85–90%) and highly acidic due to the high aspartic acid residues and very high phosphate content. DPP has a very high affinity for calcium and hydroxyapatite surfaces and may function in mineral deposition due to its acidic nature and high calcium ion-binding properties.
- DSP is also acidic, with a high carbohydrate content (sialic acid 10%), and is phosphorylated. It is present in odontoblasts, predentine and dentine, and is considered to be tooth-specific.

Growth factors

Dentine contains a cocktail of bioactive proteins called growth factors. Such growth factors are sequestered into the dentine during dentinogenesis and are thought to be held within the mineralized matrix, bound to proteoglycans or latency-associated peptides. Such factors include TGF-β1, BMP-2, 4 and 7, IGF and the angiogenic growth factor VEGF. Such factors have been shown to be important in regulating dentinogenesis and tooth development, and it is possible that release of these factors during trauma or disease (and possibly cavity lining) directs the tertiary dentinogenic response which the pulp-dentine complex exhibits.

Dentinal tubule

The basic repeatable unit in dentine is the dentinal tubule. This runs through the dentine and is widest at the pulp surface, with a diameter of about 3 μm.

Intertubular and circumpulpal dentine

Initially, the tubule contains an odontoblast process surrounded by the mineralized intertubular dentine. The dentine tubules follow a curved, sigmoid course (primary curvature) that is most prominent at the sides of the crown. In the root and beneath the cusps, the tubules run a straighter course. Along the length of each primary curvature, minor undulations of the tubule constitute the secondary curvatures. Occasionally, adjacent secondary curvatures may coincide, giving rise to a feature called a contour line (of Owen). The dentinal tubules branch along their course, this being particularly evident at the enamel–dentine junction. In the root, just beneath the cementum, the terminal branching is exaggerated and the dentinal tubules also appear to loop. These features are thought by some to be responsible for the appearance of the granular layer (of Tomes) seen in ground sections. In the bulk of the dentine (circumpulpal dentine), the collagen fibrils of the mineralized matrix are aligned parallel to the enamel–dentine junction and transverse to the dentinal tubules.

Peritubular (intratubular) dentine

Soon after the dentinal tubules have been formed, another type of dentine is deposited on the walls of the tubule, narrowing the size of the lumen. This explains why the dentinal tubule is narrower (about 1 µm) in the outer part of the dentine. This type of dentine is known as peritubular (intratubular) dentine and may eventually lead to the complete obliteration of the tubule. Peritubular dentine differs from intertubular dentine in lacking a collagenous fibrous matrix and may be considered as representing mineralized ground substance. It is hypermineralized when compared with intertubular dentine, being 10–15% more mineralized; although containing hydroxyapatite crystals, other forms of calcium phosphate may be encountered. Peritubular dentine is present in unerupted teeth. In demineralized sections, the peritubular dentine is completely lost, as it lacks a residual collagenous framework, and the tubule is restored to its original dimensions.

Associated with physiological ageing, especially in root dentine, the dentinal tubules become completely occluded by peritubular dentine formation. The contents of the tubule acquire the same refractive index as the intertubular dentine. When a ground section of a root is placed in water (which has a refractive index different from that of dentine), regions blocked by peritubular dentine will appear translucent ('translucent dentine'), while regions with patent tubules will fill with water and appear opaque. Translucent dentine forms initially near the root apex and extends both cervically and apically with age. There is a good correlation between the amount of translucent dentine and the age of the patient, and this feature is used in forensic odontology to help age teeth.

Contents of dentinal tubules

The contents of dentinal tubules may include the odontoblast process, afferent nerve terminals and processes from antigen-presenting cells. The tubule is also bathed in 'dentinal' fluid. Movement of this fluid is thought to be involved in dentine sensitivity.

Odontoblast process

The odontoblast process contains vesicles, microtubules and intermediate filaments. The main organelles associated with protein synthesis (e.g. rough endoplasmic reticulum Golgi material) are present in the odontoblast cell body but do not extend into the process. The extent of the odontoblast process inside the dentinal tubule has not been established with certainty due to considerable technical difficulties. Evidence suggests that, with age and with the formation of peritubular dentine, it is limited to the inner third of dentine. A thin, proteinaceous membrane termed the lamina limitans may be seen lining the wall of the dentinal tubule and its presence may give rise to the erroneous impression of an odontoblast process.

Sensory nerve terminals

Sensory nerve terminals may be seen adjacent to the odontoblast processes. They are limited mainly to the dentine of the crown beneath the cusps (where they may be found in 50–80% of the tubules) and project up to 200 µm from the pulp. Fewer tubules are innervated in the midcoronal dentinal regions and fewer than 5% of tubules are innervated in the cervical and root dentine. The axon is narrower than the odontoblast process and often contains mitochondria; there is no evidence of any specialized contacts between the nerve and the odontoblast process.

Regional variations in dentine structure and composition

The structure and composition of mineralized dentine varies in different parts of the tissue and one can distinguish the following zones: mantle dentine, interglobular dentine, granular layer, hyaline layer and predentine.

Mantle dentine

The outermost thin (about 20 µm) layer of dentine in the crown is termed mantle dentine. It differs from the bulk of the circumpulpal dentine in that its collagen fibrils are largely oriented perpendicular to the enamel–dentine junction rather than parallel to it, and is generally 5% less mineralized than the rest of the circumpulpal dentine. It contains no dentine phosphoprotein and the dentinal tubules show considerable branching in this region. During the initial mineralization of dentine, mantle dentine exhibits the presence of matrix vesicles. The mantle dentine lies adjacent to the three-dimensional, scalloped architecture of the enamel–dentine junction and some odontoblast processes initially extend into the enamel and give rise to enamel spindles.

Interglobular dentine

Much of dentine is deposited as calcospherites, with the hydroxyapatite crystallites arranged radially. These normally fuse to form a uniformly calcified tissue. However, in some areas, usually beneath the mantle layer in the crown, the fusion may be incomplete, giving rise to uncalcified, interglobular dentine.

Hyaline layer

In ground sections, the outermost layer of root dentine is a clear hyaline layer, whose precise origin is in dispute. This narrow band (up to 20 μm wide) appears to be non-tubular and therefore structureless. The hyaline layer may serve to bond cementum to dentine and may be of considerable clinical significance when considering periodontal regeneration.

Granular layer (of Tomes)

Immediately beneath the hyaline layer when viewed in ground sections is a narrow, dark zone called the granular layer (of Tomes).

Predentine

As it is formed throughout life, the inner surface of dentine adjacent to the pulp is lined by an unmineralized zone of dentine matrix called predentine. In demineralized sections, predentine stains differently to that of the matrix of the rest of the (mineralized) dentine matrix. This reflects a difference in the composition of its matrix. Predentine contains type I collagen which provides an organic scaffold for eventual mineralization. Non-collagenous proteins (such as decorin and biglycan) direct matrix organization and prevent premature mineralization, and this matrix is modified by proteolytic enzymes prior to mineral deposition at the mineralization front. Such remodelling includes removal of inhibitors to mineral nucleation and the processing of proteins for new functions. The presence of matrix metalloproteinases indicates that proteolytic processing occurs as predentine is modified. The mineralizing front may show a globular or linear outline, reflecting two different mineralization processes. The width of the predentine can vary from 10 to 40 μm, depending on the rate at which dentine is being deposited.

Incremental lines

Like enamel, dentine has regularly spaced incremental lines. There are two types: short-period and long-period markings. They have been attributed to:

- circadian fluctuations in acid–base balance that affect both the mineral content and the refractive index of forming hard tissues
- changes in collagen fibril orientation.

Short-period markings (von Ebner lines) may be seen as alternating dark and light bands, each pair reflecting the diurnal rhythm of dentine formation and lying approximately 3 μm apart. The coarser, long-period lines (Andresen lines) are approximately 20 μm apart. Between each

long-period line there are 6–10 pairs of short-period lines. The cause of this periodicity is unknown. A similar periodicity exists in enamel, making it likely that a common mechanism exists. As with enamel, an exaggerated line, the neonatal line, can be seen in the dentine of teeth mineralizing at birth.

Age-related and posteruptive changes

Once the tooth is erupted and fully formed, dentine can undergo a number of changes that either are related to age or occur as a response to a stimulus applied to the tooth, such as caries or attrition.

Secondary dentine

Secondary dentine is the term given to the dentine that starts to form once the root is complete, about 3 years after the tooth erupts. Its structure is very similar to that of primary dentine and it may be difficult to distinguish between the two. However, primary and secondary dentine are often delineated as a result of a change in direction of the dentinal tubules with coincidence of secondary curvatures, producing a contour line (of Owen). The increased crowding of odontoblasts as secondary dentine formation continues throughout life, together with the slower rate of deposition, make secondary dentine a little less regular than primary dentine and the incremental markings somewhat closer together. The overall result is the smaller pulp chambers and narrower root canals in the teeth of older patients.

Tertiary dentine

With more severe stimuli, such as attrition and dental caries, the dental pulp may be induced to produce a less regular form of dentine known as tertiary dentine. It may have a tubular structure or it may be relatively atubular.

Reactionary dentine

Reactionary dentine refers to the tertiary dentine forming in response to an insult in which, although some damage has been sustained, the existing odontoblasts upregulate their synthetic and secretory functions and continue to form dentine.

Reparative dentine

Reparative dentine relates to the tertiary dentine forming after a stimulus in which the original odontoblasts in the associated region have been destroyed and new calcified tissue (reparative dentine) has been formed by newly differentiated cells (referred to as 'odontoblast-like' cells). This matrix is rapidly deposited and has a dysplastic, irregular structure. No DPP is present and high levels of bone-associated proteins can be identified. This reparative dentine has also been referred to as osteodentine.

Sclerotic dentine

In addition to infilling with peritubular dentine as a physiological response to ageing, dentinal tubules commonly fill in as a response to an external stimulus such as surrounding a slowly advancing carious lesion. This type of dentine is termed sclerotic dentine and, like translucent dentine, will present as areas of dentine that lack structure and appear transparent. Little is known about the precipitated material, but it appears to differ from peritubular dentine and may not be formed by the odontoblast.

Dead tracts

If the primary odontoblasts are killed by an external stimulus, or retract before peritubular dentine occludes the tubules, empty tubules will be left. They may be sealed at their pulpal end by tertiary dentine. When ground sections are routinely prepared and mounted, the mounting medium may not enter these sealed-off tubules and they will remain air-filled. Viewed through a microscope, transmitted light will be totally internally reflected; these tubules will appear dark and are termed 'dead tracts'.

Dentine sensitivity

One of the most important clinical aspects of the dentine/pulp complex relates to the intense pain that can be generated from this site when given appropriate stimuli. Stimuli applied to dentine can be transmitted across the dentine to fire nerves at the periphery of the dental pulp. Three main hypotheses have been put forward to account for dentine sensitivity:

- One view states that stimuli are transmitted directly via nerves in dentine. However, arguing against this view is the relative scarcity of nerves and their apparent absence in the outer parts of dentine. In addition, the application of local anaesthetics to the surface of dentine does not abolish the sensitivity.
- A second hypothesis states that stimuli are transmitted via odontoblast processes. However, there is no physiological evidence to date that indicates that the odontoblast process is analogous to a nerve fibre and can similarly conduct impulses pulpwards (i.e. it has a low membrane potential). Furthermore, like nerves in dentine, the process may not extend far into dentine; nor is the application of substances designed to prevent transmission of such impulses effective. In addition, odontoblasts have not been shown to be synaptically connected to nerve fibres.
- The third and most plausible hypothesis to explain the transmission of sensory stimuli suggests that all effective stimuli applied to dentine cause fluid movement through the dentinal tubules, and that this movement is sufficient to depolarize nerve endings in the inner parts of tubules, at the pulp–predentine junction and in the subodontoblastic neural plexus. Movement in either direction would mechanically distort the terminals. This is discussed further on pages 172–173.

Dentine development (dentinogenesis)

Overview

Essential epithelial/mesenchymal interactions occur in the developing tooth germ to enable dentine formation to commence. Dentine formation, like bone and cementum, is a two-phase process, commencing with the secretion of an extracellular connective tissue matrix and its subsequent mineralization. It continues throughout life. The tissue that is produced shows regional variations in structure and well-defined age changes.

Learning objectives

You should:
- understand the process whereby dentine is formed and be able to compare and contrast it with the formation of enamel
- be able to relate the structures seen in a ground section of dentine with the development of the tissue
- be able to appreciate how age changes relate to the clinical situation.

Dentine formation begins when the tooth germ has reached the bell stage of development. In the enamel organ, the internal enamel epithelium starts to differentiate but, as yet, no enamel has been deposited. The dentine-forming cells, the odontoblasts, differentiate from the peripheral cells of the underlying dental papilla and are of neural crest origin.

Dentine formation begins, as with enamel, in the region of the cusp (or incisal margin) of the tooth and gradually extends down the slopes of the crown to the cervical margin. This represents coronal dentine. Within the dentinal tubules, peritubular dentine formation soon begins to narrow the size of the lumen. Following crown completion, root dentine then forms as the epithelial root sheath (of Hertwig) extends apically and odontoblasts differentiate from the adjacent dental papilla. Dentinogenesis continues and the thickness of dentine increases steadily until, at about the time root completion occurs, it slows down to give rise to secondary dentine.

Differentiation of odontoblasts

The differentiation of odontoblasts is the result of epithelial/mesenchymal interactions (see page 115), requiring the involvement of many signalling agents, transcription factors and growth factors (e.g. Ssh (sonic hedgehog), BMPs, fibroblast growth factors (FGFs) and TGFs). At the early bell stage of development, the cells of the dental papilla are relatively undifferentiated. As the internal enamel epithelial cells elongate to become pre-ameloblasts, the adjacent cells of the dental papilla start to differentiate. They elongate and the nucleus comes to lie in the basal part of the cell (that furthest from the internal enamel epithelium).

The Golgi material becomes pronounced and the rough endoplasmic reticulum increases in size. Cell-to-cell junctions, particularly between odontoblasts but also linking odontoblasts to subodontoblastic cells, increase in number. The odontoblasts migrate pulpwards, each trailing a number of small cell processes, one of which predominates to form the odontoblast process of the cell.

Organic matrix

From the distal end of the cell, the differentiating odontoblast secretes the initial organic matrix, the predentine of mantle dentine that surrounds the odontoblast process. This matrix is composed of small collagen fibrils (nearly all type I) embedded in its characteristic ground substance. The cell may now be referred to as an odontoblast. The collagen fibrils in mantle dentine are oriented perpendicular to the basal lamina (the site of the future enamel–dentine junction). The basal lamina soon breaks down. As the predentine thickens, it matures sufficiently to allow its matrix to mineralize.

Mineralization of mantle dentine

Mineralization of mantle dentine is thought to be initiated by matrix vesicles. These membrane-bound organelles (30–200 nm) are budded off from the odontoblast. They contain a variety of enzymes (including alkaline phosphatase) and other molecules that lead to the formation of the first mineral crystals of hydroxyapatite within the vesicles. The crystals then break out of the vesicles and subsequent mineralization of the remainder of the dentine occurs without the presence of matrix vesicles. Similar matrix vesicles have been implicated in the initial mineralization of bone and calcified cartilage.

Circumpulpal dentine

Once the initial thin layer of mantle dentine has formed, the fully differentiated odontoblasts continue retreating pulpwards, trailing out an odontoblast process around which the odontoblast continues to secrete the predentine associated with circumpulpal dentine. Compared with that of mantle dentine, the collagen fibrils are now oriented parallel to the enamel–dentine junction. When the predentine reaches a thickness of about 10–20 μm, it attains a state of maturity that will allow it to mineralize. At the mineralizing front, degradation of some molecules in predentine may occur, while other molecules may be added (e.g. dentine phosphophoryn) after being transported along the odontoblast process, thereby bypassing the bulk of the predentine layer. As the biochemistry of predentine will differ when compared with that of the organic matrix associated with mineralized dentine, predentine will stain differently.

The main path of the retreating odontoblasts will give rise to the outline of the primary curvatures, whilst minor undulations in the odontoblast process will give rise to the secondary curvatures.

Interglobular dentine

The outline of the mineralizing front indicates that two distinct patterns of mineralization can occur (and in the absence of matrix vesicles): a linear or a spherical (calcospheritic) pattern. In calcospherites, the crystallites are arranged in a radial pattern and, despite complete mineralization of dentine, this pattern can still be discerned using polarized light. Failure of calcospherites to fuse may result in the appearance of interglobular dentine, representing small regions of unmineralized matrix.

Biochemical aspects of dentine mineralization

Concerning biochemical aspects of dentine mineralization, collagen fibril formation proceeds, with alignment of tropocollagen molecules being guided by non-collagenous proteins such as decorin. Pyridinoline cross-link formation between lysine and hydroxylysine residues increases as predentine is modified, allowing for mineralization to dentine. The collagen fibril orientation, along with the presence of proteoglycans, can be said to be the scaffold on which mineral can be deposited, and collagen itself is a good nucleator of hydroxyapatite. Hydroxyapatite crystals are initially deposited at the gap zone within collagen fibrils of mineralized dentine.

Proteoglycans

Two pools of proteoglycans are synthesized as dentine is formed. One pool is found in predentine and the other pool is found in dentine. This reflects different roles that these molecules may play in dentine formation.

Decorin and biglycan, with dermatan sulphate glycosaminoglycan side-chains, and versican are synthesized in predentine. These forms of the molecules are also predominant in soft connective tissues. They are found bound to collagen fibres in the gap zone and are involved with initial matrix formation, collagen fibril formation and prevention of premature mineralization. Versican has a high proportion of GAG chains attached to core protein and has also been implicated in the inhibition of mineralization. All of these proteoglycans are removed or remodelled as predentine matures.

At the mineralization front, a second pool of decorin (and biglycan) with chondroitin sulphate glycosaminoglycan side-chains is secreted. These proteoglycans, (together with acidic proteins) may be transported intracellularly along the odontoblast process, bypassing most of the predentine layer. Levels of these proteoglycans are lower than those found in predentine; they are distributed in mineralized connective tissues interfibrilly and are associated with the gap zones of the collagen fibrils. This second pool may be associated with directing mineral deposition, as the chondroitin sulphate may be involved in transport of Ca^{2+} and HPO_4^{2-} to the gap zones in the collagen fibrils.

Acidic proteins

Acidic proteins such, as γ-carboxyglutamate-containing proteins (Gla-proteins), are found in dentine in low amounts. It is not known what their function is, but their acidic nature allows them to bind strongly to hydroxyapatite crystallites and therefore they may play some role in directing or guiding mineral deposition as predentine matures through to dentine. The other acidic proteins, osteopontin and osteonectin, may also be important in directing mineralization and these are classically associated with bone. Dentine matrix protein is another acidic phosphorylated protein found in dentine and bone, and may also be involved in regulating nucleation of mineral crystals.

Dentine phosphoproteins

The two dentine phosphoproteins, dentine sialoprotein (DSP) and dentine phosphoprotein (DPP), are post-transcriptionally cleaved from the same gene product from the dentine sialophosphoprotein (DSPP) gene. The two proteins may have similar, but slightly different roles:

DPP:

- is secreted at the mineralizing front and is not present in predentine
- is highly phosphorylated (85–90%)
- is highly acidic due to the high aspartic acid residues and very high phosphate content
- has a very high affinity for calcium hydroxyapatite surfaces
- may function in mineral deposition due to its acidic nature and high calcium ion-binding properties.

DSP:

- is acidic
- has a high carbohydrate content (sialic acid 10%)
- is phosphorylated
- is present in odontoblasts, predentine and dentine
- is considered to be tooth-specific.

Growth factors

Dentine is considered to be a bioactive matrix, as it contains a cocktail of bioactive proteins called growth factors. Such growth factors are sequestered into the dentine during dentinogenesis and are thought to be held within the mineralized matrix, bound to proteoglycans or latency-associated peptides. Such factors include TGF-β1, BMP-2, 4 and 7, IGF and the angiogenic growth factor VEGF. Such factors have been shown to be important in regulating dentinogenesis and tooth development, and it is possible that release of these factors during trauma or disease (and possibly cavity lining) directs the tertiary dentinogenic response which the pulp/dentine complex exhibits.

Dentinogenesis in the root

The basic process of dentinogenesis in the root does not differ fundamentally from that occurring in the crown. However, differences are evident in the earliest stages.

Epithelial root sheath

Following crown formation, the external enamel and internal enamel epithelia proliferate apically as the epithelial root sheath to map out the shape of the root. Internal to the root sheath lies the dental papilla, while the dental follicle is situated externally. As in the crown, epithelial/mesenchymal interactions induce the peripheral cells of the dental papilla to differentiate into odontoblasts, which commence laying down the initial root dentine. Unlike dentinogenesis in the crown, the cells of the epithelial root sheath do not enlarge or become columnar, and do not differentiate into ameloblasts. Instead, they remain cuboidal. As the odontoblasts of the root migrate pulpwards, they do not initially trail behind a process and the resulting matrix contains some organic material derived from the odontoblasts (though with fewer collagen fibrils), as well as some enamel-related proteins secreted by the epithelial root sheath cells. This epithelial contribution is reflected in the structure of the internal enamel epithelial cells, which possess some of the intracellular organelles associated with protein synthesis and secretion (e.g. Golgi material and endoplasmic reticulum). The subsequent fate of the epithelial root sheath is considered further in relation to cementum formation.

Hyaline layer

This thin, initial, organic predentine layer in root dentine will mineralize to form the hyaline layer, which is continuous in the crown with the mantle layer. Unusually, mineralization begins a few microns in from the surface and continues pulpwards, allowing these outer few microns to undergo delayed mineralization outwards and provide a firm union with the initial collagen fibrils of the cementum.

Granular layer

Following the formation of the hyaline layer, the migrating odontoblasts trail behind their odontoblast processes. Initially these branch, loop and appear dilated and, when the dentine matrix around them becomes mineralized, give rise to the granular layer immediately beneath the hyaline layer. After this, the main odontoblast process is formed in a relatively straight horizontal plane as the remaining circumpulpal dentine of the root is formed.

Secondary dentine

Once the crown has erupted into the mouth and root completion has occurred, dentine continues to form throughout life, but at a slower rate. This dentine is termed secondary dentine. As the pulp volume decreases with continuing dentine deposition, odontoblasts overlap and form a pseudostratified layer, mainly in the crown.

Peritubular dentine

Peritubular dentine is slowly deposited on the wall of the dentinal tubule, commencing soon after the formation of the dentinal tubule. It differs from intertubular dentine in containing more mineral and in lacking collagen fibres, its organic matrix consisting of non-collagenous proteins such as glycoproteins, proteoglycans and lipids. The inorganic component of peritubular dentine differs somewhat to that of intertubular dentine. Peritubular dentine formation may be under the control of the odontoblast and may incorporate plasma proteins that have diffused along the cell membrane.

Peritubular dentine will slowly narrow the diameter of the lumen of the dentinal tubule, initially about 3 μm in diameter. The lumen may be completely occluded by peritubular dentine and this happens consistently in the apical third of the root, giving rise to the appearance of translucent dentine. The amount of translucent dentine correlates very well with age.

Incremental lines

The rate of dentine formation varies, producing incremental lines. There are both short-term (diurnal) and long-period rhythms:

- A diurnal rhythm of formation produces short-period lines approximately 4 μm apart (von Ebner lines), resulting from slight differences in composition/orientation of the dentine matrix.
- Long-period lines (Andresen lines), approximately 20 μm apart, are also evident, suggesting a longer rhythm (of unknown aetiology) of about 7 days.

An exaggerated line, the neonatal line, is present in all teeth mineralizing at birth and represents the dentine formed during the first few days after birth with its disturbed nutrition.

Tertiary dentine

Tertiary dentine is the tissue that is laid down in response to a stimulus, such as severe attrition or dental caries:

- If the stimulus is mild and the original odontoblasts remain alive, a tubular form of tertiary dentine termed reactionary dentine will be formed.
- If, however, the stimulus is more severe and sufficient to destroy the original odontoblasts, new odontoblast-like cells will differentiate from stem cells within the pulp and lay down another form of tertiary dentine called reparative dentine, which is more irregular and atubular.

Development of the pulp

Once the bud-stage enamel organ invaginates to become the cap stage, the cells and matrix within the invagination are recognized as the dental papilla. During growth of the tooth germ, although relatively undifferentiated, the dental papilla interacts with the overlying epithelium (epithelial/mesenchymal interactions) to drive morphogenesis and histogenesis. The cells of the dental papilla, including its neural crest cells, are densely packed, rapidly dividing and separated by relatively little extracellular matrix.

As the enamel organ surrounding the dental papilla enlarges and enters the bell stage, the cells within the dental papilla undergo cytodifferentiation into a peripheral layer of odontoblasts and a central mass of fibroblasts. As the pulp develops, the cytoplasmic component of these central cells expands and synthetic organelles appear. The organic matrix of the pulp is released into the extracellular space and forms fine collagen fibres that are embedded in an amorphous ground substance. In the early stages of pulpal development, the ground substance has a high glycosaminoglycan content and a low quantity of hyaluronan. This balance is reversed in the mature tooth. Once the odontoblasts have begun to lay down dentine, the dental papilla becomes, by convention, the dental pulp. A proportion of cells present in the dental pulp remain as stem cells, retaining the potential to differentiate into other cells in later life, especially the odontoblast-like cells associated with the formation of tertiary dentine.

Once the full length of the root is established, the development of the dental pulp can be considered complete, although dentine deposition will continue throughout life. A cell-rich zone may be evident beneath the odontoblast layer at the time of eruption, probably the result of the migration of more central cells rather than by local cell division. Between the cell-rich zone and the odontoblast layer, a cell-free zone may become apparent at the time of eruption. However, this zone may be a fixation artefact. With age, as the odontoblasts migrate pulpally, the odontoblast layer appears pseudostratified.

Vascularization of the developing pulp starts during the early bell stage, with small branches from the principal vascular trunks of the jaws entering the base of the papilla. Of these small pioneer vessels, a few become the principal pulpal vessels, enlarge and run through the pulp towards the cuspal regions, where they give off numerous branches to form the subodontoblast plexus. The vascularity of the odontoblast layer increases as dentine is progressively laid down.

Nerves do not enter the dental pulp until dentinogenesis is well under way. The first fibres to enter the developing pulp become located close to the blood vessels. These nerves, although anatomically part of the sensory nervous system, probably play an important role via axon reflexes in controlling blood flow. The autonomic, sympathetic innervation follows later. Although a large number of nerves are found in the developing pulp, the formation of the subodontoblastic nerve plexus (of Raschkow) is not established until root formation is complete.

Dental pulp

Overview

The dental pulp is the soft connective tissue occupying the core of the tooth that is responsible for nourishing and maintaining the dentine. Its peripheral cells form the odontoblast layer, from which the odontoblast processes pass into the dentine tubules. Being almost totally surrounded by mineralized tissue gives rise to a number of specialized features. As it forms dentine throughout life, the pulp undergoes a number of important age changes. Unusually for a soft connective tissue, it has a very rich blood and nerve supply. Its extreme sensitivity gives it profound clinical significance.

Learning objectives

You should:
- know the composition and structure of the dental pulp, including all cell types present
- be able to compare the dental pulp with other soft connective tissues and be aware of specializations that may relate to its position, being surrounded by dentine
- be able to describe the blood vessels and nerves of the pulp and understand the physiology of pain
- appreciate the age changes that occur in the dental pulp and how these may relate to the clinical situation.

Organization and composition of the dental pulp

The dental pulp is a loose, soft, connective tissue derived from the dental papilla and is responsible for the formation and maintenance of dentine. It is contained within the pulp chamber and root canals of the tooth. At the apical constriction of the root canal it becomes continuous with the periodontal ligament. After a tooth has erupted into the oral cavity, the pulp forms secondary dentine slowly, but regularly, throughout life so that its size diminishes. It is able to respond to strong stimuli (such as caries, trauma, tooth movement and restorative procedures) by producing tertiary dentine. Some of the more specialized properties of the dental pulp relate to its situation, being almost completely encased in, and protected by, dentine.

As with other connective tissues, the dental pulp is made up of a combination of cells embedded in an extracellular matrix of fibres in a semifluid gel. It has a very rich blood and nerve supply. It contains 75% by weight of water and 25% organic material. The pulp is a dynamic functional matrix which has an important role in controlling the activity of the cells within it. The complex framework of collagen and associated proteoglycans and glycoproteins creates a scaffold to stabilize the structure of the pulp; however, the nature of the organic molecules within it allow it to influence cell migration, proliferation, adhesion, differentiation and function.

Collagen

The collagen of the dental pulp is a combination of types I (60%) and III (40%). The collagen fibrils are about 50 nm in diameter and form thin fibres irregularly scattered throughout the tissue. A small amount of type IV collagen is present in the basement membrane of blood vessels.

GAGs and proteoglycans

The young, immature pulp has large quantities of chondroitin sulphate, with dermatan sulphate being found in much smaller amounts. GAGs are hydrophilic and form gels that fill most of the extracellular space. They swell when hydrated which may explain the high fluid pressure within the pulp, but will also contribute to the mechanical support. Hyaluronan is found unbound to protein and is thought to facilitate cell migration through the matrix. In the older, mature pulp, the ratios are reversed, with 60% of the GAG content being hyaluronan, 20% dermatan sulphate and only about 12% chondroitin sulphate (the remainder consisting of heparin sulphate).

Among the proteoglycans within the pulp are versican, syndecan and decorin, whilst among the glycoproteins are fibronectin and tenascin. The diverse nature and role of the proteoglycans found within the pulp influence its bioactivity by binding and conferring protection to growth factors, and acting as adhesion molecules to influence cell behaviour.

Cells

The pulp contains all the usual cells expected for a soft connective tissue (i.e. fibroblasts, defence cells and stem cells). However, also present at the periphery are the cell bodies of odontoblasts, a cell type unique for this tissue.

Odontoblasts

Odontoblasts are the cells responsible for the formation of dentine. They originate from neural crest (ectomesenchyme) cells. The fully differentiated odontoblast is a polarized columnar cell 50 μm long and 5 μm in width, with a very long cell process that extends into a dentine tubule. The cell has numerous smaller processes which link it to adjacent odontoblasts and adjacent pulp cells. The nucleus lies in the basal (pulpal) half of the cell, with the other organelles involved in dentine synthesis (e.g. rough endoplasmic reticulum, Golgi material and mitochondria) above it in the distal part of the cell. Initially forming a single layer of cells, odontoblasts in the crown retreat pulpwards so that, in a mature tooth, the odontoblasts overlap and give the false appearance of multiple layers ('pseudostratification'). In the root, they are commonly more cuboidal and maintain the appearance of a single layer.

Odontoblasts have numerous cell junctions on their cell membranes namely, macula adherens junctions (desmosomes), tight junctions and gap junctions. These allow for cell signalling, maintaining the integrity of the cell layer and governing its degree of permeability. The odontoblast cell layer would appear to provide a controlled barrier between the pulp and the dentine.

During their life cycle, the activity of the odontoblasts is affected by a number of signalling and growth factors. In mature odontoblasts, these include factors such as transforming growth factor (TGF)-β and bone morphogenetic protein. As mature odontoblasts express numerous membrane receptors for the TGF-β family, it has been suggested that this growth factor may be of importance in the initiation of tertiary dentine. Although some have implied that the odontoblast could act as a sensory receptor, passing on afferent information from the outer dentine to nerve fibres in the peripheral pulp, there is no evidence of specialized junctions between nerves and odontoblasts.

Beneath the odontoblast layer in the crown, a layer relatively free of cell bodies may be seen once the tooth has erupted. This has been termed the cell-free zone (although it may represent a preparation artefact). Beneath the cell-free zone there may be a zone where there appears to be an increase in the number of cell bodies, the cell-rich zone.

Fibroblasts

Beneath the odontoblast layer, the most common cell type within the dental pulp is the fibroblast; these form a loose network throughout the tissue. As elsewhere, their morphology is highly variable. Their main function is associated with the development and maintenance of the extracellular matrix that provides the framework and support for the odontoblasts and for the neurovascular elements of the pulp. As the turnover of this matrix does not appear to be particularly rapid, pulpal fibroblasts show only moderate amounts of associated intracellular organelles such as endoplasmic reticulum, Golgi material or mitochondria.

Stem/progenitor cells

A population of stem/progenitor cells must be present within the pulp to replace pulpal fibroblasts. There must also be a population of such progenitor cells that can, in response to a severe challenge, also produce tertiary dentine. Whether these two populations represent the same stem cell is not known. However, the subject has profound clinical implications. It is to be remembered that, for odontoblasts to differentiate initially during tooth development, signalling from epithelial cells is a prerequisite. However, epithelial cells are not present within the adult dental pulp during the formation of tertiary dentine. Therefore, during repair, another analogous method must take control. As dentine contains a number of growth factors which are known to be involved in the differentiation of odontoblasts during development, it is now thought that these are released during trauma to the dentine and are critical in signalling to the undifferentiated mesenchymal cells beneath the odontoblast layer and around blood vessels to differentiate into a new generation of odontoblast-like cells.

Defence cells

The typical defence cells (e.g. lymphocytes, macrophages and mast cells) exist in the healthy dental pulp. In addition, dendritic antigen-presenting cells are also an important component of the normal dental pulp. They are at least 50 μm long and have a number of branching processes. They are present particularly at the periphery of the dental pulp and around nerves and blood vessels. Some dendritic processes extend into the dentinal tubules. The cells initiate a primary immune response and migrate, with trapped antigen, to regional lymph nodes, inducing T-lymphocyte division and differentiation there.

Blood supply

The pulp has a rich blood supply. Arterioles and venules enter and leave the dental pulp via the apical foramina. The largest of the arterioles are approximately 150 μm in diameter. They run longitudinally through the root canals, within which they send off side branches to the periphery. The vessels divide and branch profusely once they are within the coronal pulp and form a rich capillary plexus beneath the odontoblast layer. Capillary loops extend towards the dentine and pass between the odontoblasts and the predentine. Returning vessels connect to venules. The capillary network beneath the odontoblasts is dense enough to be known as the subodontoblastic capillary plexus. Approximately 5% of the capillaries in the subodontoblastic zone are fenestrated. Other specializations of the pulp vascular system are evident in the form of numerous arteriovenous and venous–venous anastomoses. The pulp has a high, pulsatile, interstitial tissue fluid pressure. This pressure would allow 'dentinal fluid' to move outwards whenever the dentinal tubules were patent peripherally. The smooth muscle of the arterioles is innervated by terminals of sympathetic nerves, which maintain a vasoconstrictor tone.

Lymphatic vessels

Lymphatic vessels are also present within the dental pulp, although they are not readily demonstrated.

Nerve supply

The dental pulp has a rich nerve supply. Of these nerves, about 25% are myelinated afferents whose cell bodies lie in the trigeminal ganglion. Of these myelinated nerves, 90% are narrow Aδ fibres (1–6 μm in diameter), with the rest belonging to the wider Aß group (6–12 μm in diameter). By the time these nerves reach the region of the odontoblast cell body, they have all lost their ensheathing Schwann cells. No specialized junctions between odontoblasts (or their processes) and nerves have been identified. Most of the non-myelinated C fibres are also afferent, the remainder being vasoconstrictor sympathetic efferents that supply arteriolar smooth muscle.

The nerve bundles run centrally in the pulp of the root in close association with the blood vessels. A few fibres leave the central bundles in the root and travel to the periphery. Most, however, continue to the coronal pulp where they spread apart and branch profusely. Most of the branches end in the odontoblastic or subodontoblastic regions. In the crown there is a pronounced plexus of nerves beneath the odontoblasts (plexus of Raschkow). This plexus is not evident until after the tooth has erupted. Branches from the plexus pass into the odontoblast layer and form the marginal plexus between the odontoblast layer and the predentine. Other branches continue into the dentine to accompany odontoblast processes in the dentinal tubules.

Due to the presence of a rich innervation with large neural plexuses, a variety of neuropeptides found in the dental pulp is considerable and includes calcitonin gene-related peptide (CRGP), substance P, neuropeptide Y and vasoactive intestinal polypeptide. These molecules have important actions on blood vessels and on the inflammatory process, and in controlling the flow of sensory activity centrally, thus helping to maintain pulpal homeostasis. The most widely distributed and most significant is CRGP, a potent vasodilator and the major agent controlling blood flow locally in the periphery of the pulp. It may also have a role to play in initiating and controlling mineralized tissue secretion. Nerve growth factor (NGF) has also been identified in the peripheral pulp tissue; the expression of NGF and its receptor is increased during pulpal injury, where it may act as a chemoattractant for leukocytes. A range of other neuropeptides and transmitters has also been identified within the pulp; however, their roles are still not understood and are somewhat open to conjecture.

Pain

There is a belief that the only sensation elicited from pulp and dentine is that of pain. It is a generally held view that all pulpal afferents (even those supplied by Aβ fibres) are nociceptive and can only give rise to one type of sensation, that of pain. Pain and nociception are not synonymous:

- Pain is a subjective sensation and is defined as 'an unpleasant sensory and emotional experience associated with actual or potential tissue damage, or described in terms of such damage'.
- Nociception, on the other hand, describes a series of objective neuronal processes and is defined as the reception, conduction and central processing of noxious signals.

Nociceptors are essentially receptors that respond to harmful or potentially harmful (noxious) stimuli. Pain clearly can be a result of stimulation of nociceptors but so are some reflexes and changes in arousal state, and they do not lead to the organism sensing pain.

Neurophysiology of pain

Nociceptors are thought to be free nerve endings and appear to respond specifically to noxious heat, intense pressure or irritant chemicals, but not to innocuous stimuli such as warming, cooling or light touch. Nerve fibres innervating the head region arise from cell bodies in the trigeminal ganglion. There are considered to be three major classes of nociceptors: thermal, mechanical and polymodal:

- Thermal nociceptors, which are activated by extreme temperatures $> 45°C$ or $< 5°C$, are innervated by small myelinated Aδ fibres that conduct impulses at about 5–30 m s^{-1}.
- Mechanical nociceptors are activated by intense pressure applied to the tissues in which they lie and are also innervated by small myelinated Aδ fibres.
- Polymodal nociceptors are activated by high-intensity mechanical, chemical or thermal (both hot and cold) stimuli and are innervated by either Aδ fibres or unmyelinated C fibres with conduction velocities of less than 0.5–2 m s^{-1}.

In most parts of the body it is possible to evoke two distinctive pain sensations. A sharp, fast (first) pain is felt almost immediately, followed by a more prolonged aching, sometimes burning, slow (second) pain. The fast pain has been attributed to stimulation of the nociceptors innervated by the Aδ fibres, and the slow pain has been attributed to stimulation of the nociceptors innervated by the C fibres. The nerves that supply the tooth pulp are an exception and appear to be supplied by larger myelinated fibres in the Aβ range, with conduction velocities of between 30 and 60 m s^{-1}.

When damaged, tissues release inflammatory agents, chemicals that have effects on the blood vessels and nerves of the tissues. The effect on the blood vessel is to cause a vasodilatation and an increased permeability of the vessel. The effect on the nerves is either to excite the nociceptor nerve ending directly, or to sensitize the nociceptor fibres. Amongst these chemicals are K^+ ions, H^+ ions, serotonin, prostaglandins, adenosine, noradrenaline and various cytokines. Substances that activate nociceptors are termed algogenic. Activation of nociceptors can be effected directly by the stimulus itself or by the action of the released chemicals when the tissue is damaged. Sensitization of the nociceptor fibres leads to an activation of the receptor ending by stimuli that would not normally produce pain, a type of hyperaesthesia called allodynia. This sensitization is caused by the release of inflammatory agents and algogenic substances, when the tissues are either inflamed or damaged, in concentrations that are not necessarily sufficient to cause direct activation of the receptor, but enough to cause its depolarization just below threshold for stimulation of the receptor. When a seemingly innocuous stimulus is applied to the inflamed or damaged tissue, such as a gentle mechanical one, this causes an activation of the nociceptor, with the resulting impulses signalling a noxious stimulation.

Cell bodies of nociceptor neurones

The cell bodies of nociceptor neurones in the oral and facial regions are to be found in the trigeminal ganglion, and the central axons project via the trigeminal sensory root to synapse in the trigeminal spinal nucleus and, in particular, the subnucleus caudalis. Nociceptive neurones in the nucleus caudalis fall into two distinct types:

- Those that receive inputs specifically from nociceptors: the so-called nociceptive-specific cells
- A second group of cells that receive inputs from a wide range of receptors such as nociceptors, mechanoreceptors and thermoreceptors: the so-called nociceptive-non-specific cells.

It is thought that the nociceptive-specific neurones signal the presence and location of the noxious stimulus, whilst the nociceptive-non-specific neurones may grade the overall severity of the stimulus. There is evidence of primary afferent divergence and convergence within the nucleus caudalis onto second-order neurones, with each primary afferent branching and synapsing with several second-order neurones and each second-order neurone receiving inputs from a number of primary afferent fibres. These phenomena may explain why pain appears to radiate and come from a larger area than that injured or inflamed. Convergence of primary afferent neurones can also explain the phenomenon of referred pain, where pain appears to come from structures other than the injured or inflamed tissue.

Nociceptor pathways

From the subnucleus caudalis, axons from the second-order nociceptor neurones cross the midline and project via the trigeminothalamic tract to the ventrobasal nuclei of the contralateral thalamus. These neurones are thought to be directly involved with the sensation of pain. The neurones that are believed to be involved with emotion and motor responses to nociception project to the posterior and medial groups of thalamic nuclei either directly or via intermediate synapses in the reticular formation. Neurones from the ventrobasal nuclei project to the primary somatosensory cortex; other nociceptive neurones project to the secondary somatosensory cortex, the insula and the anterior cingulated cortex.

Gate control theory of pain

In nociception the transmitters involved in the first synaptic pathway include glutamate, substance P and CGRP. These substances are all excitatory but their influence can be modulated by an inhibitory control mechanism often referred to as gate control.

The basic principle behind the gate control theory of pain is that the signals transmitted via the pathways from first- to second-order neurones have to pass through a so-called gate, controlled by small adjacent cells (interneurones): these are either inhibited (closing the gate) or excited (opening the gate). In this way, the gate is fully closed, and therefore no pain is felt, or fully open, in which case the pain would be severe. In most cases the pain would probably fall

between these two extremes. These interneurones can have an inhibitory effect either by decreasing the release of the excitatory transmitter (a process called presynaptic inhibition), or by inhibiting the second-order neurone (a process called postsynaptic inhibition). Amongst the neurotransmitters reported to be released by these interneurones are γ-aminobutyric acid (GABA), glycine, and endogenous opioid peptides such as endorphins, encephalins and dynorphins. The activation of the interneurones is brought about by impulses from larger afferent nerves from the same neural segment of the body as the nociceptor, such as Aβ mechanoreceptor neurones, which are stimulated by touch or by impulses descending from higher centres of the brain in a process called descending inhibition. This gate control mechanism most probably can occur at all synaptic levels of the pain pathway. Descending inhibition can be from a number of areas of the brain and brain stem, such as the periaqueductal or periventricular grey matter and the raphe nuclei; the neurotransmitters involved are the monoamine transmitters, serotonin (5-HT) and noradrenaline.

Besides the inhibitory properties of the interneurones, which reduce the transmission of impulses at the first synapse in the nociceptive pathway, there is a phenomenon called 'wind-up'. This is when there is an increase in activity (facilitation), resulting in an increase in the strength and/or the duration of the resulting pain. Wind-up is due to repetitive activation of nociceptive C fibres, which brings about an enhanced response to subsequent activity in these fibres. It is brought about by an increased release of substance P from the presynaptic neurone or by the enhanced response of postsynaptic receptor sites for substance P and glutamate.

Dental pain

The stimuli that cause pain when applied to intact teeth include electrical currents and intense heating or cooling applied to the enamel. The stimuli that cause dental pain when applied to exposed dentine and/or pulp are much more varied and include, not only electrical current, heating and cooling, but also mechanical probing, drying, application of hypertonic solutions, hydrostatic pressure and, in pulp only, the application of algogenic chemicals. Some of these stimuli may directly stimulate the intradental nerves, but it is generally believed that most will excite the pulpal or dentinal nerves indirectly via a hydrodynamic mechanism. Stimuli that cause pain when applied to human dentine have been shown to increase fluid movement through dentine either by increasing fluid flow outwards from the pulp or by producing inward fluid flow towards the pulp. Both result in the generation of action potentials in intradental nerves. It would appear that intradental nerves are more easily excited by fluid flow outwards from the pulp than inwards towards the pulp. How this fluid flow excites the nociceptive nerve terminals is not yet fully understood, but it may involve mechanosensitive channels in the intratubular part of the nerve terminal; however, it is possible that the odontoblast itself may have a role in the transduction process.

Intense heating or cooling, electrical stimuli and the application of algogenic substances directly to pulp will probably act directly on the nerves in the inner dentine or pulp. It is assumed that transient pain arising from dentinal stimulation is mediated by Aβ and Aδ myelinated fibres when nerve endings have been activated via the hydrodynamic mechanism, as the effects are localized and the pain persists for the length of time the stimulus is applied. In the case of chronic pulpal inflammation and where the stimulus persists for hours, there are obvious changes in the haemodynamics of the pulp and in nerve excitability that can be attributed to the release of algogenic chemicals in the pulp. It is assumed that these chemicals stimulate pulpal afferent, unmyelinated C fibres and give rise to the persistent, less well localized, slow pain characteristic of nociceptor C fibre activation.

Age-related changes

A number of age-related changes are seen in the pulp:

- It gets smaller with age, as secondary dentine deposition continues throughout life.

- The older pulp is less vascular and, apparently, more fibrous than the young pulp.
- There are changes in composition of the ground substance so that, in older teeth, there is more hyaluronan and less chondroitin sulphate.
- The innervation is reduced.
- The pulp often mineralizes in the form of pulp stones. These may be localized as discrete pulp stones either singly or in small groups, or be diffusely scattered throughout the pulp. Pulp stones may resemble dentine in being, at least partially, tubular ('true' denticles) or resemble bone by having cells embedded within them. In some (lamellated pulp stones), accretion by layers is evident. Some larger pulp stones may be attached to the dentine.

Self-assessment: questions (Structure and composition of dentine)

True/false statements

Which of the following statements are true and which are false?

a. On a wet weight basis, dentine contains 70% inorganic material, 20% organic material and 10% water.

b. The hydroxyapatite crystallites in dentine are the same size as those in enamel.

c. The primary curvatures in dentine represent daily incremental lines.

d. The mature dentinal tubule contains an odontoblast process that passes from the pulp–dentine border to the enamel–dentine junction.

e. In demineralized sections, predentine stains differently from the rest of the (mineralized) dentine matrix.

f. Collagen fibrils in the circumpulpal dentine are oriented parallel to the dentinal tubules.

g. Peritubular dentine is hypomineralized compared to intertubular dentine.

h. Peritubular dentine increases in thickness with age.

i. Interglobular dentine results from incomplete fusion of calcospherites.

j. Nerves have not been identified in dentine.

k. Dentine phosphophoryn is a highly acidic protein unique to dentine.

l. The granular layer (of Tomes) at the cement–dentine border is an effect produced by terminal dilatations and branching of dentinal tubules.

m. Von Ebner lines are long-period incremental lines.

n. A dead tract occurs when the dentinal tubules in that region become completely obliterated by peritubular dentine.

o. Reactionary dentine is formed by newly differentiated odontoblast-like cells.

p. Regular secondary dentine may be demarcated from primary dentine by an Owen's line.

q. Reparative dentine closely resembles secondary dentine with a regular tubular structure.

r. Dentine sialoprotein is post-transcriptionally cleaved from the same gene product as dentine phosphophorin.

Extended matching questions

Theme: Dentine structure

Lead-in

Select the most appropriate option to answer items 1–6. Each option can be used once, more than once or not at all.

Item list

1. An incremental line reflecting a diurnal rhythm of dentine secretion during development
2. A structural feature that may be present separating primary and secondary dentine

3. Hyaline layer
4. Granular layer
5. Mantle dentine
6. Translucent dentine

Option list

A. A layer containing 20% type III collagen
B. The first-formed layer in root dentine
C. Andresen line
D. A layer where the collagen fibrils are orientated parallel to the enamel–dentinal junction
E. Owen's line
F. Von Ebner line
G. A region where the dentinal tubules show considerable branching and looping
H. A layer where the collagen fibrils are orientated perpendicular to the enamel–dentinal junction
I. A region where the tubules are completely occluded by peritubular dentine
J. A region where the odontoblasts have degenerated and the tubules remain empty
K. A layer formed by tertiary dentine
L. A primary curvature

Picture questions

Figure 13.1 (Courtesy of Professor M. M. Smith)

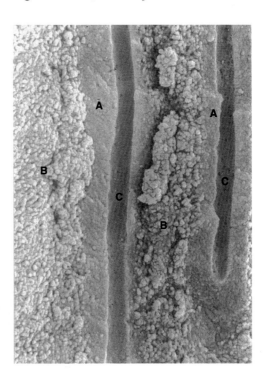

Self-assessment: questions (Structure and composition of dentine)

In this scanning electron micrograph of dentine:
a. Identify the features labelled A–C.
b. Where in the dentine is branching of the dentinal tubules particularly marked?
c. List the possible contents of a dentinal tubule.

Figure 13.2

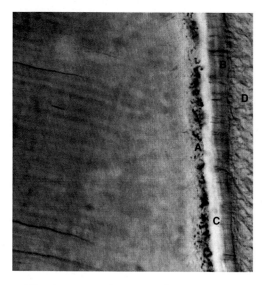

This is a ground section of a root in which part of the periodontal ligament (label D) has been retained.
a. Identify the features labelled A–C at the cement–dentine junction.
b. What is the approximate thickness of layer C?
c. Is there anything unusual about the mineralization of layer C?

Figure 13.3 (Courtesy of Professor A. G. S. Lumsden)

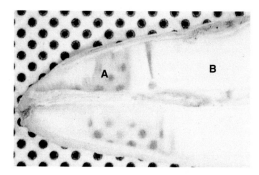

This micrograph is of a ground section of the root of a tooth immersed in water.
a. Is this section of a young or an old tooth?

b. Account for the difference in appearance between areas A and B.

Figure 13.4 (Courtesy of Mr R. V. Hawkins)

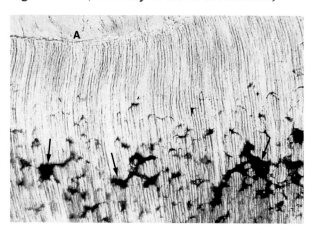

This is a ground section of outer dentine in the crown, a section of the enamel–dentine junction (A) being visible.
a. Identify the dark areas (arrows).
b. Account for their formation.
c. Will there be any peritubular dentine in these areas in older patients?
d. Name one condition in which this feature may be particularly conspicuous.

Figure 13.5 (Courtesy of Dr B. A. W. Brown)

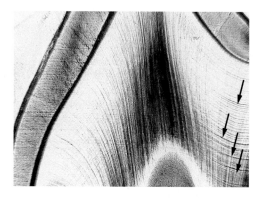

In this ground section of the crown of a tooth:
a. Identify the horizontally disposed lines arrowed, indicating their approximate distance apart.
b. Do these lines have the same spacing in primary and secondary dentine?
c. How would you account for the fact that a carious lesion reaching the enamel–dentine junction in a

Self-assessment: questions (Structure and composition of dentine)

tooth which has just erupted into the mouth is likely to be associated with a pulpal response, whilst such a lesion in the tooth of an aged individual will often be without a pulpal response?

Figure 13.6

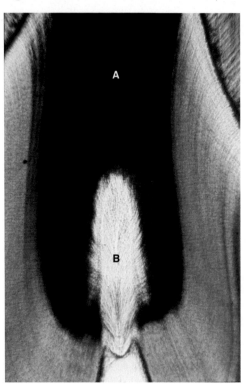

This is a micrograph of a longitudinal section of the crown of a tooth mounted in Canada balsam.
  a. Is this a ground or a demineralized section?
  b. Identify zone A; account for its appearance.
  c. Identify zone B.
  d. What might you expect to see on the occlusal surface of this tooth?

Figure 13.7 (Courtesy of Professor N. W. Johnson)

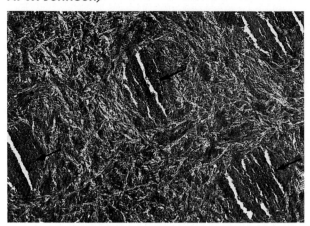

This is an electron micrograph of a cross-section of dentine bordering a carious lesion.
  a. Explain what it demonstrates.

Essay questions

1. List the three main hypotheses proposed to explain dentine sensitivity, indicating arguments for and against each one.
2. How is the structure of dentine related to its functions?
3. What are the major proteoglycans found in dentine? Explain how they may function in dentine mineralization.

Self-assessment: answers (Structure and composition of dentine)

True/false answers

a. **True**. Thus, dentine has more inorganic material than bone or dental cementum, but less than dental enamel. By volume, dentine has 50% inorganic material.

b. **False**. The crystallites of enamel are much larger in all dimensions. This is related to the fact that the organic matrix of enamel is largely removed during development, whereas collagen in dentine remains behind.

c. **False**. Primary curvatures are broad, sinuous curvatures of the dentinal tubules produced by the odontoblasts as they migrate inwards and become crowded during dentinogenesis. The tubules are relatively straight in the root.

d. **False**. There is still controversy regarding the extent of the odontoblast processes within the dentinal tubules. This relates mainly to the difficult technical problem of fixing and preserving the very long, delicate process in the tubule. Ultrastructural evidence suggests that cell processes gradually withdraw from the peripheral dentine (i.e. nearest the enamel–dentine junction) and come to occupy only about the inner third of the tubule in the adult.

e. **True**. This is due to biochemical differences that occur at the mineralizing front. A similar feature occurs in osteoid and precementum.

f. **False**. The collagen fibrils in circumpulpal dentine are oriented perpendicular to the long axis of the tubules.

g. **False**. Peritubular dentine is hypermineralized compared to intertubular dentine. It also differs from intertubular dentine in that it has no collagen.

h. **True**, although there is variation. A relationship also exists between the amount of peritubular dentine formed and the degree of attrition.

i. **True**. Calcospherites are the 'circular' form of mineralization that occurs within much of the dentine. Where regions between adjacent calcospherites fail to mineralize, hypomineralized interglobular dentine is seen.

j. **False**. The presence of sensory intratubular axons has been confirmed by studies involving axonal transport of radioactive amino acids injected initially into the trigeminal ganglion. They are more numerous over the cusps or incisal edges of teeth, and little evident in root dentine.

k. **True**. Indeed, it is said to be the most acid protein known and is thought to be involved in mineralization.

l. **True**. The granular layer has also been related to the presence of minute interglobular areas produced as a result of incomplete mineralization. It is not seen in demineralized sections.

m. **False**. Von Ebner lines are short-period lines that reflect the presence of a diurnal rhythm. They appear perpendicular to the long axis of the dentinal tubule and are about 3 μm apart.

n. **False**. Dead tracts occur because of the loss of the odontoblast processes within tubules, which then are sealed at their ends, the tubules being empty. Obliteration of the tubules with peritubular dentine results in translucent/sclerotic dentine.

o. **False**. Reactionary tertiary dentine is formed by odontoblasts that survive the initial trauma.

p. **True**. An Owen's line is the result of a coincidence of secondary curvatures.

q. **False**. Reparative dentine is atubular and dysplastic in structure and is an irregular repair tissue. It is secreted by a new generation of odontoblast-like cells derived from pulpal progenitor cells and has been known as osteodentine in other texts.

r. **True**. DSP is post-transcriptionally cleaved from the DSPP gene. The other product is DPP.

Extended matching answers

Item 1 = Option F. The von Ebner lines run perpendicular to the longitudinal axis of the dentinal tubules and are approximately 3 μm apart.

Item 2 = Option E. An Owen's line results from the coincidence of secondary curvatures in adjacent dentinal tubules.

Item 3 = Option B. During its development, the hyaline layer is thought to contain enamel-related proteins derived from the epithelial root sheath; it also undergoes delayed mineralization thought to improve the bonding between cementum and dentine.

Item 4 = Option G. An alternative explanation to account for the granular layer is that it represents a zone of deficient mineralization in the form of numerous regions of interglobular dentine.

Item 5 = Option H. Due to the orientation of its collagen fibrils, mantle dentine can be distinguished from circumpulpal dentine by the use of polarized light microscopy.

Item 6 = Option I. The blockage of the lumen of the dentinal tubules commences near the root apex and the amount formed is a useful guide to the age of a tooth.

Picture answers

Figure 13.1

a. A = peritubular dentine. B = intertubular dentine. C = dentinal tubule.

b. Branching of the dentinal tubules is particularly marked near the enamel–dentine junction.

Self-assessment: answers (Structure and composition of dentine)

c. The dentinal tubule may contain: an odontoblast process, a terminal sensory axon, the dendritic process of an antigen-presenting cell, dentinal fluid and an organic sheath (lamina limitans). In addition, peritubular dentine may be considered as an addition to the wall of the original dentinal tubule.

Figure 13.2

a. A = granular layer (of Tomes). B = cementum. C = hyaline layer.
b. Label C, the hyaline layer, is approximately 10–20 µm. In the crown, it is continuous with the mantle layer.
c. The hyaline layer does not mineralize from its outer surface inwards. There is delayed mineralization. Thus, it initially starts to mineralize a few microns in from its surface, enabling the outermost few microns to slowly mineralize outwards towards the cementum. This allows for close bonding of the hyaline layer with the cementum.

Figure 13.3

a. This section is obtained from an old tooth as the apex of the root shows a conspicuous area of translucent dentine (A).
b. In association with physiological ageing, the dentinal tubules, especially in the region of the root apex (zone A), become occluded by peritubular dentine. The contents of the tubules in this region acquire the same refractive index as the intertubular dentine. When a ground section is placed in water (which has a different refractive index to dentine), areas of affected dentine at the root apex appear translucent (as there are no patent tubules for the water to fill) compared with the more opaque normal dentine (zone B) cervically (whose patent tubules become filled with the water).

Figure 13.4

a. Interglobular dentine.
b. A considerable proportion of the mineral in dentine is normally laid down in the form of globules, the calcospherites. Where the calcospherites do not completely fuse, hypocalcified areas persist between the globules (particularly in the coronal, circumpulpal dentine close to the enamel–dentine junction). Hence the particular shape of the boundaries of interglobular dentine.
c. No. Peritubular dentine does not form in regions of interglobular dentine, these regions remaining unmineralized.

d. Conspicuous areas of interglobular dentine are seen in conditions in which the process of mineralization or collagen formation is affected, such as hypophosphatasia, renal rickets, dentine dysplasias and Ehlers–Danlos syndrome.

Figure 13.5

a. Andresen lines, which are of the order of about 20 µm apart.
b. As secondary dentine is formed more slowly, the lines in it will be closer together.
c. In the young tooth, the dentinal tubules are open and without much peritubular dentine. This, together with the large size of the pulp (and relative thinness of the dentine), would enable noxious agents from an early, carious lesion to pass along the dentinal tubules and into the dental pulp with minimum delay. In the aged tooth, the thickness of the dentine and the obliteration of tubules by peritubular dentine would deny access to such noxious agents in the early lesion.

Figure 13.6

a. Because of the general lack of staining, the presence of enamel (at the extreme upper left and right margins of the dentine) and the empty pulp chamber shown at the central lower margin of the picture, we can deduce that this is a ground section.
b. A = dead tract. It is thought that in those regions where the odontoblasts die (usually because of noxious stimuli), the ends of the associated dentinal tubules become sealed by calcific material. The blackened appearance seen in routine ground sections may be related to the retention of air in the 'emptied' tubules, which have not been penetrated by the viscous mounting medium.
c. B = tertiary dentine. This can be considered as a protective response of a vital pulp to seal off the dead tract. In this site, the newly formed dentine has a tubular structure, though this may be less regular than normal dentine. It is therefore likely that this dentine is reactionary tertiary dentine that has formed from surviving odontoblasts.
d. Dead tracts are often found beneath areas of attrition. Therefore one might find a region of exposed dentine on the crown of this tooth associated with considerable attrition.

Figure 13.7

a. The dentinal tubules have become completely occluded by mineral deposition (arrows). In such

Self-assessment: answers (Structure and composition of dentine)

regions, tubules are not evident in routine ground sections, producing a tissue known as sclerotic dentine. It is analogous to the translucent dentine seen in the root. However, the mineral components may be slightly different, as salivary components may have access to the tubules in sclerotic dentine.

Outline essay answers

Question 1

Three main hypotheses have been put forward to account for its sensitivity, implicating:

- nerves in dentine
- the odontoblast processes
- fluid movements in the dentinal tubules (hydrodynamic theory).

Arguments against the view that pain is due to direct stimulation of nerves in the dentine relate to the presence of nerves in the inner part of the dentine only, and their absence in the outer parts. In addition, the application of local anaesthetics to the surface of dentine does not abolish the sensitivity and nerves only reach dentine after tooth eruption.

Referring to the second hypothesis, there is no physiological evidence to date that indicates that the odontoblast process is analogous to a nerve fibre and can similarly conduct impulses pulpwards. Indeed, it has a low membrane potential. Furthermore, the odontoblast process may not extend to the enamel–dental junction; nor is the application of substances designed to prevent transmission of such impulses effective in eliminating pain. Odontoblasts or their processes have not been shown to be synaptically connected to nerve fibres.

The most plausible hypothesis to explain the transmission of sensory stimuli suggests that all effective stimuli applied to dentine cause fluid movement through the dentinal tubules, and that this movement is sufficient to depolarize nerve endings in the inner parts of tubules, at the pulp–predentine junction and in the subodontoblastic neural plexus. Some stimuli, such as cooling, evaporation, hypertonic solutions, decreased hydrostatic pressure and drying, would tend to cause fluid movement outwards, while others, such as heating and mechanical and increased hydrostatic pressure, would cause movement inwards. Movement in either direction would mechanically distort the terminals, fluid movement outwards resulting in greater stimulation. These stimuli have been shown to cause such fluid movement in vitro. Chemicals (in strong solution) and thermal stimuli induce a response much more quickly than can be explained by conduction or diffusion. This, too, is consistent with the hydrodynamic hypothesis. In animal experiments, however, the response of intradental nerves to chemical stimuli is often slow and

may be more readily explained by diffusion. It may be that both 'direct' and 'hydrodynamic' mechanisms operate, but that the hydrodynamic force predominates whenever there is pulpal inflammation and a lowering in threshold of intrapulpal nerves to the small mechanical forces generated by fluid flow.

Question 2

The two main functions of dentine are to resist wear at the surface of the tooth and to protect the soft tissues of the dental pulp. To resist wear during mastication when the covering enamel may be lost, dentine presents a hard surface due to the presence of mineral in the form of hydroxyapatite crystals. These comprise 70% by weight of the tissue. If it were entirely composed of mineral, dentine would be brittle and liable to fracture. To strengthen it, it is provided with a matrix of collagen fibrils throughout the tissue, around (and within) which hydroxyapatite crystals are deposited. The presence of collagen also provides the dentine with a degree of flexibility that complements enamel during loading, as enamel is extremely hard but lacks any flexibility. Indeed, the highly ordered structure of dentine comprising the tusks of elephants (and known as ivory) was so perfectly elastic as to be the prime choice for the manufacture of snooker balls.

The presence of tubules within the dentine makes the tissue permeable. The tubules contain odontoblast processes and nerves. The cell bodies of the odontoblasts line the predentine surface of the pulp. Dentine is deposited continually throughout life so that any dentine lost peripherally can be compensated for by new dentine formation at its pulpal surface. The presence of vital structures within the tubules may provide some signalling for this process.

Although it might seem that patent tubules would allow the rapid access of toxic agents into the dental pulp, dentinal tubules soon narrow and may eventually be completely occluded by the formation of peritubular (intratubular) dentine. This differs from the adjacent intertubular dentine by being hypermineralized and lacking collagen.

Dentine is exquisitely sensitive, the possible mechanisms for which are discussed in the previous question. This property is related to structural components within the dentine, such as dentinal fluid, nerves and the odontoblast processes, although the dental pulp must also participate. However, it is not clear how this sensory modality can be perceived in terms of function.

Trauma, in the form of severe attrition or dental caries, may result in the formation of tertiary dentine at the pulpal surface. Tertiary reparative dentine is formed by newly differentiated odontoblast-like cells that are derived from stem cells in the dental pulp. As dentine contains bound growth factors, such as transforming growth factors and

Self-assessment: answers (Structure and composition of dentine)

bone morphogenetic proteins, it is possible that these bio-active molecules could be released into the pulp and contribute towards the stimulation of stem cells.

The presence of dentinal fluid under positive pressure may provide a defence against toxins produced during dental caries trying to pass through dentine to infect the dental pulp.

Question 3

The major proteoglycans in dentine are decorin and big-lycan. In predentine they are rich in dermatan sulphate (DS) side-chains and inhibit the formation of mineral, but as predentine is remodelled, these species are replaced by the secretion of chondroitin sulphate (CS)-rich deco-rin and biglycan, which facilitate mineral deposition. Versican is another proteoglycan present within the pre-dentine and has a hydroxyapatite-binding region. Versi-can has a high proportion of glycosaminoglycan (GAG) chains attached to core protein and is said to be involved in the inhibition of mineralization. There appear to be two pools of proteoglycans synthesized in association with dentinogenesis. One pool (DS-rich) is associated with the predentine and is inhibitory with respect to mineraliza-tion, and another (CS-rich) is associated with mineral-ized dentine. Those synthesized within the predentine are enzymatically degraded or remodelled as predentine matures. The second pool of CS decorin (and biglycan) secreted at the mineralization front is transported intra-cellularly up the odontoblast process and, in general, the proteoglycans are found in levels lower than those in predentine. They are distributed in mineralized con-nective tissues interfibrally and associated with the gap zones of the collagen fibres; they appear to be involved in the transport of calcium and phosphate to gap zones in the collagen fibrils. The very acidic glycoproteins, pres-ent within dentine only and not predentine, have a high affinity for calcium and hydroxyapatite surfaces and may induce hydroxyapatite nucleation and control crystal growth. This acidic nature of the glycoproteins in dentine appears to be important in regulating hydroxyapatite crystal nucleation and growth.

Self-assessment: questions (Dentine development)

True/false statements

Which of the following statements are true and which are false?

a. Both the dentine and the dental pulp originate from the dental follicle of the tooth germ.

b. Dentinogenesis commences immediately after amelogenesis.

c. The first-formed dentine, the mantle dentine, may contain some components derived from subodontoblastic cells.

d. The cells forming the dentine and pulp are mesodermal in origin.

e. Unlike the fully formed dental pulp, the developing dental pulp has little glycosaminoglycan (GAG).

f. The pattern of innervation of the dental pulp is established during the cap stage of tooth development.

g. Mineralization of dentine occurs initially by the budding off of matrix vesicles from the odontoblast cell.

h. Like enamel, maturation of dentine commences when the full thickness of the dentine has been formed.

i. There is both a spherical and a linear pattern of mineralization of dentine.

j. Dentinogenesis imperfecta is an autosomal dominant genetic condition.

k. Predentine maintains a constant thickness throughout life.

l. Levels of dentine phosphophoryn are highest in predentine.

m. To reach the mineralizing front, hydroxyapatite crystals pass through the odontoblast cells.

n. A pool of chondroitin sulphate proteoglycans is secreted at the mineralization front and guides mineral deposition.

Extended matching questions

Theme: Dentine formation

Lead-in

Select the most appropriate option to answer items 1–5. Each option can be used once, more than once or not at all.

Item list

1. Hyaline layer
2. Predentine
3. Circumpulpal dentine
4. Matrix vesicle
5. Calcospherite

Option list

A. It stains differently compared with the organic component of mineralized dentine

B. Its collagen fibrils are aligned parallel to the enamel–dentine junction

C. It contains enamel-related proteins produced by epithelial root sheath cells

D. It initiates the process of mineralization in secondary dentine

E. It is budded off from odontoblasts

F. It can be visualized in light microscopy using polarized light

G. Its collagen fibrils have a mean diameter of 5 nm

H. Its collagen fibrils are aligned parallel to the long axis of dentinal tubules

I. Its odontoblast processes contain Golgi material

J. It may contain interglobular dentine

K. Its crystallites are approximately 70 nm thick

Picture questions

Figure 13.8

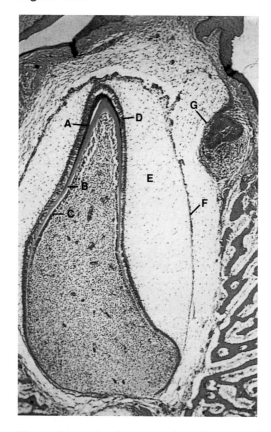

Pictured is a developing tooth at the late bell stage of development, stained with Masson's trichrome.

a. Identify the red tissue (A), the blue tissue (B), and the cell layers C–F.

b. Account for the difference in the staining properties of A and B.

c. Identify structure G.

Self-assessment: questions (Dentine development)

Figure 13.9

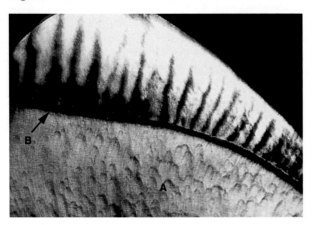

a. Some developmental features can be seen in the dentine of a fully formed tooth viewed under polarized light. Identify the rounded/arcade outlines (A) and the dark line (B) and explain their significance.

Figure 13.10 (Courtesy of Professor M. C. Dean)

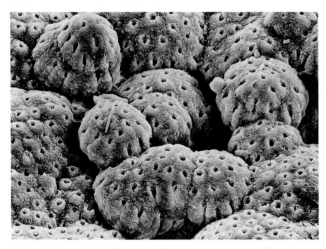

a. This is a scanning electron micrograph of the surface of dentine after it has been treated with hypochlorite. What is it demonstrating?

Figure 13.11

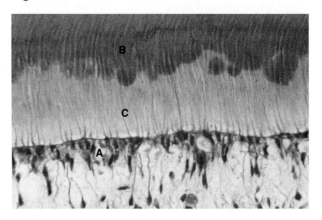

a. Identify the features of the pulpodentinal complex labelled A–C.
b. Why do layer A and layer B stain differently?
c. How does dentine initially mineralize?

Figure 13.12 (Courtesy of Dr B. A. W. Brown)

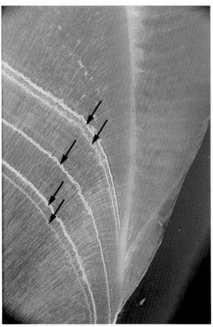

This is a ground section of a crown viewed in fluorescent light.
a. Account for the appearance of the lines arrowed.

Essay questions

1. Compare and contrast enamel and dentine formation.
2. How do structures seen in a ground longitudinal section of dentine relate to the development of the tissue?
3. What are the main features of dentine formation in the root that are not seen in the crown?

Self-assessment: answers (Dentine development)

True/false answers

a. **False**. They both arise from the dental papilla. This partly explains why some oral biologists refer to the two tissues collectively as the pulpodentinal complex.

b. **False**. Dentinogenesis precedes amelogenesis. Indeed, it is thought that the initially formed dentine has an inductive influence, resulting in the differentiation of ameloblasts from the pre-ameloblasts of the internal enamel epithelium.

c. **True**. As the odontoblasts are not yet fully mature, traces of components from the underlying dental papilla (such as type III collagen) may pass between the cells into the mantle dentine.

d. **False**. The dental papilla is mainly ectomesenchymal (neural crest) in origin.

e. **False**. In the early stages of pulpal development, the ground substance has a high GAG content relative to that in the mature tooth. The GAG level increases until the time of eruption and then decreases. The chondroitin sulphates are the main GAGs during development, with little hyaluronan. This balance is reversed in the mature pulp.

f. **False**. Although nerves are present close to the tooth germ from the very earliest stages of development, they do not enter the dental papilla until later. The final pattern is not established until root formation is complete.

g. **True**. These vesicles contain all the necessary factors (e.g. alkaline phosphatase, calcium-binding proteins) to allow the first minerals to be formed inside them.

h. **False**. Dentine maturation is obtained soon after a predentine layer is formed. The predentine layer may vary from 10 μm to 40 μm in thickness.

i. **True**. The outline of the mineralization front in dentine is often seen as a combination of both types of mineralization.

j. **True**. Dentinogenesis imperfecta is associated with 'opalescent' dentine and rapid obliteration of the pulp chambers and canals. There is often much attrition and the condition is generalized across all teeth in the dentition. The disease is not sex-linked and, when present in one parent, is transmitted by chance to about half the offspring.

k. **False**. The thickness of predentine is related to the speed of dentine formation. It is thus likely to be thicker in young teeth where the speed of formation is rapid, and thinner in the teeth of older patients where the speed of formation is slower.

l. **False**. Dentine phosphophoryn (thought to be important in mineralization) is transported along the odontoblast process, bypassing the predentine, and is deposited at the mineralizing front.

m. **False**. Calcium and other elements pass separately through (or between) the odontoblasts in their ionic state. As calcium is potentially toxic to cells, the odontoblast cell possesses various mechanisms to transport this element through the cell without causing harm.

n. **True**. CS proteoglycans are highly acidic and have a high affinity for calcium. They are thought to direct mineral deposition and are secreted by odontoblasts at the mineralization front only.

Extended matching answers

Item 1 = Option C. The presence of enamel-related proteins during normal root dentine formation underlies the reason for applying similar proteins to root surfaces in attempts to improve the success rate of periodontal regeneration.

Item 2 = Option A. This difference in staining is the result of biochemical changes occurring at the mineralizing front, involving the addition of new biochemical molecules and the degradation of others.

Item 3 = Option J. These areas of interglobular dentine are commonly present in outer dentine. They may be significantly increased in pathological conditions affecting mineralization, such as hypophosphataemia.

Item 4 = Option E. The matrix vesicles have many molecules favouring the initiation of mineralization within them, such as alkaline phosphatase and calcium-binding proteins.

Item 5 = Option F. Due to the radial orientation of the enamel crystallites in calcospherites, the extent of this pattern of dentine mineralization can be distinguished from the linear form by viewing a ground section in polarized light.

Picture answers

Figure 13.8

a. A = enamel matrix. B = dentine matrix. C = odontoblast layer. D = ameloblast layer. E= stellate reticulum. F= external enamel epithelium.

b. Unlike the adult condition, developing enamel matrix is retained in demineralized sections because of its higher organic content. The two tissues stain differently due to their different compositions, dentine being mainly collagenous, while enamel matrix consists of enamel proteins (mainly amelogenins and non-amelogenins).

c. Permanent tooth bud.

Figure 13.9

a. Polarizing microscopy can reveal differences in the orientation of collagen and hydroxyapatite crystals. The rounded/arcade outlines (A) indicate the radial orientation of hydroxyapatite crystals found in

Self-assessment: answers (Dentine development)

calcospherites, while the dark line (B) identifies mantle dentine, the first-formed dentine which, in polarized light, shows a birefringence different from the circumpulpal dentine and thus indicates different collagen fibre orientations. The collagen fibrils in mantle dentine are oriented perpendicular to the enamel–dentine junction, while those in circumpulpal dentine are oriented parallel to the enamel–dentine junction.

Figure 13.10

a. The application of hypochlorite removes the organic material (predentine) covering the mineralizing dentine. That it is dentine is evident from the presence of the numerous tubules viewed in cross-section. The tubules are gathered together as spherical clusters, indicating that we are viewing numerous calcospherites at the mineralizing front of developing dentine.

Figure 13.11

a. A = odontoblast layer. B = predentine. C = circumpulpal dentine.
b. The difference in staining properties between dentine and predentine in decalcified sections occurs because, at the time of mineralization, there is a modification of the composition of the organic matrix.
c. The first-formed dentine (mantle dentine) mineralizes within matrix vesicles budded off from the odontoblast.

Figure 13.12

a. This is a section of the crown from a patient who, due to illness, has received five separate injections of tetracycline. This drug is taken up and then localized at the mineralizing front of dentine (arrows) on each occasion, which can be visualized using fluorescence microscopy. Many other markers can be incorporated into the mineralizing front, such as alizarin red, as well as autographic techniques (using tritiated glycine or proline that becomes incorporated into developing collagen).

Outline essay answers

Question 1

The main features to be mentioned are as follows:

- There are reciprocal interactions between enamel- and dentine-forming cells during development.
- Dentinogenesis and amelogenesis both show evidence of phasic deposition, indicated by the presence of short- and long-period incremental lines.
- Both enamel and dentine formation result in the production of a repeatable unit structure: in enamel the prism, and in dentine the tubule.

- The forming cells, odontoblasts and ameloblasts, are both columnar in shape and present features of protein-synthesizing and secreting cells (e.g. rough endoplasmic reticulum, Golgi material).
- The forming cells both produce processes, although the odontoblast process is left behind in the dentine to occupy the tubule. The Tomes process of the ameloblast remains at the mineralizing enamel front and is responsible for producing the prismatic structure.
- Both processes produce a tissue composed of calcium hydroxyapatite crystallites, an organic matrix and water, although the quantities vary between the two tissues. The organic matrix of dentine is principally collagen, which is little changed during formation. However, the organic matrix of enamel is comprised of unique enamel proteins that undergo degradation and are largely lost during the maturation of enamel. In this manner, enamel reaches a higher degree of mineralization and its crystals are larger.
- There is a lag period between the initial deposition of dentine matrix and its mineralization, resulting in a layer of predentine at the dentine–pulp interface. Enamel matrix is mineralized immediately, so there is no equivalent 'pre-enamel' layer.
- As odontoblasts are retained at the periphery of the dental pulp, dentine is formed throughout life. Enamel, being limited to the crown, has completed its formation well before the tooth erupts, although some post-eruptive maturation occurs in the surface layers as a result of ionic exchange with saliva. The ameloblast layer is lost from the surface of enamel when the tooth erupts.
- Whereas enamel has a more or less uniform structure, apart from non-prismatic zones, dentine shows more variation to produce regions such as the mantle, granular and hyaline layers, and peritubular and translucent dentine.
- Being vital, sensitive and reactive, dentine can respond to external stimuli, producing sclerotic dentine, dead tracts and tertiary dentine. Enamel, being non-vital, shows little response, though small initial carious lesions may remineralize under suitable conditions.

Question 2

The basic unit of dentine seen in a ground section is the dentinal tubule. As odontoblasts at the periphery of the pulp migrate pulpwards (centripetally), they trail behind them the odontoblast processes. From their distal surfaces, the odontoblasts secrete the organic matrix of dentine around the processes. This matrix consists of collagen fibrils and the associated ground substance, and constitutes the predentine layer. In the initial mantle layer, the collagen fibrils are oriented perpendicular to the enamel–dentine junction. This contrasts with the rest of the circumpulpal dentine where the collagen is oriented parallel to

Self-assessment: answers (Dentine development)

the enamel–dentine junction. Thus, the mantle layer can be distinguished if a ground section of the crown is viewed in polarized light. When this predentine matures, mineralization occurs, resulting in tubule formation. In mantle dentine, mineralization is initiated in matrix vesicles. The odontoblasts in the crown migrate centrally (centripetally) and gradually occupy a smaller surface area; in doing so, they trace out a sinusoidal path, giving the primary curvatures of the tubules. In the root, the path of the migrating odontoblast is straighter so that the tubules are more horizontal. Smaller-scale undulations along the odontoblast process give rise to the secondary curvatures.

The first-formed dentine in the crown, mantle dentine, is about 20 μm thick and differs from the rest of the dentine (circumpulpal dentine). The immature odontoblasts at this stage have a number of smaller branching processes, rather than a single main one, accounting for the rich branching in the mantle dentine.

The first-formed dentine in the root also differs from the rest of the underlying dentine. The retreating odontoblasts in the outermost layer (10–20 μm thick) do not initially trail odontoblast processes behind, so that this layer appears relatively structureless and is termed the hyaline layer. Following formation of the hyaline layer, the odontoblast cell bodies trail behind them their odontoblast processes, which initially show considerable looping and present numerous dilations. When the dentine matrix mineralizes around these processes, the effect is seen as the granular layer.

Dentine mineralizes either along a linear front or in the form of small spherical clusters, the calcospherites. In calcospherites, the calcium hydroxyapatite crystallites are arranged radially. If a ground section is viewed in polarized light, the calcospheritic nature of mineral development is readily seen. Where calcospherites do not completely fuse together, the unmineralized matrix between the calcospherites can be seen as areas of interglobular dentine.

Dentine formation is not a continuous and homogeneous process. It shows periodic phases of activity and rest (i.e. it is incremental in nature). The dentine formed in different phases of activity possesses a slightly different structure related to features such as collagen and crystallite orientation. This results in structural lines within the tissue running somewhat transverse to the longitudinal axis of the tubules. The short-period lines have a periodicity of about 4 μm and are termed von Ebner lines, while the long-period lines have a periodicity of about 20–30 μm and are called Andresen lines. Teeth mineralizing at birth show an exaggerated line representing the dentine formed during the first few days after birth when nutrition is disturbed. Although evidence of some incremental lines can sometimes be seen in normal transmitted light, they can be more readily seen in polarized light.

After root completion, which normally occurs about 3 years after the permanent teeth erupt, secondary dentine formation occurs at a slightly slower rate compared with primary dentine. At the site of separation there is often a coincidence of secondary curvatures that produces a line known as an Owen's line evident in ground section.

With time, peritubular dentine is deposited, narrowing the lumen of the dentinal tubule. In the apical region of the root, the tubules may be completely filled with peritubular dentine. If a ground section of such a tooth is placed in water, the affected area becomes translucent (translucent dentine).

Question 3

The basic process of root dentinogenesis does not differ fundamentally from coronal dentinogenesis. However, differences are seen in the early stages, with the formation of the hyaline and granular layers. Initial collagen deposition does not begin immediately against the basal lamina of the epithelial cells of the root sheath. The space between the initial collagen and the epithelial cells becomes filled with an amorphous ground substance and a fine, fibrillar, non-collagenous material that appears to be formed from the root sheath (and may thus be a form of enamel matrix). These elements form a hyaline layer which is approximately 15 μm thick. The initial collagen fibres deposited in the root lie approximately parallel/oblique to the cement–dentine junction. This contrasts with the mantle dentine in the crown, where the collagen fibres are deposited perpendicular to the enamel–dentine junction. Odontoblasts in the root differ slightly from those in the crown, developing several fine branches which loop in 'umbrella' fashion. This gives rise to a granular layer (of Tomes), although a large part of this is also thought to be due to the presence of many small, uncalcified, interglobular areas. The different character of peripheral root dentine presumably relates to the difference between the cells of the internal enamel epithelium (which in the crown will differentiate and continue as ameloblasts) and the cells of the root sheath (which lose their continuity soon after dentinogenesis has begun). The loss of continuity of the epithelial cells results in larger numbers of interglobular areas and possibly also in the incorporation of some epithelial remnants in the peripheral dentine. Root dentine forms at a slightly slower rate than coronal dentine. Its pattern of mineralization is similar, although its initial calcospherites are smaller and its interglobular areas are more numerous. In general, mineralization of root dentine proceeds as a continuation of that in the crown, although in multirooted teeth separate areas of mineralization may occur. As the root odontoblasts trace out a straighter path in migrating inwards, the distinct primary curvatures seen in the crown are not evident.

Self-assessment: questions (Dental pulp)

True/false statements

Which of the following statements are true and which are false?

a. The pulps of deciduous teeth are relatively larger than those in permanent teeth.
b. The only sensation appreciated from the pulp is pain.
c. With age, the odontoblasts lining the pulp–dentine border become pseudostratified.
d. Lymphatic vessels in the pulp are readily visualized.
e. Pulp stones have a tubular, dentine-like appearance.
f. The majority of nerves entering the pulp are myelinated.
g. The majority of unmyelinated nerve fibres in the pulp are autonomic fibres controlling blood vessels.
h. Tissue fluid pressures in the pulp are low.
i. The pulp may be considered a soft, dense, fibrous connective tissue.
j. Approximately 40% of collagen in the pulp is type II.
k. Dendrites of antigen-presenting cells in the pulp may be present within dentinal tubules.
l. Calcitonin gene-related peptide (CGRP) is produced by sensory nerves of the dental pulp.

Extended matching questions

Theme: Dental pulp

Lead-in

Select the most appropriate option to answer items 1–6. Each option can be used once, more than once or not at all.

Item list
1. Type III collagen
2. Myelinated nerve fibres
3. Dendritic antigen-presenting cells
4. Pulpal fibroblasts
5. Pulp tissue fluid pressure
6. Capillaries in the pulp

Option list
A. Comprises about 10% of pulp collagen
B. The majority are Aβ fibres (diameter 6–12 µm)
C. They form a pseudostratified layer in the crown of the aged pulp
D. This pressure is comparatively high compared with most other connective tissues
E. They synthesize both collagen and non-collagenous proteins
F. Their processes may enter the dentinal tubules
G. Their cells stain for cytokeratins
H. This pressure is low compared with most other connective tissues
I. Comprises about 40% of pulp collagen
J. Their walls show some fenestrations

K. Like the periodontal ligament, they show high amounts of rough endoplasmic reticulum indicating a rapid turnover of collagen
L. Their cell bodies lie in the trigeminal ganglion

Theme: Pain

Lead-in

Select the most appropriate option to answer items 1–6. Each option can be used once, more than once or not at all.

Item list
1. Cell bodies of nociceptive neurons from the oral and facial region are to be found in the
2. Primary afferent nociceptive neurones diverge and converge on to second-order neurones in the
3. Second-order nociceptive neurones project to the contralateral thalamus via the
4. Nociceptive neurones from the ventrobasal nuclei of the thalamus project to the
5. The nociceptive non-specific cells are to be found in the
6. Second-order nociceptive neurones project to the

Option list
A. Primary somatosensory cortex
B. Trigeminal main sensory nucleus
C. Spinothalamic tract
D. Subnucleus caudalis
E. Trigeminal spinal nucleus
F. Mesencephalic nucleus
G. Trigeminal ganglion
H. Ventrobasal nuclei of the thalamus
I. Insula
J. Trigeminothalamic tract
K. Secondary somatosensory cortex
L. Orbitofrontal cortex

Self-assessment: questions (Dental pulp)

Picture questions

Figure 13.13

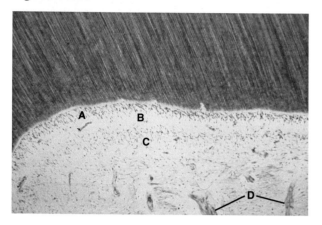

a. Identify the features of the dental pulp labelled A–D.
b. What are the main features of an odontoblast?
c. What types of nerve are found in the pulp?

Figure 13.14 (Courtesy of Dr J. Potts)

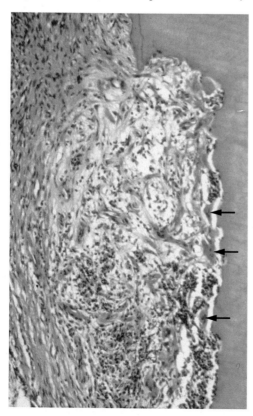

a. What process is occurring in the pulp shown here?

Figure 13.15

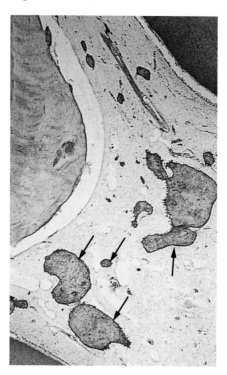

In this micrograph of the pulp:
a. Is this a ground or a demineralized section? State your reasons.
b. Identify the structures in the pulp that are arrowed.
c. How would you classify such structures?
d. Would you expect to see these structures on radiographs, and can they produce any symptoms?

Self-assessment: questions (Dental pulp)

Figure 13.16

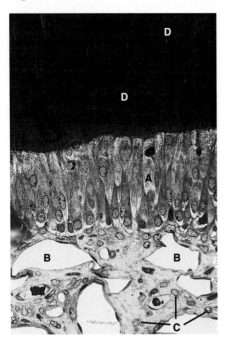

In this micrograph of the pulp:
  a. Identify the structures labelled A–D.
  b. Is this more likely to be a young or an old tooth?
  c. Are the structures labelled B typical of those found in other soft connective tissues?

Essay questions

1. Discuss the nature and origin of tertiary dentine.
2. What features does the dental pulp exhibit that are unusual for a typical connective tissue?
3. Compare and contrast the dental pulp and periodontal ligament.
4. Describe the main age changes that occur in the dental pulp, indicating some of the clinical consequences.

Self-assessment: answers (Dental pulp)

True/false answers

a. **True**. Extra care must therefore be taken over cavity preparation within deciduous teeth to avoid exposure of their pulps.

b. **True**. However, some physiological evidence is available suggesting that temperature changes may also be perceived by the dental pulp.

c. **True**, because of crowding within the considerably reduced dimensions of the ageing pulp.

d. **False**. Although lymphatic vessels are present in the pulp, they are difficult to visualize and require special techniques to demonstrate their presence.

e. **False**. Most pulp stones lack tubular structures and are not surrounded by an odontoblast layer.

f. **False**. Only about 25% of fibres are myelinated, the remaining 75% being non-myelinated.

g. **False**. As there are only a few arterioles in the pulp, there are few sympathetic efferent fibres. The majority of unmyelinated fibres are sensory.

h. **False**. Tissue fluid pressures in the pulp appear to be high (though experimental techniques for recording these values are difficult). These pressures may account for the movement of dentinal fluid along dentinal tubules and may reflect the vascular specializations.

i. **False**. The pulp is not a dense fibrous connective tissue. The collagen fibrils in the pulp, especially in young patients, are in the form of a delicate network of thin fibres.

j. **False**. Type II collagen is limited to cartilage, such as the spheno-occipital synchondrosis.

k. **True**. Such cells may be considered similar to the Langerhans cells found in oral epithelium.

l. **True**. This is probably the most widely distributed of the many neuropeptides produced in the pulp. It is a potent vasodilator and quite possibly the principal agent controlling blood flow locally in the periphery of the pulp.

Extended matching answers

Theme: Dental pulp

Item 1 = Option I. The presence of such a high percentage of type III collagen is unusual for adult connective tissues, generally being more common in younger tissues exhibiting a high turnover rate. Its significance is not known.

Item 2 = Option L. Such nerve fibres are thought to be associated with the rapid conduction of sharp pain modalities.

Item 3 = Option F. These cells are associated with the immunological system, similar to Langerhans cells in oral epithelium.

Item 4 = Option E. Like other connective tissues, pulp fibroblasts are responsible for the synthesis and secretion of both the fibres and ground substance of the extracellular matrix. Unlike tissues with a rapid turnover rate, such as the periodontal ligament, intracellular collagen profiles have not been reported within pulpal fibroblasts.

Item 5 = Option D. Compared with other connective tissues where tissue fluid pressures are low (and may even be subatmospheric), the values reported for pulp are high. Although the reasons for this are not known, it may be related to the enclosed nature of the tissue and/or the need to circulate dentinal fluid.

Item 6 = Option J. The presence of fenestrated capillaries may be related to the high tissue-fluid pressure reported for this tissue.

Theme: Pain

Item 1 = Option G. The trigeminal ganglion contains the cell bodies of most of the trigeminal afferents, including those of mechanoreception. It is equivalent to the dorsal root ganglion of the spinal cord.

Item 2 = Option D. The central axons of the trigeminal neurones project via the trigeminal sensory root to synapse in the trigeminal spinal nucleus and in particular subnucleus caudalis.

Item 3 = Option J. Axons from the second-order nociceptor neurones cross the midline and project via the trigeminothalamic tract to the ventrobasal nuclei of the contralateral thalamus. These neurones are thought to be directly involved with the sensation of pain. The neurones that are thought to be involved with emotion and motor responses to nociception project to the posterior and medial groups of thalamic nuclei either directly or via intermediate synapses in the reticular formation.

Item 4 = Option A. Neurones from the ventrobasal nuclei project to the primary somatosensory cortex; other nociceptive neurones project to the secondary somatosensory cortex, the insula and the anterior cingulated cortex.

Item 5 = Option D. Nociceptive non-specific cells in the nucleus caudalis receive inputs from a wide range of receptors such as nociceptors, mechanoreceptors and thermoreceptors; they may grade the overall severity of the stimulus.

Item 6 = Option H. Axons from the second-order nociceptor neurones cross the midline and project via the trigeminothalamic tract to the ventrobasal nuclei of the contralateral thalamus.

Picture answers

Figure 13.13

a. A = odontoblast layer. B = cell-free layer (of Weil) of the pulp. C = cell-rich layer of pulp. D = neurovascular bundles.

Self-assessment: answers (Dental pulp)

b. The odontoblast cell is an elongated columnar cell. It is highly polarized with a narrow odontoblast process arising from the distal end of the cell that enters each dentinal tubule. The odontoblast process lacks organelles and is comprised mainly of microfilaments, microtubules and vesicles. The nucleus of an odontoblast is located basally. In the supranuclear region are to be found numerous organelles associated with protein synthesis (i.e. Golgi material, rough endoplasmic reticulum and mitochondria). There are cell contacts in the form of gap junctions, tight junctions and desmosomes that link adjacent odontoblasts or link odontoblasts to underlying fibroblasts.

c. The nerves represent both afferent (sensory) and efferent (motor). There are both myelinated and unmyelinated nerves. About 25% are myelinated afferents, mainly Aδ fibres (1–6 μm in diameter), but with some larger Aβ fibres (6–12 μm in diameter). About 75% of nerve fibres are unmyelinated C fibres, the majority representing afferent fibres, the remainder being vasoconstrictor, autonomic nerves. The only modality sensed by the sensory fibres is that of pain. The afferent nerve groups also play a role in axon reflexes. A variety of neuropeptides are produced by the nerves of the pulp, including calcitonin gene-related peptide, substance P, neuropeptide Y and vasoactive intestinal polypeptide. These molecules have important actions on blood vessels and on the inflammatory process, and in controlling the flow of sensory activity centrally, thus helping to maintain pulpal homeostasis.

Figure 13.14

a. The specimen shown is of the pulp chamber of a tooth with adjacent dentine showing resorption. Note the large, multinucleated cells (odontoclasts) (arrows) lying within resorption lacunae. Although resorption occurs in the roots of deciduous teeth from the external surface of the root, and the pulp tissues appear relatively normal, in certain instances it may occur in permanent teeth, sometimes associated with trauma, as illustrated here. In these instances, the pulp becomes transformed into granulation tissue and dentine begins to be resorbed internally at the pulp–dentine surface. This condition is known as internal resorption of the pulp. If it proceeds far enough, the crown may have a pinkish coloration, as the vascular granulation tissue is seen beneath the translucent enamel.

Figure 13.15

a. As the section is stained and because of the presence of cells, this is a demineralized section.

b. Pulp stones (denticles).

c. Pulp stones may be classified as true (if consisting of tubular dentine surrounded by an odontoblast layer) or false (when generally consisting of concentric layers of calcified material with no odontoblast layer). Free pulp stones lie within the pulp, while attached pulp stones become incorporated into the dentine wall.

d. Large pulp stones are evident on radiographs. Pulp stones are nearly always symptomless. Their only clinical significance is that, if large, they may complicate root canal treatment.

Figure 13.16

a. A = odontoblast cell layer. B = subodontoblast capillaries. C = fibroblasts. D = dentine.

b. As the odontoblast layer is pseudostratified, the tooth is likely to be an older tooth.

c. Unlike capillaries in most typical soft connective tissues, those in the pulp are extremely numerous, forming complex networks, and possess fenestrations.

Outline essay answers

Question 1

The dental pulp may be induced to produce calcified material in addition to its usual primary and secondary dentine by a variety of external stimuli, including dental caries attrition and cavity preparation. Stimuli of different types and extent may be applied to teeth at different stages of development or ageing, resulting in a response tissue that may vary considerably in appearance and composition. It may resemble secondary dentine in having a regular tubular structure; it may have few and/or irregularly arranged tubules; or it may be relatively atubular. It is known as tertiary dentine and continuity of dentinal tubules between normal dentine and tertiary dentine may be lost.

Tertiary dentine may be classified into two forms: reactionary and reparative. Reactionary dentine refers to the dentine formed in response to an insult in which, although some damage has been sustained and some odontoblasts die, the existing odontoblasts recover and continue to form dentine. There will be some irregularity in dentine structure depending on the strength of the stimulus and the dentine will have an irregular appearance with fewer tubules.

The term reparative dentine relates to dentine formed after a stimulus in which the original odontoblasts in the associated region have been destroyed and new calcified tissue has been formed by newly differentiated cells referred to as 'odontoblast-like' cells. The newly differentiated cells responsible for tertiary dentine formation are very similar to odontoblasts in that they produce

Self-assessment: answers (Dental pulp)

type I collagen and dentine sialoprotein, a dentine-specific protein.

In the consideration of the origin of odontoblasts during normal tooth formation, reciprocal epithelial–mesenchymal interactions are an essential feature. However, it is clear that odontoblast-like cells arising from the adult dental pulp after a suitable stimulus do so in the absence of epithelial cells. There are two possible explanations for this. It might be that during initial dentine formation in the developing tooth germ, epithelial–mesenchymal interactions guide some cells on the path to becoming odontoblasts, but that these cells remain dormant in the pulp, awaiting a later stimulus for them to complete their life cycle and form reparative dentine. A more likely explanation, however, is that odontoblast-like cells are differentiated from a stem cell population in the adult dental pulp in the absence of any epithelial contribution. It is envisaged that the appropriate bioactive molecules necessary for such differentiation (e.g. cytokines, growth factors) are locally synthesized and released during the inflammatory process accompanying the stimulus (such as dental caries). To this effect, a number of factors have been shown to induce the formation of reparative dentine in the pulp of experimental animals, such as pieces of native dentine, pieces of demineralized dentine, crude extracts of dentine matrix, fibronectin products and bone morphogenetic protein. In the case of a carious lesion, the decalcification of dentine might release growth factors from the dentine matrix that pass to the pulp and contribute to differentiation of odontoblasts.

Question 2

Like other connective tissues, the dental pulp consists of cells embedded in a matrix of fibres and ground substance that also contains blood vessels and nerves. The cells represent fibroblasts/fibrocytes and the fibres are primarily collagen. In these features the dental pulp is a typical connective tissue. However, the dental pulp also has features not shared by other connective tissues, some of which relate to the fact that it is protected, and surrounded, by a hard and unyielding material: namely, dentine. A question that needs to be addressed is how many unusual features does a tissue need to possess before it can be considered unusual?

The dental pulp contains a cell type not found anywhere else in the body: the odontoblast. The odontoblast secretes collagen that later becomes mineralized to form dentine. Its uniqueness lies in its morphology; it is highly polarized with a thin odontoblastic process of inordinate length compared with the length of the cell body.

As an important function of connective tissues is to lend support, most possess a conspicuous network of collagen fibres. In the pulp, however, only a very delicate network of collagen is present, as little support is needed due to

the protection given by the surrounding dentine. In the majority of connective tissues, the collagen is mainly type I. In the dental pulp, however, of the little collagen present, only about 60% is type I, the remainder being type III. The reason for this is unknown, although type III collagen is often associated with young, fetal-like tissue.

For a tissue supporting the formation of dentine that does not form at a particularly fast rate, the dental pulp has an extremely rich and complicated vascular supply. Although the vessels entering and leaving the pulp are few, their branching beneath the odontoblast layer is profuse, with complex capillary loops. A number of the capillaries are fenestrated and blood flow rates can be considerable. This suggests that the vascular specializations are not just related to providing nutrition for odontoblasts. There appears to be a comparatively high tissue fluid pressure present within the dental pulp, which might be concerned with the production and flow of dentinal fluid.

For a connective tissue, the dental pulp has a particularly rich nerve supply. Although some of these nerves are autonomic nerves that have a vasoconstrictor effect on the vascular system, the great number are sensory nerves, both myelinated and unmyelinated. They mainly terminate as free nerve endings in a nerve plexus beneath the odontoblast layer, with many passing a short distance into the dentinal tubules beneath the cusps or incisal edges.

No specialized nerve endings have been seen and, regardless of the type of stimulus, the pulpal nerves only carry the modality for pain. The precise function of perceiving this modality is unknown. In addition to the usual transmitters, the dental pulp nerves also release a large variety of neuropeptides, the most widely distributed being calcitonin gene-related peptide (CGRP). The continual release of such peptides is assumed to play an important role in the homeostasis of the dental pulp.

Unlike other soft connective tissues, the dental pulp shows major age changes including the appearance of calcified pulp stones. This is probably associated with the presence in the dental pulp of a population of stem cells that can be stimulated to give rise to odontoblast-like cells capable of forming tertiary dentine. Age changes may result in the obliteration of the dental pulp.

Question 3

The dental pulp and periodontal ligament, both being soft fibrous connective tissues, have many basic structural features in common. They both consist of cells, principally fibroblasts, embedded in a fibrous matrix of collagen, surrounded by a ground substance principally composed of proteoglycans and glycoproteins that bind water. In addition, both have a rich vascular and nerve supply.

They differ in their origin, situation and functions. Though both contain components derived from neural crest (ectomesenchymal cells), the dental pulp is derived

Self-assessment: answers (Dental pulp)

from the dental papilla, whereas the periodontal ligament is derived from the dental follicle. The dental pulp is concerned with the formation, support and maintenance of dentine, and lies in the centre of the tooth surrounded by dentine. The periodontal ligament, which is the main tissue supporting the tooth, lies between the alveolar bone and the cementum, and is responsible for the production and maintenance of these two mineralized tissues. Additional functions of the periodontal ligament include its role in tooth eruption, and reflex jaw activity that is related to the presence of mechanoreceptors.

Concerning their fibroblasts, those in the periodontal ligament show much more synthetic activity than pulpal fibroblasts, as turnover of collagen and ground substance is far higher in the ligament. Thus, periodontal ligament fibroblasts have a higher cytoplasmic:nuclear ratio and show much more of the organelles associated with protein synthesis. They also possess intracellular collagen profiles, indicative of the fact that they are involved in the degradation of collagen. The fibroblasts of the periodontal ligament are also rich in the enzyme alkaline phosphatase.

Both the dental pulp and periodontal ligament possess cells that produce mineralized tissue. The pulp possesses a layer of specialized cells, the odontoblasts, at its periphery. The periodontal ligament, however, has a layer of cells both at its alveolar surface, the osteoblast layer, and at its cementum surface, the cementoblast layer. As bone and, less readily, cementum are resorbed, multinucleated osteoclasts and odontoclasts are found in the periodontal ligament. Only very occasionally are odontoclasts found resorbing dentine in the pulp.

The dental pulp and periodontal ligament both possess the defence cells associated with fibrous connective tissues, such as macrophages. The dental pulp also possesses many antigen-presenting dendritic cells, particularly in the regional of the odontoblasts. Such cells have not been described in such abundance in the periodontal ligament. The periodontal ligament possesses a cellular feature not found in the dental pulp, namely, epithelial cell rests. These are derived from the epithelial root sheath, which plays an important role in root formation.

Both the dental pulp and periodontal ligament have undifferentiated stem cells that provide replenishment for fibroblasts. In addition, the periodontal ligament must also have stem cells to provide a continuing source for osteoblasts and cementoblasts incorporated into alveolar bone and cementum as osteocytes and cementocytes. Although odontoblasts may last throughout life, their destruction due to dental caries, severe attrition and other traumatic events may be followed by the formation of tertiary reparative dentine due to the differentiation of new odontoblast-like cells. The dental pulp therefore also has a stem cell population that can provide new odontoblast-like cells.

The extracellular fibrous network of the dental pulp and periodontal ligament is composed of collagen fibres, though those in the periodontal ligament are present in much greater amounts. The majority of the collagen is type I, but both have a high proportion of type III. The periodontal ligament seems to have higher traces of other types of collagen, such as type XII. Whereas the collagen fibres are loosely organized into fine bundles in the dental pulp, which is considered a loose connective tissue, those in the periodontal ligament are gathered together in significantly larger bundles that are highly ordered and run in specific directions. These form the dento-alveolar, horizontal oblique, apical and inter-radicular principal fibre groups that attach as Sharpey fibres to the alveolar bone and cementum to help support the tooth. The periodontal ligament is considered a dense fibrous tissue. The fibres of the periodontal ligament may also show crimping, a feature that may be important in considering the biomechanical properties of the ligament. As stated above, these collagen fibres have a very rapid turnover compared with those of the dental pulp. In addition to collagen, the periodontal ligament also contains a small percentage of pre-elastin oxytalan fibres.

As the dental pulp is a loose connective tissue, the ground substance will occupy a greater volume than that of the periodontal ligament and contains more water. The components of the ground substance will differ, the chief glycosaminoglycan in the adult pulp being hyaluronan, while that of the periodontal ligament is dermatan sulphate. In the young pulp, the chief glycosaminoglycan is chondroitin sulphate, indicating a change with age. A similar change has not been described for the periodontal ligament.

Both the dental pulp and periodontal ligament have rich blood supplies. Whereas the blood supply for the dental pulp is derived from just a few vessels entering through the apical foramen, the blood supply for the periodontal ligament is derived from a large number of vessels originating from the apical region, from the alveolar bone and from gingival vessels. The pulpal vessels pass centrally through the pulp and form a complex of arcades and capillary loops in the subodontoblastic region. In the periodontal ligament, the main blood vessels are located towards the alveolar bone surface. Both the dental pulp and periodontal ligament have fenestrated capillaries and this may be associated with the comparatively high tissue fluid pressure recorded in both tissues.

The dental pulp and periodontal ligament both have a rich innervation which, like the blood vessels, enters the pulp through the apical foramen, though having a wider origin in the periodontal ligament via the root apex, alveolar bone and gingiva. Both tissues have myelinated and unmyelinated nerves that subserve sensory as well as autonomic functions. The autonomic nerves are vasoconstrictor to blood vessels. The sensory nerves in the pulp appear solely to subserve the modality of pain, whereas periodontal nerves are sensitive to both pain and pressure.

Self-assessment: answers (Dental pulp)

Unlike the sensory endings in the dental pulp, which are free nerve endings, the mechanoreceptors in the periodontal ligament have a more complex morphology in the form of Ruffini-like endings.

The nerves of the dental pulp and periodontal ligament both release many neuropeptides (such as calcitonin gene-related peptide and substance P), whose function is to maintain the integrity of the tissues (homeostasis).

The dental pulp undergoes significant age changes, the most obvious being a reduction in size as a result of continued dentine deposition. It is said to become more fibrous and less cellular with age, with a reduction in the number of blood vessels and nerves. In addition, calcific deposits known as pulp stones are seen in the dental pulp. Few similar age changes have been reported for the periodontal ligament. Indeed, the periodontal ligament has been considered to have many features in common with fetal connective tissues.

Question 4

With age and following the deposition of secondary dentine, the pulp becomes reduced in size. As the odontoblasts, particularly in the crown, retreat centripetally and occupy a smaller volume, the cells form a pseudostratified layer. With age, the rate of synthesis of dentine tends to be slower, so that the intracellular organelles associated with the synthesis and secretion of the organic matrix (e.g. Golgi material,

roughened endoplasmic reticulum) within the odontoblasts become reduced in amount. The odontoblasts tend to be cuboidal rather than columnar. It is stated that the pulp becomes more fibrous and less cellular with age. Quantitative changes in the nature of the glycosaminoglycans have been reported, with an increase in the amount of hyaluronan and a decrease in the amount of chondroitin sulphate. A decrease in the number of both blood vessels and nerves has also been reported. With age, the pulp often mineralizes in the form of pulp stones. Pulp stones may be either discrete or diffuse, free or attached, and may resemble dentine (true pulp stones) or be amorphous (false pulp stones).

Concerning the clinical consequences of dealing with older patients, the first feature is that the teeth are less sensitive. This is probably due to the combination of:

- the thicker layer of dentine
- the presence of peritubular dentine that reduces the diameter of dentinal tubules and therefore the permeability of dentine
- possibly, the reduced innervation of the pulp.

The second feature relates to the reduction in size of the pulp. An advantage of this situation means that a considerable part of the crown may be removed without fear of exposing the dental pulp. A disadvantage is that the reduced size of the root canals, and the presence of pulp stones, will make endodontic treatment more difficult.

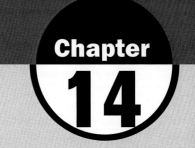

Dental tissues. III
Cementum: structure and composition

Chapter 14

Physical properties   **194**
Chemical composition   **194**
Classification   **195**
Resorption   **196**
    Self-assessment: questions   **197**
    Self-assessment: answers   **200**

Overview

Cementum is the mineralized connective tissue that covers the root of the tooth, helping to attach it, via the periodontal ligament, to alveolar bone. Although a thin layer, it is formed continuously throughout life, allowing for readjustment of attaching periodontal ligament fibres. Different systems of classification of cementum exist depending on the presence or absence of cells and/or the nature of origin of its collagen fibres. Unlike bone, it is devoid of blood vessels and nerves and has only a very limited capacity for remodelling.

Learning objectives

You should:
* know the composition and main structural features of cementum
* be familiar with the various types of cementum and be able to compare and contrast it with bone, with which it has a number of similarities
* be aware of its clinical importance during orthodontic tooth movement and its significance in periodontal disease and regeneration.

Cementum is the thin layer of calcified tissue covering the dentine of the root. It is one of the four tissues that support the tooth in the jaw (the periodontium), the others being the alveolar bone, the periodontal ligament and the gingiva. It is thickest at the root apex (up to 200 µm, although it may exceed 600 µm) and thinnest cervically (10–15 µm). Its prime function is to give attachment to collagen fibres of the periodontal ligament. Cementum is formed slowly throughout life and this allows for continual reattachment of the periodontal ligament fibres. Developmentally, cementum is said to be derived from the investing layer of the dental follicle. Similar in chemical composition and physical properties to bone, cementum is, however, avascular and has no innervation. It is also less readily resorbed than bone, a feature that is important for permitting orthodontic tooth movement. The development of cementum is described in Chapter 10.

In any single section of a tooth, three arrangements of the junction between cementum and enamel may be seen:

* In the most common (60%), the cementum overlaps the enamel for a short distance.
* In 30% of cases, the cementum and enamel meet at a butt joint.
* In the remaining 10% of specimens, the cementum and enamel fail to meet and the dentine between them is exposed.

All three patterns may be present in a single tooth

Physical properties

Cementum is pale yellow with a dull surface. It is softer than dentine. Permeability varies with age and type of cementum, the cellular variety being more permeable than the acellular.

Chemical composition

The chemical composition of cementum is somewhat similar to that of bone and comprises on a wet weight basis 65% inorganic material, 23% organic material and 12% water.

Inorganic component

The principal inorganic component is hydroxyapatite, the crystals being thin and plate-like and similar to those in bone. Other trace elements can be found within the hydroxyapatite and such substitutions are particularly found towards the external surface of the cementum. Fluoride is the most common ionic substitution, and is found in higher levels in acellular cementum than in cellular cementum. Calcification of cementum is possibly initiated by the root dentine and continues on and around the collagen fibres found in cementum.

Organic matrix

The organic matrix is collagen, with non-collagenous proteins being thought to be the same as those found in alveoar bone (see page 221). Collagen accounts for 90% of the organic matrix, the majority being type I collagen with some trace amounts of type III, mainly at the insertion points of the extrinsic Sharpey fibres. Trace amounts of other types of collagen have also been reported. The non-collagenous matrix accounts for 10% of the organic matrix. Important non-collagenous molecules found in cementum are the proteoglycans decorin and biglycan, bone sialoprotein (BSP), osteonectin, osteopontin, tenascin and fibronectin. It has been claimed that there may be present a cementum-specific glycoprotein called cementum attachment protein (CAP) that promotes the attachment of mesenchymal cells to the extracellular matrix.

Classification

The various types of cementum encountered may be classified according to the presence or absence of cells and/or the nature and origin of the organic matrix.

Acellular and cellular cementum

Acellular cementum

Acellular cementum is the first-formed cementum and usually covers the cervical two-thirds of the tooth. Acellular cementum is formed more slowly than cellular cementum. It is more highly mineralized than cellular cementum and usually lacks a layer of precementum (cementoid). Into acellular cementum the periodontal ligament fibres pass roughly perpendicularly to insert as Sharpey fibres.

Cellular cementum

Cellular cementum is found mainly in the apical and interradicular areas, overlying the acellular cementum. However, deviations from the normal arrangement are common and sometimes several layers of each variant alternate. Cellular cementum contains cells (cementocytes), representing entrapped cementoblasts. The spaces that the cementocytes occupy in cellular cementum are called lacunae, and the channels that their processes extend along are the canaliculi. Adjacent canaliculi are often connected, and the processes within them contact at gap junctions. Cementocytes are relatively inactive. Their cytoplasmic/nuclear ratio is low and they have sparse, if any, representation of the organelles responsible for energy production and for protein synthesis and secretion. In ground sections, the cellular contents are lost, air and debris filling the voids to give the dark appearance seen in transmitted light. Unlike osteocytes in bone, cementocytes:

- are not arranged circumferentially around blood vessels in the form of osteons
- are more widely dispersed
- are more randomly arranged

- have canaliculi that are preferentially oriented towards the periodontal ligament, their chief source of nutrition.

Incremental lines

Cementum is deposited rhythmically, resulting in unevenly spaced incremental lines (of Salter). Some believe the lines represent an annual cycle:

- In acellular cementum, incremental lines tend to be close together, thin and even.
- In the more rapidly formed cellular cementum, the lines are further apart, thicker and more irregular.

Extrinsic, intrinsic and mixed fibre cementum

Cementum has also been classified according to the nature and origin of its fibrous matrix:

- When the collagen is derived from the periodontal ligament as Sharpey fibres, the cementum is referred to as extrinsic fibre cementum. These Sharpey fibres continue into the cementum in the same direction as the principal fibres of the ligament (i.e. perpendicular or oblique to the root surface).
- When collagen fibres are derived from cementoblasts, the cementum is referred to as intrinsic fibre cementum. The fibres run parallel to the root surface and approximately at right angles to the extrinsic fibres.
- When both extrinsic and intrinsic fibres are present, the tissue may be termed mixed fibre cementum.

Acellular extrinsic fibre cementum

Incorporating the source of origin of the collagen as well as the presence or absence of cells, two main varieties of cementum can be classified. Acellular extrinsic fibre cementum (AEFC) is located mainly over the cervical two-thirds of the root and constitutes nearly all of the cementum in some teeth (e.g. incisors and premolars). AEFC is the first-formed cementum and layers attain a thickness of approximately 15 μm. For this type of cementum all the collagen is derived as Sharpey fibres from the periodontal ligament (the ground substance itself may be produced by the cementoblasts). This type of cementum corresponds with primary acellular cementum. It is therefore formed slowly and the root surface is smooth. The fibres are generally well mineralized.

Cellular intrinsic fibre cementum

Cellular intrinsic fibre cementum (CIFC) contains cells and is composed only of intrinsic fibres running parallel to the root surface. The absence of Sharpey fibres means that intrinsic fibre cementum has no role in tooth attachment. It is found in the apical and inter-radicular region of molars. It may be a temporary phase, with extrinsic fibres subsequently gaining a reattachment, or may represent a permanent region

Fourteen

without attaching fibres. It generally corresponds to secondary cellular cementum and, as it is formed more rapidly, has a cementoid seam on its outer surface.

Cellular mixed stratified cementum

Towards the root apex, and in the furcation areas of multi-rooted teeth, the acellular extrinsic fibre cementum and the cellular intrinsic fibre cementum commonly may be present in alternating layers known as cellular mixed stratified cementum.

Chemical differences exist between the different forms of cementum. For example, dentine sialoprotein, fibronectin and tenascin are not present in acellular extrinsic fibre cementum, but are found in cellular intrinsic fibre cementum.

Afibrillar cementum

A further type of cementum can be identified that contains no collagen fibres. This afibrillar cementum is sparsely distributed as a thin, acellular layer (difficult to identify at the light microscope level) that covers cervical enamel or intervenes between fibrillar cementum and dentine. It consists of a well-mineralized ground substance that may be of epithelial origin.

Intermediate cementum

It is often reported that an 'intermediate layer' can sometimes be visualized between cementum and the hyaline layer of dentine. This is referred to as intermediate cementum; it is said to be characterized by wide, irregular branching spaces and is most commonly found in the apical region of cheek teeth. The spaces may interconnect with dentinal tubules. The nature, origin and function of this layer are controversial. Some differences in glycoprotein species can be found in this intermediate layer. In rats, the intermediate layer is rich in the bone-related glycoproteins bone sialoprotein and osteopontin. In many human teeth, the collagen fibres from the AEFC intermingle with the dentine matrix with no increase in glycoprotein levels.

The clinical significance of the interface between cementum and dentine relates to regeneration of the periodontium following periodontal surgery. Although a layer of cementum may regenerate, subsequent histological examination may show a 'space' between regenerated cementum and surface dentine, perhaps indicating an absence of a true union.

Resorption

Although cementum is less susceptible to resorption than bone under the same pressures, most roots of permanent teeth still show small, localized areas of resorption. The resorption is carried out by multinucleated odontoclasts and may continue into the root dentine. Resorption deficiencies may be filled by deposition of mineralized tissue from a layer of cementoblast-like cells. A reversal line may be seen separating the repair tissue from the normal underlying dental tissues. Where repair is slow, the repair tissue may be acellular. However, where the repair tissue is formed rapidly it may be cellular.

Self-assessment: questions

True/false statements

Which of the following statements are true and which are false?

a. Cementum consists of 65% mineral, 25% organic matrix and 12% water on a volume basis.

b. Cementoblasts are all derived from cells of the dental follicle.

c. The incremental lines in cellular cementum are further apart than those in acellular cementum.

d. Cervical enamel may be covered by a type of cementum lacking any collagen fibres.

e. The formation of cementum ceases following removal of the pulp.

f. The uncalcified matrix of cementum is termed intermediate cementum.

g. Sharpey fibres in cementum have a similar diameter to those in alveolar bone.

h. Like the adjacent periodontal ligament, cementum contains about 20% type III collagen.

i. Acellular and cellular cementum can be distinguished using polarized light microscopy.

j. The canaliculi in cementum and bone have a similar orientation.

k. Cellular cementum is usually the first-formed layer of cementum.

l. The fibres in intrinsic fibre cementum are derived from the periodontal ligament.

m. Unlike bone, cementum does not undergo resorption.

n. A neonatal line is present in the cementum of the deciduous incisors.

o. Like dentine, cementum is sensitive.

p. The non-collagenous portion of cementum is minimal and accounts for less than 1% of the organic matrix.

Extended matching questions

Theme: Cementum

Lead-in

Select the most appropriate option to answer items 1–6. Each option can be used once, more than once or not at all.

Item list

1. Spaces containing cell bodies in cellular cementum
2. A layer of unmineralized matrix on the surface of cementum
3. Cementum attachment protein (CAP)
4. Incremental lines
5. A multinucleated cell responsible for the resorption of cementum
6. Intrinsic fibres in cementum

Option list

A. Canaliculi
B. A collagenous protein unique to cementum
C. The mineralizing front of cementum
D. Odontoclast
E. A non-collagenous protein unique to cementum
F. Closer together in acellular than cellular cementum
G. Results from the fusion of cementoblasts
H. Lacunae
I. Precementum
J. Approximately 10 μm apart
K. Represent a weekly rhythm
L. Intermediate cementum
M. Oriented parallel to the root surface
N. Responsible for the formation of interglobular cementum

Picture questions

Figure 14.1

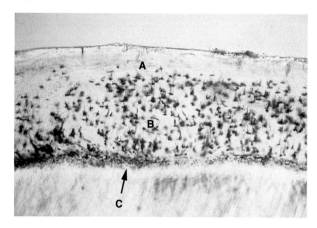

a. Identify the structures labelled A–C.
b. Is this the typical arrangement of the tissues?
c. Classify tissues A and B based on the nature and origin of the organic matrix.

Self-assessment: questions

Figure 14.2

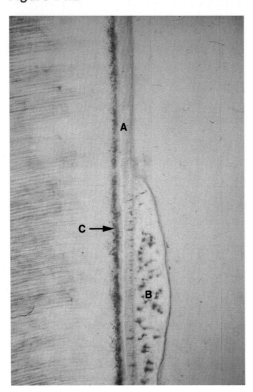

Figure 14.3

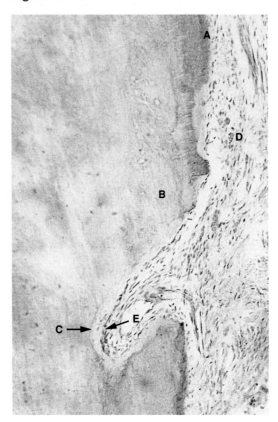

This is a ground longitudinal section of a tooth viewed in polarized light.

a. Identify the tissues labelled A–C.
b. Account for the reason for the different appearance of tissues A and B in polarized light.
c. Is the position of the root apex of this tooth more likely to be beyond the top or the bottom of the micrograph?

In this decalcified section of a root:

a. Indicate the process that is taking place by identifying the structures labelled A–E.
b. Is the process illustrated here common?

Self-assessment: questions

Figure 14.4 (Figure A courtesy of Dr J. Potts)

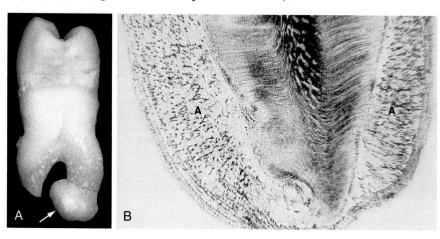

Figure 14.4A shows the root of a tooth. Figure 14.4B is a ground section of the region arrowed in Figure 14.4A.
  a. Name the condition that could account for the appearance of the increased thickness of layer A in this micrograph.
  b. What might one often find associated with the incisal edge of a tooth that has the appearance seen in Figure 14.4A?
  c. What local pathological condition may be responsible for producing the increase in thickness of layer A?
  d. Name the rare condition that may produce a generalized increase in the thickness of layer A in all the teeth.
  e. What clinical problem may arise as a result of this condition?

Figure 14.5 (Courtesy of Professor A. G. S Lumsden)

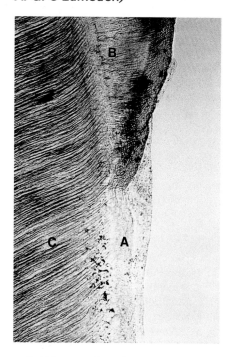

In this ground section:
  a. Identify the layers labelled A–C.
  b. Is this the normal distribution of the three tissues?
  c. What is the clinical significance of this junctional region?

Essay questions

  1. Compare and contrast cementum and alveolar bone.
  2. Indicate some features of cementum that may be of clinical relevance.
  3. Compare and contrast acellular and cellular cementum.

True/false answers

a. **False**. These values are composition by weight (not volume).

b. **False**. Recent evidence suggests that some cemento-blasts associated with the formation of acellular cementum have a different origin: namely, from cells of the epithelial root sheath.

c. **True**, as cellular cementum is formed at a faster rate. Unlike incremental lines in enamel and dentine, the incremental rhythm for those in cementum is not known but must be much longer, some people suggesting an annual separation.

d. **True**. This type of cementum is called afibrillar cementum and consists of a mineralized ground substance. Its formation may require loss of the reduced enamel epithelium, so that cells of the adjacent dental follicle come to lie against the surface enamel, which helps to induce it.

e. **False**. In addition to apical blood vessels that are destroyed during endodontic treatment, cementum also receives nutrition from the periodontal ligament, allowing it to function following removal of the pulp.

f. **False**. Uncalcified cementum matrix is termed precementum. Intermediate cementum is a calcified layer adjacent to the dentine surface which is characterized by its wide, irregular branching spaces.

g. **False**. Sharpey fibres in alveolar bone are larger (and fewer).

h. **False**. Collagen in cementum is virtually all type I collagen, although it has very small traces of type III collagen.

i. **True**. This is because the collagen fibres in the matrix show different orientations in the two tissues and these can be detected using polarized light. Collagen in acellular cementum is classified as extrinsic and is oriented perpendicular to the root surface. Collagen in cellular cementum is mainly intrinsic and is oriented parallel to the root surface.

j. **False**. Canaliculi in cementum are preferentially oriented towards the periodontal ligament, their source of nutrition, while those in bone are more uniformly oriented.

k. **False**. Acellular cementum forms first. Indeed, anterior teeth may show little, if any, cellular cementum. Cellular cementum forms later than acellular cementum and is found particularly at the root apex of cheek teeth.

l. **False**. In intrinsic fibre cementum, the collagen fibres are derived from cementoblasts lying on the surface and are oriented parallel to the root surface.

m. **False**. Cementum does undergo resorption, although this is limited to small areas on the root surface. These appear to increase with age.

n. **False**. No teeth exhibit a neonatal line in cementum, as no roots have started to form before birth.

o. **False**. Cementum has no innervation. Hypersensitivity associated with exposed root is due to the presence of exposed dentine that possesses patent dentinal tubules.

p. **False**. The non-collagenous matrix accounts for 10% of the organic matrix and contains varied proteoglycan species, including decorin and biglycan, along with osteopontin and bone sialoprotein.

Extended matching answers

Item 1 = Option H. The lacunae in cementum are less regularly arranged than those in bone, whilst the canaliculi are preferentially oriented towards the periodontal ligament.

Item 2 = Option I. The unmineralized precementum layer is barely evident in acellular cementum owing to its slow rate of formation.

Item 3 = Option E. The uniqueness of CAP may be used as a marker to distinguish bone from cementum and may possibly allow for the attachment of cementoblasts to the surface of cementum.

Item 4 = Option F. The closeness of incremental lines in acellular cementum compared with cellular cementum is a reflection of the slower rate of formation of acellular cementum.

Item 5 = Option D. The multinucleated odontoclast appears to have the same origin and structure as the osteoclast.

Item 6 = Option M. The intrinsic fibres oriented parallel to the root surface are produced by cementoblasts, in contrast with the extrinsic fibres that lie roughly perpendicular to the root surface and are produced by periodontal ligament fibroblasts.

Picture answers

Figure 14.1

a. A = acellular cementum. B = cellular cementum. C = granular layer (of Tomes).

b. No. Typically, cellular cementum overlies acellular cementum.

c. Acellular cementum is mainly extrinsic fibre cementum while cellular cementum is primarily intrinsic fibre cementum.

Figure 14.2

a. A = acellular cementum. B = cellular cementum. C = granular layer (of Tomes) in root dentine.

b. The differences reflect the differences in orientation of collagen fibres in acellular and cellular cementum. In acellular cementum, the fibres are extrinsic and are oriented perpendicular to the root surface. In cellular cementum, the intrinsic

Self-assessment: answers

collagen fibres are oriented parallel to the root surface.

c. As the first-formed cementum is acellular and later becomes overlaid more apically with cellular cementum, the root apex is more likely to be located beyond the bottom of the micrograph.

Figure 14.3

a. This section illustrates a small area of root resorption that is undergoing repair. A = cementum layer. B = dentine. C = reversal line. D = periodontal ligament. E = reparative cementoblast layer.
b. The roots of all deciduous teeth undergo widespread resorption. Most roots of permanent teeth show small localized areas of root resorption. This tends to increase with age. Root resorption may also accompany orthodontic tooth movement if the loading is not very carefully controlled.

Figure 14.4

a. Hypercementosis.
b. The increased thickness of cementum at the root apex may be a response to attrition of the crown of the tooth with resulting compensatory eruption.
c. Localized hypercementosis at the root apex may be a response to chronic pulp inflammation.
d. Generalized hypercementosis is associated with Paget's disease.
e. Hypercementosis may cause difficulty during tooth extraction, necessitating surgical removal of the overlying bone. Two adjacent teeth (mainly second and third permanent molars) may even become fused by union of their cement, a condition referred to as concrescence. This will complicate the extraction of one of the teeth.

Figure 14.5

a. A = cementum. B = enamel. C = dentine.
b. Yes. In about 65% of sections, cementum overlaps enamel. In about 25% of sections, cementum and enamel meet at a butt joint. In the remaining 10% of sections, cementum fails to reach enamel, exposing dentine.
c. Where dentine is exposed in the mouth, hypersensitivity may result if the dentinal tubules are patent.

Outline essay answers

Question 1

Bone and cementum may both be derived from neural crest cells (ectomesenchyme). They have similar compositions, both being comprised of hydroxyapatite crystals embedded in an organic matrix comprised of collagen (mainly type I), non-collagenous proteins and water. Cellular cementum and bone have similar cell types, forming (cementoblasts and osteoblasts), maintaining (cementocytes and osteocytes) and resorbing (odontoclasts and osteoclasts) the tissues, as well as a stem cell population. Bone and cementum are formed throughout life and, when forming, have an unmineralized surface layer (cementoid, osteoid). Both tissues have a supportive role for the teeth and give attachment to Sharpey fibres derived from the periodontal ligament.

Among the major differences, cementum has an acellular variety lacking cells and an afibrillar variety lacking collagen fibres. Whereas both cellular cementum and bone have intrinsic collagen fibres, these are lacking in acellular cementum. Although they have similar compositions, differences do exist, such as the presence of cementum attachment protein in cementum. The arrangement of the osteocytes is more regular than that of cementocytes, while the canaliculi of cementocytes are preferentially oriented towards the periodontal ligament, their chief source of nutrition. Unlike cementum, bone possesses both nerves and blood vessels and, in compact bone, the osteocytes are arranged in a circular manner around the central blood vessel, forming the Haversian system (osteon). The arrangement of the collagen is far more complex in bone, changing direction from one lamella to the next. Although cementum can undergo some resorption, this is very limited and localized in permanent teeth. Bone, however, shows widespread remodelling throughout life. Alveolar bone, like bone elsewhere, has functions other than that of tooth support. Thus, it can generate blood cells from its bone marrow spaces, its cells are involved in calcium homeostasis and it can provide attachment for muscles (e.g. buccinator). Whereas initial bone mineralization may involve the participation of matrix vesicles, such organelles are absent from cementum.

Question 2

The junction between cementum and enamel may be clinically significant as, in a small number of instances, the two tissues do not meet and the intervening dentine may be exposed. If the dentinal tubules in this region are patent, the patient may exhibit hypersensitivity and experience pain from stimuli, such as cold, that would not normally produce such a reaction. As cementum is comparatively soft and also present as a thin layer in the cervical region, incorrect toothbrushing may remove cementum and result in exposed dentine. Exposed cementum is also liable to dental caries.

Cementum is less readily resorbed than alveolar bone, a feature that is important for permitting orthodontic tooth movement. The reason for this feature is unknown but it may be related to:
- differences in physicochemical or biological properties between bone and cementum

Self-assessment: answers

- the properties of the precementum
- the increased density of Sharpey fibres (particularly in acellular cementum)
- the proximity of epithelial cell rests to the root surface
- the closer proximity of blood vessels in the periodontal ligament to the bone rather than the cementum.

However, if excessive orthodontic loads are applied to a tooth, the cementum and dentine may be resorbed, resulting in irreversible loss of root length.

Root fractures may repair by the formation of a cemental callus. Unlike the callus that forms around fractured bone, the cemental callus does not usually remodel to the original dimensions of the tooth.

Cementum continues to be deposited slowly throughout life, its thickness increasing about threefold between the ages of 16 and 70, although whether this proceeds in a linear manner is not known. Cementum may be formed at the root apex in much greater amounts as a result of compensatory tooth eruption in response to attrition (wear) at the occlusal surface. Where there has been a history of chronic periapical inflammation, cementum formation may be substantial, giving rise to local hypercementosis. This may cause problems during tooth extraction. If interdental bone is lost, continued cementum formation may result in fusion of the roots of adjacent teeth. Such a condition is known as concrescence and will lead to difficulties during tooth extraction. It seems to affect permanent second and third molars in particular, even when the latter fail to erupt. Extraction of just one of the teeth will require prior separation. Hypercementosis affecting all the teeth may be associated with Paget's disease.

Hypophosphatasia is a rare condition in which there is a reduction in the activity of tissue non-specific alkaline phosphatase. The condition is characterized by a significant reduction in the amount of cementum formed and affects both acellular and cellular cementum. As a result, the attachment of the principal fibres of the periodontal ligament is compromised, with premature loss of the deciduous teeth. Permanent teeth are similarly affected.

Where the root canal exits at the apex of the tooth, cementum is deposited not only over the apex, but also for a short distance (usually 0.5–1.5 mm) internally from the anatomical apex. This results in a narrowing of the root canal at this point, the apical constriction. This represents the junction of the pulp and periodontal tissue (although there is no visible demarcation in the soft tissue). In clinical procedures of root canal therapy that call for the removal of a diseased or decayed pulp, this is the point to which the cleansing should be extended.

Following the onset of periodontal disease, alveolar bone and periodontal ligament fibres may be broken down, resulting in exposure of cervical cementum in the oral cavity. This cementum is susceptible to dental caries and will provide a surface for the attachment of plaque and, subsequently, dental calculus. Once exposed in the mouth, its surface will react with the oral environment and render it an unsuitable surface for subsequent periodontal regeneration.

Question 3

Acellular and cellular cementum both cover the root of a tooth. Whereas acellular cementum is the first-formed cementum and is found over the cervical two-thirds of the root, cellular cementum is formed later in the apical third (and in the inter-radicular region), especially in molar teeth.

Acellular and cellular cementum are both calcified connective tissues, the organic component being collagen and the mineral component hydroxyapatite crystals. The mineral component in both comprises about 65% by weight, although acellular cementum, being formed more slowly, is likely to be slightly more mineralized. The collagen in both is mainly type I, with traces of other types, such as III and V. However, the orientation and origin of the collagen differ between the two types. In acellular cementum, the collagen is derived from fibroblasts in the periodontal ligament (extrinsic collagen) and inserts as Sharpey fibres into the cementum, perpendicular to the long axis of the root. In this context, acellular cementum has the important function of tooth support. In cellular cementum, the collagen fibres are produced by the cementoblasts themselves (intrinsic collagen) and are oriented parallel to the root surface. As it does not attach Sharpey fibres in significant numbers, cellular cementum plays little role in tooth support.

Although both acellular and cellular cementum have many similar components in common in their ground substances, differences do exist. Dentine sialoprotein, fibronectin and tenascin are not present in acellular cementum but are found in cellular cementum. Furthermore, acellular cementum is deficient in other non-collagenous proteins (such as lumican, versican, decorin, biglycan and fibromodulin).

Both acellular and cellular cementum exhibit incremental lines. As cellular cementum is formed more rapidly, its incremental lines are more widely spaced. This difference in rate of formation also accounts for the presence of a thin layer of precementum on the surface of cellular cementum, but not usually associated with the surface of acellular cementum.

A main difference between acellular and cellular cementum is the presence of cells, the cementocytes, in cellular cementum. The cementocytes lie in lacunae while numerous processes from the cells lie in fine channels (canaliculi) within the cementum.

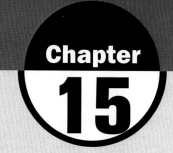

Periodontal ligament (including oral and periodontal mechanoreception and the tooth support mechanism)

Chapter 15

Fibres **203**
Non-collagenous matrix or ground substance **204**
Cells **205**
Blood supply **206**
Nerve fibres **206**
Mechanoreception **207**
Periodontal ligament as a specialized connective tissue **210**
Development of the root and periodontal ligament **210**
Tooth support mechanism **210**
    Self-assessment: questions **212**
    Self-assessment: answers **216**

Overview

The periodontal ligament is a fetal-like connective tissue that is the tissue of 'attachment' of the tooth to the alveolar bone. It is involved in the tooth support mechanism (resisting masticatory loads) and in the generation of the force(s) of eruption (see page 120). It is a highly vascular and well-innervated tissue. The mechanoreceptors within the periodontal ligament convey sensory information to the brain stem and the trigeminal nuclei, and they are also involved in the reflexes of mastication and salivation. Clinically, the ligament is involved in inflammatory periodontal disease and is the tissue that reacts to orthodontic loads. Being fetal-like, it could be a source of embryonic stem cells.

In terms of the tooth support mechanism, the periodontal ligament is often thought of as a 'suspensory ligament' whereby masticatory loads are resisted by the periodontal oblique collagen fibres, being placed in tension. The evidence, however, suggests a more multifactorial mechanism with the tissue being placed under compression with masticatory loads.

Learning objectives

You should:
- know the structural components (including vasculature and innervation) and biochemical composition of the periodontal ligament, and be able to relate these to the functions of the tissue (particularly the tooth support and tooth eruptive mechanisms; see also page 120)
- be able to describe the development of the periodontal ligament and understand the 'specialities' of the tissue.

The periodontal ligament is the dense fibrous connective tissue that occupies the periodontal space between the root of the tooth and the alveolus. It is derived from the dental follicle (see page 114). The average width of the periodontal space is 0.2 mm. Functionally, the periodontal ligament is:

- the tissue of attachment between the tooth and alveolar bone; it is thus responsible for resisting displacing forces (the tooth support mechanism) and for protecting the dental tissues from damage caused by excessive occlusal loads (especially at the root apex)
- responsible for the mechanisms whereby a tooth attains, and then maintains, its functional position; this includes the mechanisms of tooth eruption (see page 120), tooth support (particularly the recovery response after loading) and drift
- involved in the formation, maintenance and repair of alveolar bone and cementum
- via its mechanoreceptors, involved in the neurological control of mastication.

Fibres

The fibres of the periodontal ligament are mainly collagenous but there may be small amounts of oxytalan, reticulin fibres and, in some species, elastin fibres.

Collagen

There are two main types of collagen in the periodontal ligament, type I and type III. These are categorized as fibrous collagens:
- The major type is type I, accounting for approximately 70% of the periodontal ligament collagen. It contains

two identical α1 chains and a chemically different α2 chain. It is low in hydroxylysine and glycosylated hydroxylysine.

- Type III collagen represents approximately 20% of the periodontal ligament collagen. This molecule consists of three identical α1 III chains and is high in hydroxyproline but low in hydroxylysine, and contains cysteine. The function of type III collagen is not properly understood, although it is associated in other sites of the body with rapid turnover.
- Small amounts of type V, VI and XII collagens have also been identified in the periodontal ligament, along with trace amounts of basement membrane collagens (types IV and VII).

Principal fibres of the periodontal ligament

Much of the collagen is gathered together to form bundles approximately 5 mm in diameter. These bundles are termed the principal fibres of the periodontal ligament. The principal collagen fibres are comprised of:

- dento-alveolar crest fibres
- horizontal fibres
- oblique fibres
- apical fibres
- inter-radicular fibres.

Within each collagen bundle, subunits of structure called collagen fibrils can be seen. The collagen fibrils are formed by the packing together of individual tropocollagen molecules. The collagen fibrils of the periodontal ligament are small and of uniform diameter (approximately 40–45 nm). This pattern is reminiscent of collagen in connective tissues placed under compression and differs markedly from the bimodal distribution with large fibrils usually associated with tissues under tension (e.g. tendon).

Although controversy has existed concerning the extent to which individual fibres across the width of the periodontal ligament, it is now known that the fibres cross the entire width of the periodontal space and there are no separate tooth-related and bone-related fibres merging at an intermediate fibre plexus. The principal fibres of the periodontal ligament do not run a straight course as they pass from the alveolar bone to the tooth, being 'wavy'. A specific type of waviness seen in the fibrils of collagenous tissues (including the periodontal ligament) is crimping, and it has been proposed that the crimps are gradually pulled out when the ligament is subjected to mechanical tension. The principal fibres of the periodontal ligament that are embedded into cementum and the bone lining the tooth socket are termed Sharpey fibres.

Functional roles of the collagens

The periodontal ligament connective tissue architecture is regulated by collagen type XII, interacting with the periodontal cells. This collagen is a non-fibrous collagen and may function by linking together the other collagens within the periodontal ligament. Evidence suggests that type XII is present only when the periodontal ligament is fully functional. The rate of collagen turnover is faster than other connective tissues and differs in different parts along the root of the tooth. The high rate of turnover is probably associated with the functional demands of the periodontal ligament in terms of remodelling in response to occlusal loads. However, turnover from teeth subjected to greater masticatory loads is not much different from teeth subjected to normal loads. Furthermore, the rate of turnover may not reflect total protein turnover and there may be several protein pools which have different turnover rates. Additionally, matrix turnover may be dependent on extracellular processing, rather than rate of synthesis.

Oxytalan

Depending upon species, the periodontal ligament contains either oxytalan fibres or elastin fibres. The ultrastructural characteristics of oxytalan suggest that they are immature elastin fibres (pre-elastin). Oxytalan fibres are attached into the cementum of the tooth and course out into the periodontal ligament in various directions, rarely being incorporated into bone. In the cervical region, they follow the course of gingival and trans-septal collagen fibres but, within the periodontal ligament proper, they are more longitudinally oriented, crossing the oblique fibre bundles more or less perpendicularly. In the outer part of the ligament, they are said often to terminate around blood vessels and nerves. Unlike collagen, oxytalan fibres are not susceptible to acid hydrolysis. The functions of the oxytalan fibres remain unknown. Elastin fibres are restricted to the walls of the blood vessels, although in some animals (e.g. herbivores) they replace the oxytalan fibres. Reticulin fibres are related to basement membranes within the periodontal ligament (i.e. associated with blood vessels and epithelial cell rests) and are a variety of collagen.

Non-collagenous matrix or ground substance

Concerning the non-collagenous matrix or ground substance of the periodontal ligament, little detailed information about this important component is available because of its relative inaccessibility and complex biochemical nature. Although we are used to thinking of the ligament as a collagen-rich tissue, in reality it is a tissue rich in ground substance. The ground substance of the periodontal ligament consists mainly of hyaluronate glycosaminoglycans, proteoglycans and glycoproteins. All components of the periodontal ligament ground substance are presumed to be secreted by fibroblasts. The two proteoglycans identified within the PDL are proteodermatan sulphate and a proteoglycan containing chondroitin sulphate/dermatan sulphate hybrids, designated PG1.

The ground substance of the periodontal ligament is thought to have many important functions (ion and water binding and exchange, control of collagen fibrillogenesis and fibre orientation). Tissue fluid pressure is high in the periodontal ligament, about 10 mmHg above atmospheric pressure, and the tissue fluid has been implicated in the tooth support and eruptive mechanisms (see page 121).

Fibronectin

Fibronectin is a glycoprotein that is thought to promote attachment of cells to the substratum, especially to collagen fibrils. Furthermore, cells also preferentially adhere to fibronectin and it may be involved in cell migration and orientation. Fibronectin is uniformly distributed throughout the periodontal ligament (in both erupting and fully erupted teeth) and is localized over collagen fibres and at certain sites on the cell–collagen interface. It is known that loss of fibronectin expression is a marker of tissue maturation in many connective tissues, and the fact that the periodontal ligament retains fibronectin expression may be indicative of the ligament's perceived fetal-like characteristics.

Tenascin

Tenascin is another glycoprotein found within the periodontal ligament and, like fibronectin, is more characteristic of a fetal-like connective tissue than a fully 'mature' connective tissue. Unlike fibronectin, tenascin is concentrated adjacent to the alveolar bone and the cementum. The role of this glycoprotein in the functions of the periodontal ligament awaits clarification.

Cells

The predominant cell in the periodontal ligament is the fibroblast.

Fibroblasts

The periodontal ligament fibroblasts are responsible for regeneration of the tooth support apparatus and have an essential role in the adaptive responses to mechanical loading of the tooth (including orthodontic loading). The periodontal ligament fibroblasts appear as flattened, disc-shaped cells with many fine cytoplasmic processes. Periodontal fibroblasts are rich in the intracytoplasmic organelles associated with the synthesis and export of proteins: rough endoplasmic reticulum, Golgi apparatus and mitochondria. There is evidence, however, that, in addition to synthesizing and secreting proteins, the cells are responsible for collagen degradation. This contrasts with earlier views that degradation was essentially an extracellular event involving the activity of proteolytic enzymes such as collagenases. The main evidence indicating that the periodontal fibroblasts are also 'fibroclastic' is the presence of organelles termed intracellular collagen profiles. These profiles show banded collagen fibrils within an elongated membrane-bound vacuole. It is thought that the intracellular collagen profiles are associated with the degradation of collagen that has been 'ingested' from the extracellular environment. Nevertheless, the degradation of collagen may be expected to include both extracellular and intracellular events (see below).

The periodontal ligament fibroblasts have cilia and many intercellular contacts, a feature that is not common in the fibroblasts of other fibrous connective tissues. The significance of the cilia in fibroblasts is unknown. The intercellular contacts comprise simplified desmosomes and gap junctions. There is little information concerning the functional significance of these organelles in the periodontal fibroblast.

Role of the periodontal fibroblasts in tissue remodelling

Because of the high rate of turnover of collagen in the periodontal ligament, any alteration in fibroblast cell function will produce a loss of this tissue. Evidence exists that not only do fibroblasts synthesize and secrete collagen but also that they are responsible for collagen degradation; however, it is more widely accepted that periodontal fibroblasts secrete matrix metalloproteinase-1 (MMP-1), which degrades extracellular matrix collagen, and can also secrete tissue inhibitors of metalloproteinases (TIMPs). These TIMPs are found in high concentrations in healthy periodontal tissues. Collagenase secretion can be upregulated in response to cytokine exposure. Because fibroblasts are induced to secrete cytokines (including prostaglandin) in response to applied mechanical loads (such as orthodontics), the periodontal fibroblasts may have intrinsic mechanisms for remodelling the matrix. Importantly, inflammation associated with periodontal disease may cause increased expression of MMPs and aggressive loss of collagen within the periodontal ligament, leading to tissue destruction.

Cementoblasts, cementoclasts, osteoblasts and osteoclasts

In addition to fibroblasts, the connective tissue cells of the periodontal ligament also include cementoblasts and cementoclasts, and osteoblasts and osteoclasts:

- Cementoblasts are the cement-forming cells lining the surface of cementum. They are squat cuboidal cells; they are rich in cytoplasm and have large nuclei. Like fibroblasts, they contain all the intracytoplasmic organelles necessary for protein synthesis and secretion.
- Osteoblasts are the bone-forming cells lining the tooth socket, closely resembling cementoblasts. The layer of osteoblasts is prominent only when there is active bone formation. When bone is not forming, its surface is occupied by flattened, inactive bone-lining cells. Like the periodontal fibroblasts, active osteoblasts contain an extensive rough endoplasmic reticulum and numerous mitochondria and vesicles, although their Golgi material appears more localized and extensive.
- Osteoclasts and cementoclasts (or odontoclasts) are found in areas where bone and cementum are being resorbed. These cells arise from blood cells of the macrophage type. When osteoclasts resorb alveolar bone, the surface of the alveolar bone shows resorption

concavities termed Howship's lacunae, in which lie the osteoclasts. Osteoclasts show considerable variation in size and shape, ranging from small mononuclear cells to large multinuclear cells. The part of the cell that lies adjacent to bone often has a striated appearance, the so-called 'brush border'. The brush border comprises many tightly packed microvilli which may be coated with fine, bristle-like structures. The cytoplasm contains large numbers of vesicles of different sizes and types; some contain acid phosphatase.

Epithelial cell rests

Aggregations of epithelial cell rests, the rests of Malassez, are a normal feature of the periodontal ligament. They are said to be the remains of the developmental epithelial root sheath of Hertwig (see page 116). The rests lie about 25 μm from the cementum surface. In cross-section, the epithelial cells appear cluster-like, though tangential or serial sections show a network of interconnecting strands parallel to the long axis of the root. The cluster arrangement of the cells is reminiscent of a duct-like structure. The cells are separated from the surrounding connective tissue by a basal lamina. Studies reveal little activity in the epithelial cells and cell turnover is slow.

Defence cells

Defence cells within the periodontal ligament include macrophages, mast cells and eosinophils. These are similar to defence cells in other connective tissues. Macrophages are responsible for phagocytosing particulate matter and invading organisms, and for synthesizing a range of molecules with important functions such as interferon (the antiviral factor), prostaglandins and factors that enhance the growth of fibroblasts and endothelial cells. Macrophages are derived from blood monocytes. Mast cells are often associated with blood vessels. They show a large number of intracytoplasmic granules. Other cytoplasmic organelles are relatively sparse. Numerous functions have been ascribed to the mast cell, including the production of histamine, heparin and factors associated with anaphylaxis. Eosinophils are only occasionally seen in the normal periodontal ligament. Characteristically, they possess granules called peroxisomes. The cells are capable of phagocytosis.

Blood supply

The rich blood supply to the periodontal ligament is derived from the appropriate superior and inferior alveolar arteries, although arteries from the gingiva (such as the lingual and palatine arteries) may also be involved. The arteries supplying the periodontal ligament are not primarily derived from those entering the pulp at the apex of the tooth, but from a series of perforation arteries passing through the alveolar bone. The major vessels of the periodontal ligament lie between the principal fibre bundles, close to the wall of the alveolus. The volume of the periodontal space occupied by blood vessels and by blood may be so great that we should perhaps think of the periodontal ligament as a 'blood space' as much as a 'connective tissue'!

Specialized features of the vasculature of the periodontal ligament vasculature are:

- a crevicular plexus of capillary loops
- the presence of large numbers of fenestrations in the capillaries.

A crevicular plexus of capillary loops completely encircles the tooth within the connective tissue beneath the region of the gingival crevice. The functional significance of this is not fully understood, although it may be related to the provision of a dentogingival seal.

Fenestration of capillaries within the periodontal ligament is unusual because fibrous connective tissues usually have continuous capillaries. It is possible that the fenestrations are related to the high metabolic requirements of the periodontal ligament (high rate of turnover). The number of fenestrations also relates to the stage of eruption.

The veins within the periodontal ligament do not usually accompany the arteries. Instead, they pass through the alveolar walls into intra-alveolar venous networks. Anastomoses with veins in the gingiva also occur. A dense venous network is particularly prominent around the apex of the alveolus.

Nerve fibres

The nerve fibres supplying the periodontal ligament are functionally of two types: sensory and autonomic:

- The sensory fibres are associated with nociception and mechanoreception.
- The autonomic fibres are associated mainly with the supply of the periodontal blood vessels.

Compared with other dense fibrous connective tissues, the periodontal ligament is well innervated. The nerve fibres entering the periodontal ligament are derived from two sources. Some nerve bundles enter near the root apex and pass up through the periodontal ligament; others enter the middle and cervical portions of the ligament as finer branches through openings in the alveolar walls.

Periodontal nerve fibres are both myelinated and unmyelinated:

- The myelinated fibres are on average about 5 μm in diameter (although some are as large as 15 μm) and are sensory fibres only.
- The unmyelinated fibres are about 0.5 μm in diameter and are both sensory and autonomic.

At the light microscope level, a plethora of forms that are assumed to represent nerve endings have been described within the periodontal ligament. These forms vary from simple free endings to more elaborate arborizing structures, although they still only mediate two sensory modalities — pain or pressure.

Mechanoreception

Most attention has been paid to the periodontal mechanoreceptors (the detection of mechanical stimuli being the modality of mechanoreception). There are a number of different morphological types of mechanoreceptor nerve ending, each responding to a different type of mechanical stimulus. Mechanoreceptors in and around the mouth perform a major role in the transmission of touch and textural information when eating. The sensations of texture, such as smoothness, crunchiness, crispiness and chewiness are all transduced by mechanoreceptors situated on the tongue and oral mucosa and within the periodontal ligament. Mechanoreceptors also provide afferent feedback essential in the control of mastication, swallowing and salivation. Much of the work on mechanoreceptors has been carried out on hairy and non-hairy skin and the adjacent subcutaneous connective tissues, and comparatively little has been carried out on the oral tissues. Nevertheless, the literature reveals many morphological and functional similarities between mechanoreceptors found in the mouth and those found in non-hairy skin and related connective tissues.

Like cutaneous mechanoreceptors, oral mechanoreceptors may be classified on the basis of their response properties into two main categories: slowly adapting (SA) types and rapidly adapting (RA) types. These two categories are associated with the sensations of touch-pressure (SA types) and flutter-vibration (RA types). Slowly adapting receptors discharge repetitively for as long as the stimulus is maintained and rapidly adapting receptors discharge only when the stimulus is applied (and sometimes when it is removed). This selectivity of the mechanoreceptors to different types of stimuli depends mainly on their structure. Anatomically, the structures that mediate mechanosensation in the mouth include Merkel cell complexes, Ruffini type endings, Meissner endings and possibly Pacinian corpuscles:

- The Merkel cell complex and Ruffini type endings are associated with slowly adapting responses and in the cutaneous tissues have been designated slowly adapting type I (SAI) and slowly adapting type II (SAII) receptors respectively.
- The Meissner endings are associated with rapidly adapting responses and, in the glabrous cutaneous tissues, have been designated rapidly adapting type I (RAI) receptors.
- Pacinian corpuscles appear to be rare in oral tissues; however, in cutaneous tissues these receptors are associated with very rapidly adapting responses and have been designated rapidly adapting type II (RAII) receptors.

Neurones involved in mechanoreception are usually myelinated fibres of the Aβ type with axons ranging between 5 and 14 μm in diameter which conduct impulses at a velocity of 30–70 m sec^{-1}. If these receptors are classified according to their functions, they can be divided into:

- intensity and duration detectors (SA types)
- velocity detectors (RA and SA types)
- acceleration and vibration detectors (RA types).

Although each of the types of receptor has a unique morphological and physiological characteristic, any mechanical stimulus applied to the oral cavity could simultaneously excite some, or all, of these receptor types to varying degrees. The few studies that have been carried out on the mechanoreceptors within the mouth lead us to believe that these receptors do not have any particular properties that are unique to their location in the oral tissues. Even those within the unique periodontal tissues appear to be typical Ruffini-like, slowly adapting receptors.

SAI receptors

SAI receptors signal information about the intensity and duration of the mechanical stimulus applied to the tissues in which they are located. Because of both their dynamic and static sensitivities they are also able to signal the velocity of the applied stimulus. They respond with an irregular frequency of firing and adapt slowly to a sustained force. These very slowly adapting receptors are associated with Merkel cell neurite complexes, they respond to perpendicular ramp-and-hold-type displacements of the tissues as low as 15 μm or constant force-type stimuli of as low as 1 mg. They signal an initial velocity-dependent nervous discharge followed by a slowly adapting discharge of action potentials in the afferent nerve. They do not, however, respond to horizontal stretching of the tissues. Their frequency of firing can be greater than 1 kHz when excited by their optimal surface pressure. They have been found in the oral mucosa, the epithelium of the fungiform papillae of the tongue, hard palate, incisive papilla, attached gingivae, and unattached oral mucosa. SAI-type responses have been recorded from mucous membranes of the tongue, lips and cheeks of human beings.

SAII receptors

SAII receptors are slowly adapting receptors that signal information about the intensity and direction of mechanical stimuli to the tissues in which they are located, as well as the velocity of the applied stimulus. Unlike SAItype receptors, they respond with a regular frequency of firing but, in common with SAI types, they also display both dynamic and static sensitivities. These low-threshold, slowly adapting receptors have been identified as Ruffinilike endings. They not only respond to perpendicular lowforce indentations of the tissues (threshold approximately 15 μm), but can also be stimulated by stretch of the tissues in which they lie. There is generally one low-threshold spot for each fibre innervating the SAII receptor. They can follow vibration stimuli of up to 400 Hz. The Ruffinilike endings are sometimes encapsulated by fibroblast or perineural cells; however, the presence of a capsule depends on the structure of the surrounding tissues. Those in the skin, and particularly those associated with hairs, mucosa and some joints, appear to be encapsulated, whilst those in the periodontium lack a capsule. The presence or lack of a capsule appears to have no effect on the function but may be associated with whether or not the connective tissue in which they lie is already aligned or not. Ruffini-like endings have been found in the oral tissues, including hard palate, incisive papillae, periodontal ligament and oral mucosa.

Periodontal ligament mechanoreceptors (Ruffini-like SAII receptors)

Concerning periodontal ligament mechanoreceptors, when a horizontal force is applied to the tooth crown, the whole tooth rotates about a fulcrum and mechanoreceptors, which lie in the periodontal ligament, are stimulated. If recordings are made from afferent nerve fibres from these mechanoreceptors, the response properties range from very rapidly adapting to very slowly adapting. Many studies have attributed the response properties to many of the morphological types of receptor described in other tissues. However, there is now compelling evidence that there is not a range of receptor types within the periodontal ligament, but that there is only one single type, whose response characteristics depend on its position in the ligament as well as on the rate, magnitude and direction in which the stimulating force is applied to the tooth. Rapidly adapting responses are seen from receptors found close to the fulcrum of the tooth, and slowly adapting responses are seen from receptors close to the apex of the tooth. There appears to be a grading of adapting properties for receptors lying between these two extreme locations. Furthermore, the thresholds of the receptors also appear to be related to their position in the ligament, with those found close to the fulcrum of the tooth having higher thresholds and those found closer to the apex having very low thresholds, again with a graded force threshold between the two sites. When morphological studies have been made on receptors that have been located in relation to their position relative to the fulcrum and apex of the tooth, only Ruffini-like endings have been identified. The characteristics of these endings were that they were branched, unencapsulated and incompletely surrounded by terminal Schwann cells with extensions projecting towards the collagen bundles. The Ruffini-like ending is considered to be the primary mechanoreceptor in the periodontal ligament. The physiological response characteristics of the periodontal ligament mechanoreceptors are consistent with them being type II slowly adapting (SAII) receptors. Given optimal stimulation, the receptors located at the apex of the tooth exhibit typical slowly adapting type II dynamic and static responses with a regular discharge of impulses. On the other hand, the receptors located close to the fulcrum exhibit responses typical of a slowly adapting receptor that is receiving a stimulus that is just above threshold, and they give what appears to be a rapidly adapting response. The

lower thresholds exhibited by those closer to the apex can also be explained by the degree of stimulation being greater at the apex than at the fulcrum of the tooth. Periodontal ligament mechanoreceptors respond maximally when the area in which they lie is put into tension (i.e. stretch). They exhibit directional sensitivity in response to forces applied to the crown of the tooth and this can be explained by their discrete receptive fields. Both the morphological and the physiological evidence supports the view that periodontal ligament mechanoreceptors are Ruffini type II mechanoreceptors.

Rapidly adapting type I (RAI) receptors

Rapidly adapting type I (RAI) receptors generally signal information about the velocity of the mechanical stimulus to tissues in which they are located. Classical features are that they:
- adapt rapidly
- have small receptive fields with distinct borders
- respond to low perpendicular forces applied to the tissues in which they lie.

They have amplitude thresholds lower than 0.5 mm and their velocity thresholds are between 0.4 and 40 mm^{-s}. They respond optimally to vibration frequencies of 30–90 Hz and they sometimes exhibit off responses. Although they can signal intensity, because they stop firing before the stimulus is removed, they cannot signal the duration of the stimulus, unless they respond to both on and off stimuli. These low-threshold, moderately rapidly adapting receptors are associated with a receptor ending called the Meissner corpuscle. This receptor is lamellated and sits close to the surface of the epithelium. Meissner corpuscles have been found in the oral mucosa, vermilion border and mucosal areas of the lips, hard palate and incisive papillae.

Rapidly adapting type II (RAII) receptor

The rapidly adapting type II (RAII) receptor signals information about vibration and acceleration of mechanical stimulation of the tissues in which they are located. Classically, they:

- are very rapidly adapting
- can be stimulated by vibration of receptive fields with typically ill-defined borders
- respond to step indentation with both an on and an off discharge of typically one, or maybe two, impulses.

They have low mechanical threshold with indentation thresholds of 7–10 μm. They have low-frequency thresholds in the range of 80–300 Hz, but with higher strengths of stimuli they can respond in a one-to-one fashion to frequencies over the range 30–1000 Hz. These very rapidly adapting receptors are associated with lamellated Pacinian corpuscles. It would appear from morphological studies that lamellated Pacini-like corpuscles are rarely present in the oral tissues. However, a few have been described in small numbers in the lamina propria, mainly in incisive papillae. No recordings typical of RAII-type responses have been made from oral soft tissues.

Central pathways

The cell bodies of neurones innervating mechanorecep-tors in the oral and perioral tissues mostly lie within the trigeminal ganglion. Recordings have been made in the trigeminal ganglion from neurones that respond to mechanical stimulation of hairy and non-hairy skin of the face, the oral mucous membrane, gingivae, palate, tongue and periodontal ligament. The trigeminal mesencephalic nucleus also contains cell bodies of neurones that inner-vate structures within the oral cavity. Recordings have been made from neurones that innervate the ipsilateral maxillary and mandibular periodontal ligament mecha-noreceptors, as well as from receptors that respond to forces applied to all the teeth in the maxillary arch and to forces applied to the nose and hard palate. It has been suggested that these receptors lie in the palatomaxillary sutures. The mesencephalic nucleus also contains the cell bodies of the jaw elevator muscle spindles that are involved in signalling the changes in length of the extra-fusal muscle fibres.

Neurones that respond to mechanical stimulation of the oral and perioral tissues have been located in the trigemi-nal nuclei, the thalamus and the somatosensory cortex. There are insufficient data to draw any firm conclusions about the specific pathways taken by the four basic types of mechanosensitive neurones described.

Trigeminal nuclei

Within the trigeminal nuclei, neurones that respond to mechanical stimulation of the teeth have been found in the spinal trigeminal nucleus (comprising the subdivisions oralis, interpolaris and caudalis) and the main sensory nucleus. Recordings have also been made from the nucleus supratrigeminalis, but this is regarded as an extension of the main sensory nucleus. Neurones with varying prop-erties can be observed in different parts of the trigeminal complex. Periodontal mechanoreceptive neurones in the oralis and interpolaris give sustained responses to forces applied to the teeth, similar to neurones in the trigeminal main sensory nucleus. In contrast, neurones in the sub-nucleus caudalis give transient responses. The receptive fields of neurones located in the trigeminal nuclear com-plex appear to be broader than those of the primary affer-ent neurones. Neurones that respond to forces applied to the teeth still exhibit directional sensitivity but may appear to respond to forces over a broader range of stimu-lus direction.

Recordings from first-order periodontal ligament mech-anoreceptive neurones in the mesencephalic nucleus have shown receptors with intermediate adaptation properties and intermediate threshold. It has been shown that these receptors are situated in a discrete area of the periodon-tal ligament and lie midway between the fulcrum and the apex of the tooth. The functional significance of this obser-vation is unknown.

Neurones in some parts of the trigeminal nuclear complex respond to mechanical stimulation of a number of different structures. In the interpolaris and caudalis

subnuclei, many neurones respond to forces applied to more than one tooth, although in the subnucleus oralis the majority of neurones respond to a single tooth. In the main sensory nucleus, approximately 25% of the neurones respond to forces applied to multiple teeth. In addition, some neurones have been known to respond to mechanical stimulation of more than one type of tissue within the oral and perioral region. Neurones in the main sensory nucleus respond to mechanical stimulation of the teeth and intra-oral mucosa or facial hair. Similar observations have been made in the main sensory and spinal trigeminal nuclear complex on periodontal mechanoreceptive neurones that also respond to stimulation of receptors in the oral mucosa and facial regions.

Thalamus

The majority of fibres that arise in the trigeminal sensory nuclei (principally the main sensory and spinal nuclei) cross the midline and ascend in the trigeminal lemniscus to the nucleus ventralis posteromedialis of the thalamus. From the thalamus, the fibres are relayed to the cortical postcentral gyrus (areas 3, 1 and 2). Some fibres from the trigeminal sensory nuclei ascend to the thalamus on the ipsilateral side (without crossing over). It is most likely that collateral branches of both primary and secondary afferent trigeminal neurones reach many other regions, such as the reticular formation, tectum, cerebellum, sub-thalamus, hypothalamus and other cranial nerve nuclei.

Somatosensory cortex

Recordings have been made in the nucleus ventralis pos-teromedialis of the thalamus from neurones that respond to mechanical stimulation of the teeth. Most neurones receive contralateral inputs and most neurones that respond to periodontal inputs also respond to mechanical stimulation of other oral and facial structures such as hair (vibrissae), nose, lips, tongue and palate. These large receptive field areas of the thalamus, which are greater than those in the trigeminal nuclear complex, suggest there is a considerable amount of convergence of neurones. Recordings have been made in the somatosensory cortex (S1) from neurones that respond to force applied to the teeth. As observed in the thalamus, periodontal ligament mechanoreceptors in the somatosensory cortex have receptive fields not only from multiple teeth, but also from other oral structures such as gingivae, lips and tongue mucosa. Similarly, a range of adaptations have been observed. There is some evidence that many of the mechanosensitive neurones that respond to stimuli of the oral and facial regions can be modulated by tasks such as biting or tongue protrusion.

The cell bodies of the ensheathing Schwann-type cells contain rough endoplasmic reticulum and the nucleus may be indented. Numerous vesicles may be observed within, and forming on, both the inner and outer surfaces of the ensheathing cells. These vesicles may be associated with rapid transport of materials to and from the nerve ter-minal. The collagen in the immediate vicinity of the nerve ending appears to be arranged in a lamellar pattern.

Fifteen

Nociceptors in the periodontal ligament

Little is known about nociceptor fibres within the periodontal ligament, but it is presumed that, as elsewhere in the body, they are represented by fine, unmyelinated fibres terminating as free nerve endings. A similar lack of information exists concerning the fine (0.2–1 μm diameter) autonomic fibres. These fibres are important in the control of regional blood flow, having vasoconstrictor activity. Thus, experiments affecting the sympathetic system are seen to produce changes in tooth position.

As for the pulp, sensory nerve endings in the periodontal ligament can release neuropeptides such as substance P, vasoactive intestinal peptide and calcitonin gene-related peptide. These substances can have widespread effects on blood vessels and cells and must have an important, but as yet undetermined, role in the biology of the ligament. Many of them are upregulated during orthodontic tooth movement.

Periodontal ligament as a specialized connective tissue

It has been shown that the periodontal ligament resembles immature, fetal-like connective tissues. The functional significance of the periodontal ligament being fetal-like relates to the fact that the structural, ultrastructural and biochemical features of the tissue do not depend primarily upon mechanical demands. Indeed, the high rates of turnover may have a greater role in determining the characteristics of the periodontal ligament. The fetal-like characteristics of the periodontal ligament also may aid our understanding of inflammatory periodontal disease. In addition, recent research has highlighted the possibility of extracting 'embryonic' stem cells from the connective tissues in and around the tooth.

Development of the root and periodontal ligament

For the development of the principal periodontal ligament collagen fibres, significant differences in development have been described for teeth of the deciduous/primary dentition (and also the permanent molars which lack successors) and successional or succedaneous teeth (i.e. permanent premolars). Indeed, as the tooth emerges into the oral cavity, the periodontal ligament of the permanent molar is well differentiated (the oblique fibres being the most conspicuous), whereas in the permanent premolar only the fibres in the region of the alveolar crest are becoming organized. In the periodontal ligament itself, although collagen fibres are developing, they do not yet span the periodontal space. It appears, therefore, that collagen fibres may not be well organized during eruption, and this could be significant if it is assumed that collagen has an important role in the generation of tractional forces during eruption (see page 120).

As the tooth erupts, resorption is the predominant pattern of bone activity at the base of the socket (i.e. beneath the developing root). Thus, bone deposition at this site is precluded as a cause of tooth eruption. There are species differences, however, bone deposition being found beneath the erupting permanent premolars of dogs. The different patterns of bone activity in different species may relate to the distance a tooth has to erupt; if the distance is greater than the length of the root, then bone deposition is clearly necessary to maintain the normal dimensions of the periodontal ligament at the root apex of the tooth. Remodelling of alveolar bone other than at the socket's base may also be seen during eruption, and this relates to the relocation of the teeth during jaw growth and to the establishment of occlusion.

Tooth support mechanism

The tooth support mechanism describes the manner whereby the periodontal ligament resists the axially directed intrusive loads that occur during biting. It is frequently stated that the periodontal ligament behaves as a 'suspensory ligament' during masticatory loading. Accordingly, loads on the tissue are dissipated to the alveolar bone primarily through the oblique principal fibres of the ligament, which, being placed in tension, are analogous to the guy-ropes of a tent. On release of the load, there is elastic recoil of the tissue, which enables the tooth to recover its resting position. The essentially elastic responses of the periodontal ligament during both loading and recovery imply that the tissue obeys Hooke's Law. However, present evidence argues against the notion that the periodontal ligament is a 'suspensory ligament'.

Tooth mobility studies
Physiological tooth mobility studies

Physiological tooth mobility studies provide information concerning the basic biomechanical properties of the periodontal ligament. They rely upon analysis of the patterns of mobility when loading teeth whose periodontal tissues have not been altered experimentally. These studies show that the ligament:

- does not obey Hooke's law during loading and recovery
- shows the property of hysteresis
- exhibits responses whose time dependency suggests that the tissue has viscoelastic properties.

Furthermore, the patterns of loading are not dependent on the direction of the load relative to the orientation of the principal fibres in the periodontal ligament and, for loads of similar magnitude, the amount of displacement for an axially directed intrusive load is greater than for an extrusive load.

Experimental tooth mobility studies

Experimental tooth mobility studies rely upon investigating the effects on the patterns of mobility obtained following alterations to a specific component of the periodontal ligament. Experiments with lathyrogens (drugs which specifically inhibit the formation of collagen cross-links and disrupt the fibrous network of the periodontal ligament), with vasoactive drugs, and following surgical disruption of the periodontal ligament indicate that both the periodontal collagen fibres and the periodontal vasculature are involved in tooth support.

In experiments where the apical half of the periodontal ligament was removed and the tooth loaded to assess the effects on its mobility, no effects were observed; consequently, it was argued that the ligament did not behave as a compressive structure because it was presumed that only the tissue around the root apex could behave in this manner. Subsequent experiments performed to assess the role of tension in the more cervically situated principal fibres of the ligament have shown that the periodontal ligament around the alveolar crest could also be removed without major changes in tooth mobility. These experiments therefore do not provide definitive evidence for or against tension or compression in the periodontal ligament, but do suggest that, even where there is marked trauma to a region of the ligament, the remaining tissue can still perform a supporting function in the short term.

Some morphological evidence suggesting that the periodontal collagen is placed in tension during masticatory loading comes from study of the Sharpey's fibre attachments and from the collagen crimps (see pages 204 and 224):

- Sharpey fibres appear as mineralized stubs projecting into the periodontal ligament from the wall of the alveolus. The occurrence of mineralization at approximately right angles to the long axes of the fibres has been adduced as evidence that the fibres are under tension. However, even if this were the case, the distribution of Sharpey fibres along the alveolus indicates that they are limited mainly to the region of the alveolar crest.
- Evidence from connective tissues elsewhere in the body (particularly from tendons) suggests that the collagen crimps are involved in the initial stages of loading, allowing some degree of movement before the tissue is placed under tension.

Morphological and biochemical comparisons between the periodontal ligament and other connective tissues known to be under tension or compression have been undertaken to throw some light on the role of the periodontal

Table 15.1 Relationship between the ultrastructural features of the periodontal ligament and mechanical properties

Features of the periodontal ligament suggesting tension	Features of the periodontal ligament suggesting compression
• Sharpey's fibre structure • The flattened disc shape of the fibroblasts • Dermatan sulphate-rich composition of ground substance	• Small collagen fibril diameters • Unimodal collagen size/frequency distribution • Distribution of Sharpey fibres to socket • Smooth surface of fibroblast membrane • Large amounts of ground substance

ligament in tooth support. They work on the assumption that the structure of a connective tissue is dictated by the mechanical demands placed upon it (see Table 15.1 for a comparison). Whereas some features of the periodontal ligament suggest a tensional mode of activity, many of the features indicate a compressive mode. Indeed, experiments involving relatively long-term changes in the mechanical demands placed upon the tissue (e.g. pinning a tooth to prevent tooth movements completely) produced no major changes in the structure of the periodontal ligament and provide evidence for the view that the ligament is not as affected by the mechanical demands placed upon it as tissues elsewhere in the body. Recent biochemical analysis of the proteoglycans within the periodontal ligament and under different loading regimes shows that the degree of aggregation/disaggregation of the ground substance may have a role in tooth support. Where teeth are unloaded for a period of 3 hours, a high-molecular-weight fraction within the periodontal ligament is greatly increased. On the other hand, with loads between 0.25 N and 1 N, this fraction is greatly reduced. Loads of 4 N are associated with a further decrease, followed by an increase during a 3-hour undisturbed recovery phase.

There is thus evidence that the collagen fibres, vasculature and ground substance of the periodontal ligament are all involved in tooth support. Consequently, the mechanism of tooth support should not be regarded as a property of a single component of the periodontal ligament, but as a function of the tissue as a whole.

Self-assessment: questions

True/false statements

Which of the following statements are true and which are false?

a. The normal width of the periodontal space is 0.8 mm.

b. The collagen in the periodontal ligament is arranged as 'principal fibres', the most common of which are termed the oblique fibres.

c. Within the collagen fibres are collagen fibrils; these are small in diameter for the periodontal ligament and suggest a connective tissue placed under tension.

d. All periodontal collagen fibres are attached to the alveolar bone as Sharpey fibres.

e. The Sharpey fibres from the bone often project into the periodontal ligament as calcified stubs, a feature of a connective tissue under tension.

f. Oxytalan fibres can be readily observed in the periodontal ligament using haematoxylin and eosin stains.

g. Oxytalan fibres are said to increase in number under increased loading of the tooth.

h. The periodontal ligament is rich in ground substance.

i. The fibroblasts of the periodontal ligament are myofibroblast-like, containing distinct bundles of microfilaments.

j. Most degradation of collagen in the periodontal ligament occurs extracellularly by means of the actions of metalloproteinases.

k. As for fibroblasts in all other connective tissues, the periodontal fibroblasts are 'linked' by numerous intercellular junctional organelles.

l. The cementoblasts lining the dental cement are derived from circulating monocytes.

m. The blood supply to the periodontal ligament is derived entirely from the apical vessels passing into the dental pulp.

n. The periodontal ligament is unusual in that it has numerous fenestrated capillaries.

o. The high rate of turnover of the periodontal ligament is one of its fetal-like (mesenchymal) features.

p. The periodontal ligament is richly innervated with sensory and autonomic nerves.

q. Comparisons of the periodontal ligament with other fibrous connective tissues indicate that it is mainly placed in tension during loading.

r. The types of mechanoreceptor in the mouth are unique to the oral tissues.

s. Meissner corpuscles are typical slowly adapting type I receptors found in the oral mucosa.

t. Neurones involved in mechanoreception in the mouth are usually innervated by Aβ fibres, which are myelinated fibres with a conduction velocity of between 30 and 70 m sec^{-1}.

u. Slowly adapting periodontal ligament mechanoreceptors are thought to be Ruffini-type endings (SA type II), and rapidly adapting periodontal ligament mechanoreceptors are thought to be Meissner corpuscles (RA type I).

v. During mastication, the teeth have to be supported by the periodontal tissues to resist loads of approximately 10 kg.

w. The tooth support mechanism is essentially a 'property' of the oblique fibres of the periodontal ligament that behave as a 'suspensory ligament'.

x. The size of the collagen fibrils within the collagen bundles of the periodontal ligament is characteristic of a tissue placed under tension on loading.

y. The proteoglycans of the periodontal ligament aggregate to form large-molecular-weight glycoconjugates when the teeth are not loaded and disaggregate to form much smaller molecular-weight glycoconjugates on loading.

Extended matching questions

Theme: Structure of the periodontal ligament

Lead-in

Select the most appropriate option to answer items 1–5. Each option can be used once, more than once or not at all.

Item list

1. An arrangement of collagen where tooth-related and bone-related fibres meet
2. Name given to collagen degrading by lysosomal activity
3. Attachment of principal fibres into tooth and bone
4. Epithelial cells within the periodontal ligament
5. Mechanoreceptors in the periodontal ligament

Option list

A. Cementoblasts
B. Cementoclasts
C. Collagen profiles
D. Fenestrae
E. Fibronectin
F. Gap junctions
G. Intermediate plexus
H. Myofibroblasts
I. Osteoclasts
J. Oxytalan
K. Rests of Malassez
L. Ruffini terminals
M. Sharpey fibres
N. Simplified desmosomes

Theme: Tooth support mechanism and the fibrous components of the periodontal tissues

Lead-in

Select the most appropriate option to answer items 1–5. Each option can be used once, more than once or not at all.

Self-assessment: questions

Item list

1. Fibres that are primarily responsible for resisting extrusive loading and movement of the tooth out of the socket
2. Fibrous components initially resisting loading ('toe region' of stress-strain curve)
3. Fibres that pull the teeth together (as in interproximal (mesial) drifting)
4. Fibrous components that have been implicated as a site for remodelling of the periodontal ligament as teeth move/relocate
5. Fibres running longitudinally up the human periodontal ligament that have been implicated in tooth support

Option list

A. Alveolar crest principal fibres
B. Alveolar bone-related fibres
C. Crimping of collagen fibres
D. Cross-linking of collagen
E. Elastin fibres
F. Horizontal principal fibres
G. Intermediate fibre plexus
H. Inter-radicular principal fibres
I. Oblique principal fibres
J. Oxytalan fibres
K. Reticulin
L. Tooth-related fibres
M. Trans-septal fibres

Picture questions

Figure 15.1

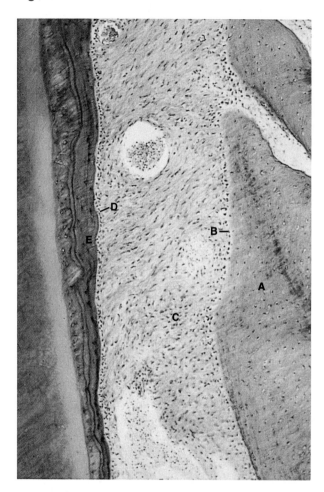

a. Identify the various components of the periodontal ligament labelled A–E.
b. What factors influence the width of the periodontal space?
c. Name the various types of fibre found in the periodontal ligament.
d. In which direction is this tooth moving?

213

Self-assessment: questions

Figure 15.2

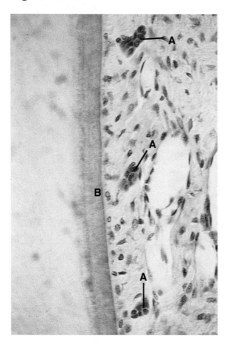

This is a section of the periodontal ligament.
a. Name the cells labelled A.
b. In relation to the adjacent tissues, what is their most unique feature?
c. What is their clinical significance?
d. Identify B.

Figure 15.3 (Courtesy of Dr R. C. Shore)

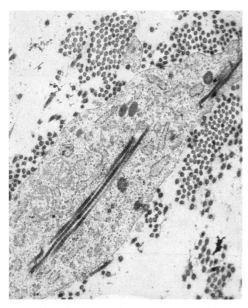

a. What does this electron micrograph showing the structure of a periodontal fibroblast tell you about its function?

Figure 15.4

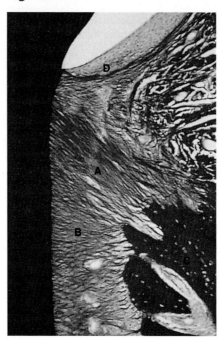

This is a longitudinal section of a tooth.
a. Identify the structures seen at A and B, indicating their composition.
b. Do these structures have a rapid or slow turnover?
c. Why are no cells evident in these regions?
d. Identify the structures labelled C and D.

Figure 15.5 (Courtesy of Dr A .D. Beynon)

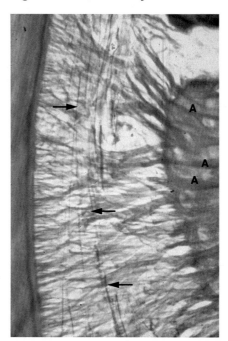

Self-assessment: questions

This is a longitudinal section of a tooth near the alveolar crest.
  a. Identify the vertically oriented lines arrowed.
  b. Describe their ultrastructural appearance.
  c. What volume of the periodontal ligament do they occupy?
  d. Identify the horizontal lines labelled A, indicating their extent.

Figure 15.6

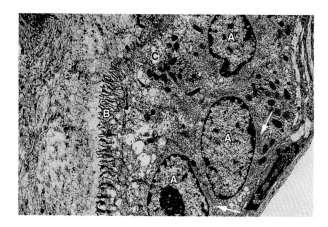

  a. What is the cell type shown in this electron micrograph from the surface of the periodontal ligament adjacent to alveolar bone?
  b. Identify the features labelled A–C.
  c. What is the function of this cell?

Figure 15.7

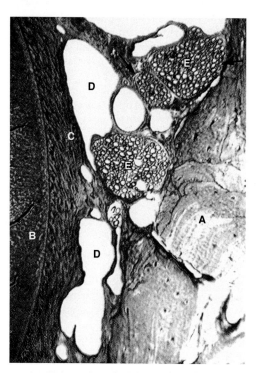

The picture shows a semithin demineralized section.
  a. Identify the features of a tooth in situ labelled A–E.
  b. What features of the periodontal vasculature may be considered unusual/specialized compared with the vasculature of a typical fibrous connective tissue?
  c. What is the evidence for and against the notion that there is an intermediate plexus/zone of shear towards the middle of the periodontal ligament?

Essay questions

  1. What are the 'specialized' features of the periodontal ligament and what is the clinical significance of the tissue being described as 'specialized'?
  2. Compare and contrast the features of the periodontal ligament which suggest that the tissue is placed under tension or compression during masticatory loading.
  3. Describe the properties and functions of periodontal ligament mechanoreceptors.
  4. Describe the composition of the extracellular matrix of the adult periodontal ligament.

Self-assessment: answers

True/false statements

a. **False.** The normal width of the periodontal space is 0.2 mm, although there is much variation between teeth and within individual teeth with age.

b. **True.** Other 'principal' fibres are the dento-alveolar crest fibres, horizontal fibres, apical fibres and the inter-radicular fibres.

c. **False.** Collagen fibrils with small diameters are associated with connective tissues under compression. Tissues under tension have two groups of fibrils with small and large diameters.

d. **False.** It is mainly near the alveolar crest that the fibres are attached into the alveolar bone as Sharpey fibres. Elsewhere, many of the fibres terminate at the bone surface or around adjacent blood vessels.

e. **True.** Furthermore, the occurrence of mineralization at approximately right angles to the long axes of the fibres is indicative of tensional forces.

f. **False.** To visualize oxytalan it is necessary to pre-oxidize the tissue and then use special stains.

g. **True.** However, decreased loading is not associated with a decrease in the number of oxytalan fibres.

h. **True.** Even the collagen fibres are composed of 60% ground substance by volume.

i. **False.** Myofibroblast-like cells are produced when periodontal cells are cultured on collagen gels but are not usually seen in vivo.

j. **True.** However, intracellular degradation of collagen resembling phagocytosis also occurs. Thus, periodontal fibroblasts are both -blastic and -clastic in terms of collagen metabolism.

k. **False.** The periodontal fibroblasts do show numerous intercellular junctional organelles but this is unusual for fibrous connective tissues in adult animals yet not uncommon in fetal mesenchyme.

l. **False.** The cementoblasts are derived directly from the periodontal connective tissues; cementoclasts (odontoclasts), which are osteoclast-like, are derived from circulating monocytes.

m. **False.** Much of the blood supply is also derived from the vessels in the alveolar bone and from the gingiva. If this were not so, apicectomies (endodontic treatment) would not be possible.

n. **True.** Most fibrous connective tissues have a vascular bed with continuous capillaries.

o. **True.** That the periodontal ligament is fetal-like (mesenchymal) is clinically important in terms of the responses to pathologies, wound healing and orthodontic loading. Recent research also indicates that embryonic stem cells can be harvested from the tissues in and around the tooth.

p. **True.** These are involved in mechanoreceptor and nocireceptor activity, as well as vasomotor control.

q. **False.** Most features are suggestive of a connective tissue placed in compression during loading.

r. **False.** Mechanoreceptor types found in the mouth are very similar to those found elsewhere in the body and in particular the non-hairy parts of the skin.

s. **False.** Meissner corpuscles are typically rapidly adapting type I receptors found in the oral mucosa. SA type I receptors are typically Merkel cell neurite complexes.

t. **True.** They are similar to most mechanoreceptors involved in the sensation of touch and pressure.

u. **False.** All periodontal ligament mechanoreceptors are thought to be Ruffini-type receptors, and both the slowly adapting and rapidly adapting properties are thought to be related to their position in the ligament rather than their morphology.

v. **True.** During mastication the periodontal tissues resist loads of approximately 10 kg. The maximum biting load is much higher (approximately 50 kg load).

w. **False.** The tooth support mechanism is a 'property' of the periodontal ligament as a whole, involving the fibrous and non-fibrous components of the ligament as well as its vasculature. There is much evidence against the notion that the oblique fibres of the periodontal ligament behave as a 'suspensory ligament' (not least that the tissue is placed under compression and not tension during loading).

x. **False.** The collagen fibrils within the collagen bundles of the periodontal ligament are uniformly small in diameter and are characteristic of a tissue placed under compression on loading. For a tissue under tension, there are small and large collagen fibrils.

y. **True.** Aggregation and disaggregation of glycoconjugates within the periodontal ligament on loading and following recovery is an important component of the tooth support mechanism.

Extended matching answers

Theme: Structure of the periodontal ligament

Item 1 = Option G. It was once believed that there were separate tooth-related collagen fibres and bone-related fibres that met in the middle of the periodontal ligament to form an 'intermediate fibre plexus'. This was an attractive concept since it explained and located the site of remodelling of the ligament with tooth movements and eruption. However, scanning electron microscopy (SEM) studies have shown that the principal collagen fibres pass uninterruptedly across the ligament and physiological studies have shown that remodelling takes place at the tooth surface.

Item 2 = Option C. Collagen profiles are sites of intracellular fibril degradation and indicate that collagen degradation and turnover might not just occur extracellularly.

Self-assessment: answers

Item 3 = Option M. Sharpey fibres are the attachments of the principal bundles into alveolar bone and cementum. However, much of the periodontal collagen does not terminate into the alveolar bone, but terminates close to the bone surface and in association with the numerous blood vessels at that location. Sharpey fibres in bone are particularly prominent near the alveolar crest.

Item 4 = Option K. Rests of Malassez are the remains of the epithelial root sheath in the developing tooth that map out the forming root. They appear as clusters of cells (with few intracellular organelles and low metabolic activity) or as a network of cells close to the tooth surface. Their function is unknown.

Item 5 = Option L. Periodontal mechanoreceptors are Ruffini-like and there is not a range of receptor types within the periodontal ligament. The response characteristics of these mechanoreceptors depend on their positions in the ligament as well as on the rate, magnitude and direction in which the stimulating forces are applied to the tooth.

Theme: Tooth support mechanism and fibrous components of the periodontal tissues

Item 1 = Option A or H. Tooth mobility studies have shown that, for loads of similar magnitude, resistance to displacement is greater for extrusive loads than for intrusive loads. The alveolar crest fibres have a directionality that indicates that they might be involved in resisting extrusive loads and SEM studies have shown that these principal fibres, unlike the oblique fibres, are well attached into the alveolar bone by Sharpey fibres. The inter-radicular principal collagen fibres (between roots for a multirooted tooth) and the apical fibres (at the root apex), also because of their direction and mode of attachment, are candidates for structures resisting extrusive loading.

Item 2 = Option C. The stress–strain curve for the periodontal ligament is sigmoid-shaped. The initial part of the curve (the 'toe' region) has been shown to be related to the 'unravelling' of the crimps in the collagen. Crimps are associated with the wavy course of the collagen fibrils in a collagen bundle.

Item 3 = Option M. There have been many hypotheses proposed to explain mesial drifting, including a vector of forces produced during mastication. However, experimental evidence suggests that the trans-septal fibres that pass within the gingival connective tissues and between adjacent teeth might generate the force required to produce mesial drift.

Item 4 = Option G. As stated in answer 1 of the previous extended matching question, the intermediate fibre plexus was once believed to be a site for remodelling of the periodontal ligament where tooth-related and bone-related collagen fibres met. However, this is now known to be an artefact of tissue preparation due to the 'waviness' of the principal periodontal collagen fibres as they cross the periodontal ligament.

Item 5 = Option J. Oxytalan fibres are immature elastin fibres that pass from the cementum of the root of the tooth up the periodontal ligament towards the alveolar crest. They terminate either in the gingival connective tissues or around the blood vessels adjacent to the surface of the tooth socket. They are rarely incorporated into the bone. They are longitudinally orientated and cross the oblique principal collagen fibres more or less perpendicularly. The functions of oxytalan are unknown. Their possible role in tooth support stems from the observation that the fibres are thicker and more numerous in teeth that are subjected to abnormally high loads. However, they do not change with a reduction in masticatory loading.

Picture answers

Figure 15.1

a. A = alveolar bone. B = osteoblast layer. C = fibroblasts and collagen fibres within the body of the periodontal ligament. D = cementoblast layer. E = cementum.

b. The width of the periodontal space in the healthy state is said to be 0.2 mm. The width is thought to be narrowed in the mid-root region, near the fulcrum about which the tooth moves when an orthodontic load (tipping load) is applied to the crown. The space is reduced in non-functioning and unerupted teeth and is increased in teeth subjected to heavy occlusal stress. With age, the periodontal space narrows. The periodontal spaces of the permanent teeth are said to be narrower than those of the deciduous teeth.

c. The collagen fibres are arranged in fibre bundles with specific orientations and names, i.e. dento-alveolar crest fibres, horizontal fibres, oblique fibres, apical fibres and inter-radicular fibres. The oxytalan fibres are analogous to pre-elastin and, in some species, may be replaced by elastin. Reticulin fibres are related to basement membranes within the periodontal ligament.

d. The tooth is undergoing physiological drift and, as bone is being deposited on this wall of the socket, the tooth must be moving to the left of the micrograph (the alveolar wall on that surface would exhibit resorption).

Figure 15.2

a. Epithelial cells rests (of Malassez).

b. Uniquely for epithelial cells, they are completely surrounded by a basement membrane and by connective tissue cells.

c. The main clinical significance of epithelial cell rests relates to their propensity to form cysts, or even

Self-assessment: answers

tumours. It has been suggested that their presence may help inhibit root resorption and ankylosis.
d. B = cementum.

Figure 15.3

a. The presence within the cell of intracellular organelles, such as rough endoplasmic reticulum, mitochondria, various vesicles and microtubules, indicates this cells is actively synthesizing and secreting proteins. The presence of what appear to be collagen fibrils sectioned transversely in the extracellular space close to the cell membrane points to the cell being a fibroblast. Furthermore, the presence in the central part of the cell of intracellular collagen profiles may indicate that the cell is responsible for degradation of this protein.

Figure 15.4

a. A = alveolar crest fibres of periodontal ligament. B = horizontal fibres of periodontal ligament. The fibres are composed of collagen (~80% type I and ~20% type III).
b. Collagen in the periodontal ligament has a very rapid turnover, probably in the order of days.
c. The reason that cells are not evident in the periodontal ligament is that a special stain has been used (van Gieson) to stain only the collagen fibres, and there is no counterstain for the cells.
d. C = alveolar bone. D = junctional epithelium.

Figure 15.5

a. Oxytalan fibres.
b. The oxytalan fibre comprises a collection of unbanded fibrils arranged parallel to the long axis of the fibre. Each fibril is about 15 nm in diameter and an interfibrillar amorphous material is present in variable amounts. In cross-section, the fibre is oval and may be up to 1 μm in diameter. It can therefore be readily distinguished from collagen.
c. The oxytalan fibres constitute about 3% by volume of the extracellular fibres of the periodontal ligament.
d. A = Sharpey fibres. In the region of the alveolar crest, where the bone type is mainly compact, Sharpey fibres may pass straight through to become continuous with similar fibres in the root of the adjacent tooth. These fibres may then be called transalveolar fibres.

Figure 15.6

a. The cell is a multinucleated osteoclast.
b. A = nuclei. B = brush border with microvilli where resorption is taking place. C = annular zone (which forms a seal).

c. The osteoclast resorbs both the inorganic and organic components of bone.

Figure 15.7

a. A = alveolar bone. B = root dentine. C = periodontal connective tissue. D = thin-walled blood vessels of the periodontal ligament. E = nerve bundles within periodontal ligament.
b. The periodontal ligament has a richer vasculature than most other fibrous connective tissues. There is a prominent cervical plexus of capillary loops around the gingival crevice. The capillaries are fenestrated.
c. An intermediate plexus implies that there are separate alveolar-related and tooth-related fibres which 'mesh' together towards the middle of the periodontal ligament. This plexus is thought to be the major site of remodelling of the ligament during tooth movement. Histologically, however, the plexus is an artefact produced by cutting across wavy periodontal collagen arranged as sheets, which ultrastructurally are seen to pass uninterruptedly across the periodontal space. Some studies using radioactive proline suggest that there is more labelling towards the centre of the ligament and this might be confirmed by an increase in intracellular collagen profiles in the fibroblasts centrally. However, there is some evidence that remodelling during tooth movements occurs close to the tooth surface.

Outline essay answers

Question 1

Introductory information should be given concerning the location of the periodontal ligament, its unmineralized nature and important functions.

There are two ways of dealing with 'specialization' of this tissue:

- Firstly, by providing a list of special features. In this regard, it is important to emphasize the features that the periodontal ligament has in common with other non-mineralized fibrous connective tissues.
- Secondly, by identifying analogues for this tissue elsewhere in the body.

Discussion can therefore evolve around a comparison between connective tissues placed under tension or under compression, or more meaningfully by showing that the periodontal ligament is a fetal connective tissue (i.e. a mesenchyme).

The clinical consequences of recognition of the periodontal ligament as a fetal connective tissue include:

- wound healing regeneration following inflammatory periodontal disease and reattachment to teeth
- periodontal grafting using appropriate tissues

Self-assessment: answers

- consequences for our understanding of orthodontic tooth movements
- harvesting of stem cells for clinical use.

Question 2

Your introduction should cover the location and basic biological characteristics of the periodontal ligament and the functions of the periodontal ligament, including the tooth support mechanism. Mention should be made of the fact that maximum biting forces are of the order of a 50 kg load and that masticatory forces are approximately 10 kg. Thus the periodontal ligament has to resist considerable loads in biting.

Discussion should follow concerning the controversy surrounding the tooth support mechanism, to include a review of the classical view of tooth support (i.e. the 'suspensory ligament hypothesis'), indicating that there is little supporting experimental evidence. According to this hypothesis, the periodontal ligament is placed into tension on loading; consequently, the oblique fibres of the periodontal ligament primary are 'stretched' and the loads are thought to be dissipated through the alveolar bone.

A basic 'law' of connective tissue biology is that the structural and biochemical characteristics of a connective tissue are based upon the mechanical demands placed upon it. However, present evidence suggests that the periodontal ligament, being a fetal connective tissue, is not significantly affected by changes in mechanical demand. Furthermore, although there are some features suggesting that the periodontal ligament is placed in tension, most of the features suggest that the ligament is placed into compression on loading. The features listed in Table 15.1 (see page 211) should be mentioned.

Question 3

When a force is applied to a tooth, the tooth rotates about a fulcrum and receptors, called periodontal ligament mechanoreceptors, are stimulated. These receptors are slowly adapting Ruffini-like stretch receptors situated in the periodontal ligament between the fulcrum and the apex of the tooth root, closer to the tooth root than the alveolar bone. They respond to stretching of the ligament when the part of the ligament in which they lie is put into tension.

The adaptation and threshold properties of individual receptors depend on their position within the ligament, with those situated just below the fulcrum of the rotating tooth having higher thresholds and more rapidly adapting responses, and those closer to the apex having lower thresholds and more slowly adapting responses. Receptors located between these extremes have graded responses, from high-threshold and rapidly adapting to low-threshold and very slowly adapting.

The thresholds range from 10 mN to 200 mN. Periodontal ligament mechanoreceptors are innervated by large Aβ fibres which have conduction velocities of between 25 and 90 m sec^{-1}. The receptive fields are restricted to a single tooth and exhibit directional sensitivity, in that they respond to a force applied to the tooth crown in one direction only. The cell bodies of periodontal ligament mechanoreceptors are found in the trigeminal ganglion or the trigeminal mesencephalic nucleus within the brain stem (along with the cell bodies of the jaw elevator muscle spindles, only primary afferent cell bodies are to be found in the central nervous system itself). The neurones with cell bodies in the trigeminal ganglion have the full range of thresholds and adaptation properties, whereas those in the mesencephalic nucleus have only intermediate thresholds and adaptation properties. The peripheral distribution of the mesencephalic receptors is different in that, instead of being evenly distributed around the tooth, as is the case for the trigeminal ganglion receptors, they are to be found in a discrete area between the fulcrum and apex of the tooth. The rationale behind these differences is unknown.

The functional roles of periodontal ligament mechanoreceptors are sensory, and they are involved in the reflex control of mastication and salivation.

When a tooth crown is mechanically stimulated, the tooth rotates and periodontal ligament mechanoreceptors will signal this movement. They will signal the movement and direction of movement of individual teeth and also, since they are slowly adapting, they will signal the duration of the movement. Perception of force, movement and when something is stuck between the teeth will be apparent.

Periodontal ligament mechanoreceptors contribute significantly to the complex series of reflexes seen in the jaw closing muscles when a force is applied to a tooth, particularly the so-called jaw-opening reflex. When stimulated, they cause a short-latency inhibition of the jaw-closing muscles; however, they are not the only receptors in the mouth that contribute to the inhibition of these muscles when forces are applied to the teeth. Receptors elsewhere, possibly in the sutures of the skull bones and in the gingiva, also contribute to the inhibition. Stimulation of nociceptors in and around the mouth can also cause inhibition of the jaw elevator muscles and lead to a reflex jaw opening.

Periodontal ligament mechanoreceptors contribute to the so-called masticatory-salivary reflex. When chewing takes place on the left side of the mouth, the flow of parotid saliva is greater from the left parotid duct than the right parotid duct, and it has been shown that there is a relationship between the chewing side and the secretory side during eating, in that 'each gland seems to be most intimately associated with the receptors of its own side' (Lashley 1916). The threshold for the masticatory salivary reflex is lower than 5% of comfortable chewing forces, which is consistent with the observed thresholds of periodontal ligament mechanoreceptors. Indeed, these mechanoreceptors have been shown to be important contributors to the masticatory-salivary reflex seen in both human beings and other animals.

Question 4

The periodontal ligament consists of principal fibre groups (dento-alveolar crest, horizontal, oblique, apical and inter-radicular). Between each group of fibres is a space termed the interstitial space. The periodontal ligament consists of a network of blood vessels, nerves and lymphatics within an extracellular matrix. The majority of connective fibres are collagenous, but some are elastic-like, such as the oxytalan fibres. The principal collagen found in the periodontal ligament is collagen type I (80%), which is low in hydroxylysine and glycosylated hydroxylysine, with type III making up 20% (high in hydroxyproline, low in hydroxylysine, and contains

cysteine). Small amounts of types V, VI and XII are also present, along with trace amounts of basement membrane collagens (IV and VII). The periodontal ligament connective tissue architecture is regulated by collagen type XII, which interacts with the periodontal cells and functions by linking together the other collagens within the periodontal ligament. Water is found within the periodontal ligament, along with a non-collagenous matrix made up principally of proteoglycans. Also known as ground substance, this proteoglycan-rich matrix surrounds and protects collagen fibres, controlling fibrillogenesis and fibre orientation, influencing ion and water binding and exchange, and providing cells with vital substances from blood capillaries and returning catabolites to these vessels. The two proteoglycans identified within the periodontal ligament are proteodermatan sulphate and PG1, a proteoglycan containing chondroitin sulphate/dermatan sulphate hybrids. Fibronectin and tenascin are present within the periodontal ligament. Fibronectin promotes attachment of cells to the collagen fibrils.

Alveolar bone: structure and composition

Chapter

16

Biochemical composition	221
Classification	222
Gross morphology	222
Histology	222
Cell types	223
Sharpey fibres	224
Structural lines	224
Resorption and deposition of bone	224
Self-assessment: questions	226
Self-assessment: answers	229

Overview

Alveolar bone is the mineralized connective tissue that supports and protects the teeth. Similar to bone elsewhere, it also provides for muscle attachment and contains bone marrow. The most important property of bone is its 'plasticity', allowing it to remodel according to the functional demands placed on it. There are five main types of bone cell and the basic unit of bone is the osteon (Haversian system). The processes of bone resorption and formation at sites of remodelling do not occur randomly. There must be tight control to ensure a balance between the two processes (coupling), as any disruption of this balance can lead to bone disease.

Learning objectives

You should:
- know the composition, classification and main structural features of bone
- be familiar with the various cell types and understand how their structure is related to function
- be aware of the principles that regulate bone formation and resorption and how these processes are coupled
- understand why a considerable knowledge of bone is necessary to appreciate the many ways it impinges on the clinical situation.

The part of the maxilla or mandible that supports and protects the teeth is known as alveolar bone. An arbitrary boundary at the level of the root apices of the teeth separates the alveolar processes from the body of the mandible or the maxilla. Like bone in other sites, alveolar bone functions as a mineralized supporting tissue, giving attachment to muscles, providing a framework for bone marrow, and acting as a reservoir for ions (especially calcium). Apart from its obvious strength, one of the most important biological properties of bone is its 'plasticity', allowing it to model/remodel according to the functional demands placed upon it. Bone depends on function (i.e. mechanical stimuli) to maintain its structure and mass.

Biochemical composition

Bone is a mineralized connective tissue. Approximately 60% of the wet weight of bone is inorganic mineral, with 25% organic matrix and the remaining 15% water. The mineral phase provides the hardness and rigidity of bone and consists of carbonated hydroxyapatite, present in the form of thin needle-like crystallites or thin plates (about 50 nm wide, up to 8 nm thick and of variable length) distributed between the gap zones of the collagen molecules. The organic matrix contributes to other aspects of its physical properties, such as tensile strength and modulus of elasticity, and is approximately 90% type I collagen. Most collagen can be regarded as intrinsic collagen secreted by osteoblasts. However, collagen inserted as Sharpey fibres from the periodontal ligament can be considered as extrinsic collagen. The non-collagenous matrix is a heterogenous group of proteins, which accounts for 10% of the organic matrix. These proteins include the proteoglycans, which incorporate chondroitin and heparan sulphate glycosaminoglycans, mainly in the form of decorin and biglycan. Glycoproteins associated with bone include osteopontin, osteonectin, bone sialoprotein (BSP), osteocalcin and fibronectin. The part played by these individual proteoglycans still requires clarification; however, they may have important roles in bone formation and subsequent mineralization. Bone also contains exogenously derived proteins that may circulate in the blood. These include albumin and also a varied cocktail of cytokines and growth factors, including interleukins, tumour necrosis factor, TGF-β, FGF, PDGF and BMPs. These bioactive molecules are stored or locked up within the bone matrix. Release of these molecules during trauma or general remodelling may play a role in controlling further bone activity.

Classification

There are a number of ways that the classification of bone can be achieved:

- Developmentally, there is endochondral bone (where bone is preceded by a cartilaginous model that is eventually replaced by bone in a process termed endochondral ossification) and intramembranous bone (where bone forms directly within a vascular, fibrous membrane).
- Histologically, mature bone may be categorized as compact (cortical) or cancellous (spongy), according to its density. As the names suggest, compact bone forms a dense, solid mass, while in spongy bone there is a lattice arrangement of the individual bony trabeculae that surround bone marrow.
- In newly formed bone, the collagen fibres have a more variable diameter and lack a preferential orientation, giving the bone a matted (basketweave) structure. This immature bone, termed woven bone, has larger and more numerous osteocytes. Woven bone is subsequently converted to fine-fibred, adult lamellar bone.

Gross morphology

The alveolar, tooth-bearing portion of the jaws is composed of outer and inner alveolar plates. The individual sockets are separated by plates of bone termed the interdental septa, while the roots of multirooted teeth are divided by inter-radicular septa. The compact layer of bone lining the tooth socket has been referred to as the cribriform plate, reflecting the sieve-like appearance produced by the numerous vascular canals (Volkmann's canals) passing between the alveolar bone and the periodontal ligament. It has also been called bundle bone because numerous bundles of Sharpey fibres pass into it from the periodontal ligament. In clinical radiographs, the bone lining the alveolus commonly appears as a dense white line and is given the name lamina dura. Between the bundle bone and the inner and outer plates of compact bone are variable amounts of spongy bone, depending on site.

Histology

Bone is deposited in layers, or lamellae, each being 3–5 μm thick.

Bone organization

In compact bone the lamellae are arranged in two major patterns:

- At external (periosteal) and internal (endosteal) surfaces, they are arranged in parallel layers completely surrounding the bony surfaces and are known as circumferential lamellae.

- Deep to the circumferential lamellae, the lamellae are arranged as small, concentric layers around a central neurovascular canal. The central canal (about 50 μm in diameter), together with the concentric lamellae, is known as an osteon or Haversian system.

There may be up to about 20 concentric lamellae within each Haversian system, the number being limited by the ability of nutrients to diffuse from the central vessel to the cells in the outermost lamella. A cement line of mineralized matrix delineates each Haversian system. The collagen fibres within each lamella are parallel to one another and spiral along the length of the lamella, but have a different orientation to those in the adjacent lamella. As a consequence of remodelling, fragments of previous Haversian systems (interstitial lamellae) may be present.

In spongy bone, the lamellae are apposed to each other to form trabeculae up to about 50 μm thick, surrounded by the marrow spaces. The trabeculae are not arranged randomly but are aligned along lines of stress so as best to withstand the forces applied to the bone while adding minimally to mass.

In young bone, the marrow is red and haemopoietic. It contains stem cells of both the fibroblastic/mesenchymal type (capable of giving rise to fibroblasts, osteoblasts, adipocytes, chondroblasts and myoblasts) and blood cell lineage (capable of giving rise to osteoclasts). In old bone, the marrow is yellow, with loss of haemopoietic potential and increased accumulation of fat cells.

Osteoid

Any surface where active bone formation is occurring will be covered by a layer of newly deposited, unmineralized, bone matrix called osteoid, having a thickness of approximately 5–10 μm. This represents an initial deposition of unmineralized matrix. Like predentine, osteoid will stain differently from the matrix associated with mineralized bone, indicating that biochemical changes take place within the matrix at the mineralizing front to enable mineralization to occur; some molecules may be added, others may be degraded. Osteoid contains a cocktail of cytokines and growth factors in a collagen matrix. Collagen is present as type I collagen arranged parallel to the bone surface. Traces of collagen type III are present at Sharpey fibre insertions. The collagen is embedded in a non-collagenous matrix rich in proteoglycans, including dermatan sulphate-substituted forms of decorin and biglycan. These two proteoglycans are thought to have roles in cell differentiation, proliferation and matrix assembly. Other glycoproteins also present within this unmineralized matrix include:

- versican, a large interstitial proteoglycan associated with capture of space
- fibronectin and tenascin, usually associated with soft connective tissues, which are evident at Sharpey's insertion points and have roles in matrix formation and cell adhesion.

Matrix metalloproteinase is also present for removal of matrix proteins, which prevent deposition of mineral, and for proteolytic processing of proteins, to yield protein with new functions.

Matrix vesicles

Initial mineralization of osteoid may be controlled by matrix vesicles, which bud off from the osteoblast cell membrane. These vesicles contain the initial mineral crystals and the membrane around these crystals breaks down to form the seed around which extensive mineralization occurs by epitaxy or heterogenous nucleation. Significant remodelling and biochemical changes occur within the osteoid prior to mineralization and that accounts for the perceived lag phase before the deepest layer of osteoid undergoes mineralization.

Cell types

Bone contains several different cell types that are responsible for the synthesis, maintenance and resorption of bone. They can be regarded as belonging to two main families, one mesenchymal and the other haemopoietic:
- The osteoblasts, osteocytes and bone-lining cells are derived from a mesenchymal (or ectomesenchymal) stem cell.
- Osteoclasts, however, are derived from a haemopoietic source, the macrophage/monocyte lineage.

Osteoblasts

A layer of osteoblasts is prominent on bone surfaces where there is active bone formation. They appear cuboidal and exhibit conspicuous amounts of endoplasmic reticulum and Golgi material. Osteoblasts are also in contact with underlying osteocytes. Osteoblasts secrete the organic matrix of bone that initially is represented by an unmineralized layer, the osteoid. Useful markers of the osteoblast phenotype include osteocalcin and osteoblast transcription factor, Runx2 (Cbfa-1). Alkaline phosphatase activity, although not entirely specific to bone, is also a reliable indicator of osteoblastic differentiation. The secreted, intrinsic collagen fibrils lie parallel to the bone surface. At the surface of alveolar bone adjacent to the periodontal ligament, extrinsic Sharpey fibres pass more or less perpendicularly into the osteoid layer. In addition to secreting the formative components of bone, the osteoblast secretes molecules controlling its own activity (such as growth factors, cytokines and prostaglandins) and that of the osteoclast.

Osteocytes

Osteocytes are postmitotic cells lying within the bone itself and represent 'entrapped' osteoblasts. However, compared with osteoblasts, they show a considerable reduction in the intracellular organelles associated with protein synthesis. Osteocytes play an important role in calcium homeostasis. They are housed in lacunae, possess numerous cell processes that run in channels (canaliculi) within bone, and

link up with the processes of neighbouring osteocytes at gap junctions. The superficially situated osteocytes are in contact with cells lining the bone surface. The cell processes in the canaliculi allow the diffusion of substances from adjacent blood vessels throughout the bone.

As a result of their widespread distribution in bone and their interconnections, osteocytes are obvious candidates to detect load-induced strains in bone and are therefore regarded as the primary mechanosensors in bone.

Bone-lining cells

When bone surfaces are in neither the formative nor resorptive phase, they are lined by a layer of flattened cells termed bone-lining cells. Like osteoblasts, the bone-lining cells are connected to underlying osteocytes. They show little sign of synthetic activity and may be regarded as post-proliferative osteoblasts. By covering the surface of bone, they may:
- play a role in calcium and phosphate metabolism
- protect the surface from any resorptive activity by osteoclasts
- participate in initiating bone remodelling.

Stem cells

In order to generate osteoblasts throughout life, a stem-cell population is required. Stem cells have the ability to maintain their numbers throughout life. They reside in the layer of cells beneath the osteoblast layer in the periosteal region, in the periodontal ligament, or in the adjacent marrow spaces.

Osteoclasts

Osteoclasts are derived from fusion of haemopoietic cells of the macrophage/monocyte lineage, giving rise to multinucleated cells. Osteoclasts are highly motile. Their lifespan is not known with certainty, although it is thought to be between 10 and 14 days, after which the cells undergo apoptosis. Resorbing surfaces of alveolar bone show typical resorption concavities (Howship's lacunae) in which the osteoclasts lie. A useful marker for osteoclasts is the enzyme tartrate-resistant acid phosphatase.

Characteristically, human osteoclasts may be up to 100 μm in diameter and have on average 10–20 nuclei. When actively resorbing, osteoclasts possess a ruffled border composed of many tightly packed microvilli adjacent to the bone surface, providing a large surface area for the resorptive process. A sealing (clear) zone surrounds the periphery of the ruffled border. Here, the plasma membrane is smooth and the organelle-free cytoplasm beneath it contains numerous contractile actin microfilaments (surrounded by two vinculin rings). The sealing zone serves to attach the cell very closely to the surface of bone, mainly due to the presence of cell membrane adhesion proteins known as integrins. The osteoclast contains numerous mitochondria and large numbers of vesicles of different sizes and types, some containing lysosomal enzymes

Sixteen

capable of degrading the organic matrix of bone. Once the osteoclast has been activated, bone resorption occurs in two stages. Initially, the mineral phase is removed and later the organic matrix.

Sharpey fibres

Extrinsic Sharpey fibres inserting into the cribriform plate are derived from the principal fibres of the periodontal ligament. Sharpey fibres are particularly prominent in the cervical portion (alveolar crest region) of the alveolar bone. Here, where bone is compact, Sharpey fibres may penetrate the bone to a considerable depth. Sharpey fibres entering alveolar bone are less numerous but thicker than those at the cementum surface. Because of the attachments of numerous bundles of collagen fibres, the cribriform plate has also been called bundle bone.

Structural lines

Structural lines are evident in bone. Bone is laid down rhythmically, which results in the formation of regular parallel lines that, because they are formed in periods of relative quiescence, are termed resting lines. Such resting lines differ biochemically from adjacent bone. These lines are prominent in bundle bone on the distal surface of the socket wall during physiological mesial drift of the teeth. Bone will also contain reversal lines, representing the site of change from bone resorption to bone deposition. Such reversal lines will show evidence of a scalloped outline, reflecting the position of Howship's lacunae.

Resorption and deposition of bone

There is close correlation between resorption and deposition of bone. The osteoclast has far fewer surface receptors than the osteoblast and is not directly responsive to the majority of hormones or growth factors. This has led to the concept that the osteoblast has a controlling influence in the development and maturation of the osteoclast. However, important receptors that the osteoclast does express are those for calcitonin (a powerful inhibitor of osteoclasis that interferes with the cell attachment mechanism to bone), prostaglandins and RANK (receptor activator of nuclear factor kappa B).

The processes of bone resorption and formation at sites of remodelling do not occur randomly. Clearly, there must be tight control to ensure a balance between the two processes, as any disruption of this balance can lead to metabolic bone disease (such as osteopetrosis and osteoporosis). This close control can be referred to as coupling. From a resting state, the sequence of remodelling consists of four main phases:

- Resorption: recruitment, migration and activation of osteoclasts, causing bone resorption.
- Reversal: cessation of resorption and disappearance of osteoclasts. The site becomes occupied by

mononuclear cells. The changeover from resorption to deposition is characterized by a reversal line.
- Formation: osteoblast recruitment, migration, differentiation and formation of new bone in the resorption site.
- Resting: formation of bone ceases and the surface is lined by a flattened layer of bone-lining cells.

There is thus a clear relationship between bone deposition and bone resorption, and this relationship is mediated biochemically. Many of the factors that result in bone resorption do not have direct effects on osteoclasts but act through osteoblasts, as most receptors to the bioactive molecules responsible for resorption are present on the osteoblast. How the osteoblast promotes resorption may be through the release of bioactive proteins such as cytokines and growth factors, including macrophage colony stimulating factor (MSC-F), osteoprotegerin, receptor activator of nuclear factor kappa B ligand (RANKL), and interleukins, which may stimulate the production of osteoclasts. Osteoblasts may release MMPs, degrading the osteoid on the bone surface, exposing the mineralized bone matrix, and allowing osteoclasts to attach themselves to the mineralized bone and begin resorption. Whilst the precise signals responsible for causing the cessation of resorption and a reversal to osteoblast differentiation and activation of bone formation are not known, the release of molecules such as growth factors, initially bound up in the bone matrix but exposed/activated by the resorption process, may be involved. For example, BMPs and IGF released from bone may stimulate osteoblastogenesis, while TGF-β released from bone may inhibit osteoclastogenesis while stimulating osteoblastogenesis. These bone-bound bioactive growth factors are activated by subsequent osteoclastic bone resorption and bind to their receptors on osteoblasts and osteoclasts, influencing bone remodelling. Ambient pH and levels of oxygen are also important factors affecting resorption.

As a reduction in the mechanical loads impinging on bone is associated with bone loss, it can be assumed that such loading is normally required to stimulate the modelling/remodelling processes of bone necessary to maintain normal bone structure. Strains need to be intermittent (rather than continuous), and the osteogenic response is dependent upon the size of the load and the frequency and rate of application. To maintain bone mass may only require the application of relatively few loading cycles.

The molecular mechanisms whereby forces impinging on the bone are transduced into bone resorption or deposition remain elusive, although many theories have been proposed. Osteocytes, together with the surface layer of osteoblasts/bone-lining cells, appear to be the most obvious candidates for detecting strain within bone. Deformation of bone following loading is thought to deform the cell processes/cell membranes either directly, or indirectly through movement of tissue fluid residing in the lacunocanalicular system. Signals are then transduced via the cell membrane at the surface (e.g. involving K^+ and Ca^{2+} ion channels and integrins) to cytoskeletal elements within the cell, with stimulation of secondary messengers. These changes eventually lead to the production and release of molecules that initiate an osteogenic response.

Osteoblast formation

Osteoblast formation is initiated from pluripotent mesenchymal stem cells. These cells give rise to intermediate progenitor cells that form osteoprogenitors (immature and mature forms) and pre-osteoblasts. It takes about eight cell divisions before an osteoblast finally differentiates to form an osteoid seam that mineralizes to produce bone. Among the earliest markers to indicate that a stem cell is progressing along an osteogenic phenotype is the expression of the nuclear transcription factor, core binding factor 1 (Cbfa1, also called Runx2). This is responsible for regulating the production of a number of important protein products in bone matrix. The induction of Cbfa1 involves the action of growth factors such TGF-β and BMP-2. Osteoprogenitor cells can be identified by the progressive expression of molecules such as type I collagen, alkaline phosphatase and osteopontin. These cells are relatively undifferentiated and there is little roughened endoplasmic reticulum. In the postmitotic osteoblast, even more activity of the markers first seen in pre-osteoblasts is present and there is marked development of roughened endoplasmic reticulum and Golgi material. In addition, new molecules related to mineralization (e.g. osteocalcin) and cell adhesion make their appearance.

Osteoclast formation

Osteoclast formation differs from the other cells associated with bone (e.g. osteoblasts, osteocytes, bone-lining cells), as they are derived from blood cells, not from stromal cells. The pluripotent stem cell is of the monocyte/macrophage lineage. Early important transcription factors indicative of its eventual fate are c-Fos and PU-1. Differentiation from the myeloid progenitor to the mononuclear osteoclast precursor involves the activity of many factors, two of the most important of which are macrophage-colony stimulating factor (M-CSF) and RANKL. These two factors are produced by osteoblast/stromal cells. As osteoclast progenitors have a receptor (c-Fms) for M-CSF and a receptor (RANK) for RANKL, close association between the two cell types drives the differentiation of the osteoclast precursors into mononuclear pre-osteoclasts. As a method of controlling the rate of formation of osteoclast precursors, the osteoblast also secretes osteoprotegerin (OPG), which acts as a soluble decoy molecule by binding with RANKL and thereby inhibiting osteoclast formation.

Fusion of mononuclear osteoclasts into multinucleated osteoclasts and their subsequent activation is also driven by the RANKL/RANK system. Initially, the cell is non-polarized; it is only on attaching to bone by cell–matrix interactions (involving transmembrane receptors such as integrins and matrix components such as collagen and osteopontin) that the osteoclast becomes polarized: it develops the ruffled border, sealing zone and the systems to demineralize bone and degrade its organic matrix successfully. Following the resorptive phase, osteoclasts are thought to be removed by apoptosis. Two additional important factors involved in the activation of osteoclasts are acidification and hypoxia.

Sixteen

Self-assessment: questions

True/false statements

Which of the following statements are true and which are false?

a. Bundle bone refers to the alveolar bone into which Sharpey fibres are embedded.

b. In the incisor region, little cancellous bone is present between inner and outer cortical plates of alveolar bone.

c. In the alveolar crest region, Sharpey fibres may extend completely through the alveolar bone.

d. A histochemical marker for osteoblasts is alkaline phosphatase.

e. The main receptors for parathormone (which leads to bone resorption) are found on osteoblasts.

f. Cancellous bone of the alveolus is haemopoietic during childhood.

g. Osteoclasts, like periodontal fibroblasts, degrade collagen in intracellular collagen profiles.

h. Mesial drift of a molar tooth is accompanied by deposition of bone mesially and resorption of bone distally.

i. The basic unit of bone, the lamella, is about 5 μm thick.

j. In cancellous bone, the trabeculae are about 500 μm thick.

k. The nuclei present in osteoclasts are derived from a single cell that undergoes numerous divisions.

l. Osteoclasts digest bone by first removing the collagen.

m. Osteoblasts on the surface of bone are not in contact with underlying osteocytes.

n. Osteoclasts are unaffected by local changes in pH.

o. Osteoblasts and osteoclasts are derived from the same cell type.

p. The canaliculi of osteocytes in alveolar bone are preferentially orientated towards the periodontal ligament.

q. In adult bone, the surface is frequently lined by bone-lining cells.

s. Osteoblasts are involved in bone resorption.

t. Bone can be considered as a reservoir of bioactive growth factors and cytokines.

Extended matching questions

Theme: Bone

Lead-in

Select the most appropriate option to answer items 1–6. Each option can be used once, more than once or not at all.

Item list

1. Interstitial lamella
2. Bone-lining cells
3. Osteoblasts
4. Osteoclasts
5. Haversian vessels
6. Woven bone

Option list

A. A specialized form of bone that lacks cells

B. Contain receptors for calcitonin

C. Cells most likely to be the main strain receptors in bone

D. Contain significant amounts of rough endoplasmic reticulum and Golgi material

E. Their canaliculi are numerous with no preferential orientation

F. Hypermineralized compared with normal bone

G. The bone initially present at the site of fractures

H. Cover most of the bone surface in old individuals

I. Surrounded by concentric lamellae

J. Osteoprogenitor cells

K. Following remodelling, it represents remnants of a previous osteon/Haversian system

L. Mineralization occurs in the form of calcospherites

Picture questions

Figure 16.1 (Courtesy of Professor T. R. Arnett)

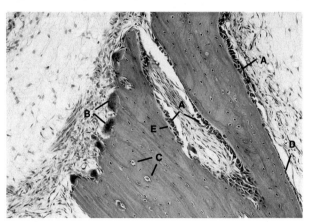

a. Is this a ground or demineralized section?

b. Identify cell types A–D.

c. Do cell types A and B have the same origin?

d. Are there any connections between the cells labelled C?

e. Account for the staining difference between the paler zone (E) immediately adjacent to cell layer A and the rest of the bone matrix.

Self-assessment: questions

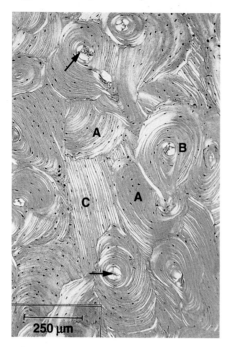

Figure 16.2 (Courtesy of Professor M. M. Smith)

a. Is this a ground or demineralized section?
b. Identify the structures labelled A–C.
c. What occupies the numerous small black spot-like areas?
d. What volume of the tissue is occupied by the organic matrix?

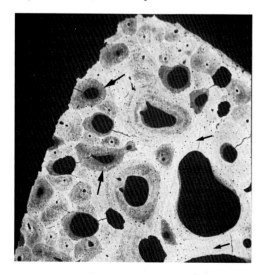

Figure 16.3 (Courtesy of Professor S. J. Jones)

This is a ground section of bone.
a. What technique has been used to produce this image?
b. Account for the variation between the lighter (small arrows) and darker (large arrows) shading.

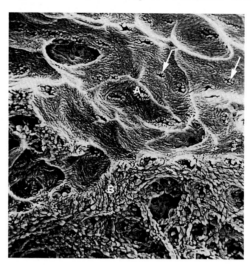

Figure 16.4 (Courtesy of Professor S. J. Jones)

This is a scanning electron micrograph of the surface of alveolar bone adjacent to the root of a tooth. The organic surface layer has been removed with hypochlorite.
a. Account for the difference seen between the upper (A) and lower part (B) of the micrograph.
b. Identify the structures arrowed.

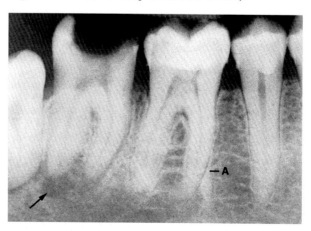

Figure 16.5 (Courtesy of Ms N. White)

In this radiograph:
a. Name feature A, the radiopaque line.
b. Account for its radiological appearance.
c. Is the appearance in the region of the alveolar crest similar throughout the jaw?
d. What feature determines whether the radiolucency at the root apex (arrow) is pathological?
e. What would be the principal radiological feature associated with chronic periodontal disease?
f. Could a fracture of a root be diagnosed on a radiograph?

Self-assessment: questions

g. When would the first radiographic signs of bony repair be evident in the socket of an extracted tooth?

Figure 16.6 (Courtesy of Professor S. J. Jones)

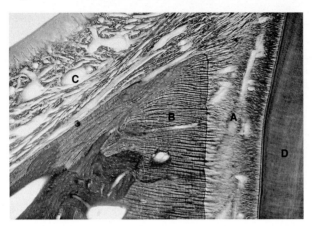

This is a demineralized section stained with van Gieson stain.

a. Identify the structures labelled A–D.
b. Why are no cells evident?
c. Account for the horizontal striations in B, giving their approximate dimensions.

Figure 16.7

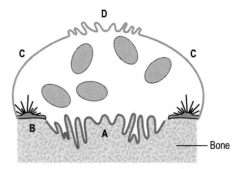

This is a diagram of an osteoclast.

a. Explain the functional significance of cell membrane areas A–D.

Essay questions

1. Describe how a Haversian system is remodelled, with particular reference to the osteoclast.
2. How does a knowledge of alveolar bone impact on the day-to-day clinical situation?
3. Discuss the main factors that control osteoclasis.

Self-assessment: answers

True/false answers

a. **True**. Bundle bone may exhibit resting lines related to physiological drift.

b. **True**. The thinness of the bone here allows for simple infiltration anaesthetic techniques to anaesthetize the incisor teeth.

c. **True**. This is because the bone here is compact. The fibres may even pass completely through the bone and, anteroposteriorly, provide a link between adjacent teeth (transalveolar fibres).

d. **True**. A marker for osteoclasts is acid phosphatase.

e. **True** (although osteoclasts appear to possess some receptors). Many of the factors eventually leading to bone resorption have their receptors on the osteoblast rather than the osteoclast.

f. **True**. In the adult this feature is lost, the marrow then being termed yellow (as opposed to the active red marrow).

g. **False**. Intracellular collagen profiles have not been found in normal osteoclasts. This implies that much collagen breakdown occurs extracellularly in bone as a result of enzymes released at the brush border of the osteoclast.

h. **False**. Bone is deposited distally and resorbed mesially. It is likely that the bone activity is an effect of the drift rather than the direct cause.

i. **True**. The orientation of the collagen will change from lamella to lamella, strengthening the bone. This change in collagen orientation can be confirmed at the light microscopic level using polarized light.

j. **False**. Individual trabeculae in cancellous bone are about 50 µm thick, this thickness being limited by the ability of nutritional molecules to diffuse through the canalicular system.

k. **False**. The nuclei present in osteoclasts are derived by fusion of many mononuclear haemopoietic cells of the macrophage/monocyte lineage.

l. **False**. Osteoclasts digest bone by first removing the mineral. This is achieved by generating protons to lower the pH via the enzyme carbonic anhydrase II. The exposed organic matrix is subsequently removed by enzymes, such as matrix metalloproteinases and cathepsins.

m. **False**. Osteoblasts on the surface of bone are in contact with underlying osteocytes. Through such contacts, the osteocytes can influence the activity of osteoblasts.

n. **False**. Lowering the pH (i.e. acidification) in the microenvironment helps activate osteoclasts, as does hypoxia.

o. **False**. Osteoblasts are derived from stromal/mesenchymal (neural crest) cells, while osteoclasts are derived by fusion of mononuclear haemopoietic cells of the macrophage/monocyte lineage.

p. **False**. Unlike cementocytes in cementum, which is avascular, osteocytes derive their nutrition via blood vessels in the bone lying in the Haversian canals.

q. **True**. As bone turnover is slower, the bone-lining cells protect a greater surface area of bone that might otherwise be a target for osteoclasts. Thus, the surface must be exposed and any osteoid removed for resorption to begin.

s. **True**. Osteoblasts promote resorption by release of cytokines and growth factors, including MSC-F, osteoprotegerin and interleukins that stimulate the production of osteoclasts.

t. **True**. Bone contains a large number of growth factors and cytokines, including TGF-β, BMP-2 and interleukins.

Extended matching answers

Item 1 = Option K. Remodelling of an osteon will commence with resorption at the surface of the central canal. With subsequent deposition back upon itself, part of the original osteon may remain isolated as an interstitial lamella.

Item 2 = Option H. Bone-lining cells cover most of the bone surface in old individuals, in whom there is less evidence of bone deposition and resorption typical of the young.

Item 3 = Option D. Osteoblasts contain significant amounts of rough endoplasmic reticulum and Golgi material, as they are actively secreting the organic matrix of new bone.

Item 4 = Option B. Osteoclasts contain receptors for the hormone calcitonin, whose action is inhibitory on bone resorption.

Item 5 = Option I. Haversian vessels lie in Haversian canals at the centre of Haversian systems (osteons). The bony lamellae surrounding the vessels are arranged concentrically. The orientation of collagen fibrils will change between adjacent lamellae.

Item 6 = Option G. Woven bone is initially present at the site of fractures. Its collagen is less well ordered and will subsequently be remodelled to adult bone.

Picture answers

Figure 16.1

a. As the section is stained and contains cellular material, it is a demineralized section.

b. A = osteoblasts. B = osteoclasts. C = osteocytes embedded in the bone matrix. D = flattened bone-lining cells.

c. No. Osteoblasts (which are also transformed into osteocytes) are cells of the connective tissue series (which may originally be of ectomesenchymal

Self-assessment: answers

origin), while osteoclasts are derived from blood cell precursors.

d. Osteocytes contact each other via gap junctions. As they are interconnected throughout bone, and are also connected with osteoblasts, they are perfectly situated to assess any deformation of bone.

e. The darker staining of the matrix associated with the mineralized bone compared with the lighter staining of unmineralized osteoid at E indicates the two areas have different biochemical compositions as a result of changes at the mineralizing front.

Figure 16.2

a. It is a ground section, as there is no staining and cellular material is absent from the Haversian canals (arrowed), which are filled with debris.

b. A = interstitial lamellae. B = Haversian system consisting of concentric lamellae surrounding a central Haversian canal. C = original circumferential lamellae now lying deep within the bone following remodelling.

c. In ground sections, cellular material (i.e. osteocytes) is lost and the black spaces represent lacunae (spaces that in life house osteocytes) filled with air or cell debris.

d. The organic matrix, consisting primarily (90%) of type I collagen and non-collagenous proteins (10%), comprises about 35% of the tissue by volume.

Figure 16.3

a. This is a radiograph of a thin section of bone. The technique is called microradiography.

b. The varying lighter and darker shades reflect the density (and therefore the degree of mineralization) of the bone. The darker the region of bone (i.e. the more radiolucent), the less the degree of mineralization. This illustrates that bone is continually turning over and remodelling. Cancellous bone turns over more rapidly than compact bone.

Figure 16.4

a. The smooth, scooped-out appearance in the upper part of the micrograph represents an area of bone resorption, the scooped-out regions corresponding to Howship's lacunae. The granular appearance in the lower part of the micrograph represents clusters of hydroxyapatite crystals being deposited on collagen fibrils in an area of bone formation.

b. The structures arrowed represent Sharpey fibres inserting into bone, whose central parts are unmineralized and therefore digested by the hypochlorite used to reveal the mineralizing surface.

Figure 16.5

a. A = lamina dura.

b. The radiopacity of the lamina dura is not due to hypermineralization, but is a consequence of super-imposition of a three-dimensional structure in this two-dimensional image.

c. No. Between the molar teeth, the alveolar crests are flat and horizontal. Between the incisors, the alveolar crests end as points or spines.

d. Discontinuity of the lamina dura here (and resorp-tion of alveolar bone) is indicative of a pathology.

e. Chronic inflammatory periodontal disease begins in the gingiva as a gingivitis, above the alveolar crest and the periodontal ligament. Radiologically, once the gingivitis has spread to involve deeper struc-tures, bone at the alveolar crest becomes involved in the disease process, and the condition moves from being a gingivitis to a periodontitis. The alveolar crests undergo resorption. This loss may be even in all areas such that the pattern of bone loss is hori-zontal or, with advanced tissue destruction, uneven, with irregular vertical bone resorption.

f. Yes. A thin crack-like radiolucent line would initially indicate the fracture site along the root. However, this could gradually disappear following repair with a cementum-like tissue.

g. About 3 weeks after extraction, evidence of new bone formation appears in the healing socket.

Figure 16.6

a. A = periodontal ligament. B = alveolar bone. C = blood vessel in lamina propria of attached gingival. D = root of tooth.

b. This section has been specially stained for collagen fibres with no separate counterstain to highlight the cells.

c. The horizontal striations are periodontal ligament fibres attaching to the alveolar bone surface as Sharpey fibres. In this buccolingual section of a tooth in the region of the apical crest where the bone is compact, the collagen fibres extend for a considerable distance and may pass completely through the alveolar bone (transalveolar fibres). The Sharpey fibres vary between 10 and 20 μm in diameter, being larger (and fewer) than those inserting into the cementum of the root.

Figure 16.7

a. A = ruffled border, that part of the cell that lies adjacent to bone and where resorption occurs. More than one ruffled border may be present at any one time. At the ultrastructural level, the ruffled border is composed of many tightly packed microvilli adjacent

Self-assessment: answers

to the bone surface, providing a large surface area for the resorptive process. Products from the osteoclast (such as protons and proteases) are discharged (exocytosed) and the resulting degraded matrix absorbed (endocytosed) in the central region of the ruffled border. This accounts for the numerous vesicles in the region. Energy for this membrane exchange is provided by the numerous adjacent mitochondria.
B = sealing zone. At the periphery of the ruffled border the sealing (annular/clear) zone separates the ruffled border from the basolateral membrane. Here, the plasma membrane tends to become smooth and the organelle-free cytoplasm beneath it contains numerous contractile actin microfilaments (surrounded by two vinculin rings). The sealing zone serves to attach the cell very closely to the surface of the bone, thus creating an isolated microenvironment in which resorption of bone can take place without diffusion of the protons and proteases produced by the cell into adjacent soft tissue. This isolated microenvironment can be considered as a specialized 'extracellular' lysosome. The attachment of the osteoclast cell membrane to the bone matrix at the sealing zone is mainly due to the presence of cell membrane adhesion proteins known as integrins (mainly $\alpha_v\beta_3$, but also $\alpha_v\beta_1$, $\alpha_2\alpha\beta_1$).
C = basolateral zone. The basolateral surface is the site of surface receptors, such as calcitonin, prostaglandin and RANK. This allows it to function as a regulatory surface for the osteoclast to receive messages from neighbouring cells that govern its activity. The osteoclast has far fewer surface receptors than the osteoblast and is not directly responsive to the majority of hormones or growth factors. This has led to the concept that the osteoblast has a controlling influence in the development and maturation of the osteoclast.
D = functional secretory domain. Opposite the ruffled border, this is a collection site of vesicles. It is believed that bone matrix, degraded at the ruffled border, passes across the cell in these vesicles to be exocytosed here (transcytosis).

Outline essay answers

Question 1

Remodelling of bone only occurs at surfaces. For a Haversian system (osteon), this will therefore commence at the surface of the central Haversian canal. The canal contains vessels and nerves surrounded by loose connective tissue. Prior to remodelling, an inactive surface is covered by a layer of flattened, inactive, bone-lining cells. The first phase in remodelling is the resorptive phase. Osteoclast precursors derived from the haemopoietic system will arrive at the surface in the form of mononuclear precursors. Here,

driven by released bioactive molecules, the mononuclear precursors will fuse to form multinucleated osteoclasts. The cells previously lining the bone surface of the Haversian system will withdraw, exposing the surface to the osteoclasts. Any unmineralized osteoid lining the surface will need to be removed so that the osteoclasts can attack the mineralized surface. Bone-lining cells may release enzymes such as matrix metalloproteinase to help remove any osteoid. Osteoclasts are then activated by further signals (including local acidification and hypoxia) and attach to the bone surface at sealing (clear) zones. Here, the plasma membrane tends to become smooth and the organelle-free cytoplasm beneath it contains numerous contractile actin microfilaments. The sealing zone serves to attach the cell very closely to the surface of the bone, due mainly due to the presence of cell membrane adhesion proteins known as integrins. The sealing zone surrounds the periphery of the ruffled border and is composed of many tightly packed microvilli adjacent to the bone surface, providing a large surface area for the resorptive process. The osteoclast will contain a variable number of ruffled borders.

Once the osteoclast has been activated, bone resorption occurs in two stages. Initially, the mineral phase is removed and later the remaining organic matrix. To provide a low pH for dissolving the mineral phase, the osteoclast secretes protons across the ruffled border by means of a V-type ATPase proton pump; the enzyme carbonic anhydrase II is involved in generating protons. The organic matrix exposed in the resorbing lacuna is then degraded by enzymes such as the MMPs and lysosomal and non-lysosomal enzymes (especially cathepsin K). The structure of the osteoclast clearly relates to its function. In addition to the annular zone and the ruffled border, the cytoplasm of the osteoclast contains numerous mitochondria and large numbers of vesicles of different sizes and types, some containing lysosomal enzymes. Being motile, osteoclasts will then move along and into the Haversian system, resorbing bone and enlarging the size of the canal. In this manner, an initial 'cutting cone' of osteoclastic resorption moves along the central canal of an osteon at about 50 μm/day.

When the appropriate amount of bone has been resorbed, the osteoclasts will receive a signal to cease their resorbing activity. This is the reversal phase. The osteoclasts migrate away from the surface and apoptose. The exposed surface will later be seen as a reversal line and is characterized by its irregular outline and its tendency to stain more deeply due to its distinct biochemistry, particularly its higher quantity of osteopontin and acid phosphatase. The surface of the bone now becomes occupied by small mononuclear cells of mesenchymal origin.

The reversal stage is followed by the formation stage, when the surface of the previously resorbing bone becomes occupied by a layer of osteoblasts. This involves the recruitment, migration and differentiation of osteoblasts from mesenchymal stem cells. Stem cells will change

Self-assessment: answers

to osteoprogenitors, then pre-osteoblasts and finally osteoblasts. The process is characterized by a decreasing proliferative capacity and an increasing degree of differentiation of the cells. Among the earliest markers to indicate that a stem cell is progressing along an osteogenic phenotype is the expression of the nuclear transcription factor, core binding factor 1 (Cbfa1). Osteoprogenitor cells can be identified by the progressive expression of molecules such as type I collagen, alkaline phosphatase and osteopontin. In the pre-osteoblast, the concentration of many of the osteogenic markers seen in the osteoprogenitor cells increases and there is still some limited proliferation. The cell is relatively undifferentiated and there is little roughened endoplasmic reticulum. In the postmitotic osteoblast, even more activity of the markers first seen in pre-osteoblasts is present and there is marked development of roughened endoplasmic reticulum and Golgi material. In addition, new molecules related to mineralization (e.g. osteocalcin) and cell adhesion molecules make their appearance. The osteoblasts will form a distinctive layer of cuboidal cells on the surface, with numerous cell contacts, and will begin to lay down new bone, starting with a layer of organic matrix called osteoid, which will subsequently mineralize. Bone will be deposited in layers (lamellae), reducing the size of the canal until the appropriate size is achieved. In each layer, the collagen fibrils will be laid down in a spiral manner, parallel to the long axis of the Haversian system and with a different angulation in each lamella, providing the bone with extra strength against displacement and fracture. This new bone will form a 'closing zone' behind the preceding 'cutting zone'.

When the appropriate amount of new bone is formed, the osteoblasts at the surface will lose many of their intracellular organelles and be converted into, or replaced by, flattened, resting bone-lining cells that will protect the bone surface until another cycle of activity is started.

Question 2

As maintenance of bone mass is dependent on suitable functional stimuli, alveolar bone tends to atrophy when occlusal loading (transmitted via the periodontal ligament) is decreased. Thus, following tooth extraction, alveolar bone will resorb unless the remaining ridge is loaded. Even the placement of a denture over the remaining alveolar ridge may retard total bone loss. However, if the prosthesis produces excessive compression, the denture-bearing area may show accelerated resorption.

The thickness and type of alveolar bone will determine whether a local anaesthetic will diffuse through to anaesthetize the tooth. Most teeth can be anaesthetized by local infiltration. However, this is precluded for lower cheek teeth, where buccal bone is thick. Here, an inferior alveolar nerve block is required. The thickness of alveolar bone in the molar region will also determine the direction in which the teeth can be extracted.

The ability of alveolar bone to remodel throughout life allows teeth to be repositioned during orthodontic treatment, with resorption of bone in front of the moving tooth matched by deposition of bone behind. However, as osteoclasts cannot fully differentiate between dentine, cementum and bone, excessive orthodontic forces can cause root resorption, ranging from blunting the apices in minor cases up to destruction of a considerable portion of the root.

Localized alveolar bone loss is found in periodontal disease (and in periapical abscesses) in response to the inflammatory process associated with the chronic presence of dental plaque and calculus at the cervical margins. Among important bioactive molecules implicated in this resorption process are cytokines, prostaglandins and protons (as inflamed tissue is generally acidic). As differences exist between the collagen and the ground substance of bone and periodontal ligament, analysis of their breakdown products in the local serum exudates contributing to gingival crevicular fluid may provide a marker to distinguish those patients who are more at risk of losing alveolar bone.

Apart from localized inflammation, more generalized conditions exist where the normal balance between bone formation and bone resorption is disturbed. A knowledge of the normal histological and radiological appearance of bone helps in diagnosing disease. For example, osteopetrosis is a heterogeneous disorder characterized by impaired osteoclast function. In one type, there is a deficiency of the enzyme carbonic anhydrase type II; although bone formation occurs, the defective osteoclasts lose their ability to resorb normally formed bone, which becomes increasingly thickened. An analogous condition in rodents prevents teeth from erupting due to the inability of osteoclasts to resorb the overlying bone. The cause of one such condition is a lack of production of macrophage colony stimulating factor. If the missing factor is replaced, osteoclasts can be switched on to allow alveolar bone resorption and normal eruption.

A clinical area where knowledge of bone biology is important concerns the field of implantology. Whereas a foreign material placed into bone is normally regarded as 'non-self' and becomes surrounded by a capsule of fibrous tissue running parallel to the foreign material surface, some materials allow for a direct structural osseous union. When inserted into the jaw to provide the basis of support for a crown, denture or orthodontic appliance, this union between the dental implant and adjacent living bone is termed osseo-integration. The materials most commonly used in the jaws are based on titanium or its aluminium/vanadium alloys, the spontaneously formed metal-oxide (ceramic) surfaces being critical to integration. A narrow interface (20–40 nm) between the bone and implant contains non-collagenous bone matrix proteins such as osteopontin and bone sialoprotein. The successful long-term retention of

Self-assessment: answers

an implant depends on initial surgical technique to ensure minimum trauma, heating and infection at the implant site and absence of excessive micromotion following implantation, and factors related to the implant (such as shape, stiffness, composition and surface chemistry).

Normally, adjacent to dental implants, bone to a depth of 1 mm may necrose and be remodelled and replaced by new bone, a period of about 17 weeks being required for the establishment of a suitable viable bone interface with the implant. Some modern implantation techniques can, however, allow immediate function if the implant is rigidly held in good-quality dense cortical bone. From a knowledge of basic bone biology, implants are being used that are coated with materials thought likely to encourage osseo-integration, such as cell adhesion molecules and hydroxy-apatite crystals, although delamination of material layers in such a hostile environment can cause long-term problems.

As fractures involving the face and jaws are common, an understanding of the principles involved in bone healing is essential in the clinical situation. Similarly, after tooth extraction, the empty socket will initially fill with a blood clot. In this clot, granulation tissue will form and stem cells and osteoprogenitor cells will soon appear. These cells will eventually differentiate into osteoblasts, the process involving cell–matrix interactions. The initial immature (woven) bone will ultimately be remodelled to form mature, fine-fibred bone, having served its purpose by achieving an initial rapid fracture repair.

In some clinical situations, in particular the replacement of bone lost in trauma or malignant disease, the need for larger amounts of bone may require additional techniques. Requirements may be met by either autologous bone grafts (taken from the patient), allografts (taken from another person) or xenografts (taken from a different species, typically BioOss-bovine bone chips). However, major advances are being made in the application of tissue engineering techniques. These employ laboratory-based materials to either substitute for bone or provide scaffolds and stimuli to promote rapid bony healing in adverse lesions (and those otherwise too large to heal themselves). The three components to be considered in tissue engineering are the scaffold, the cells and additional molecules to drive osteogenesis.

The rate of fracture repair appears to slow down with age, the precise reason for which remains to be clarified. It may be that there is a reduction in the number of viable stem cells in bone with age. An approach to speed up fracture repair in older patients is to isolate some stem cells from the patient's bone, culture them to increase their numbers and then seed them in a suitable framework, which is then placed in the fracture site.

Distraction osteogenesis refers to the technique whereby a bone is sectioned (an osteotomy) and, after an initial interval of 5–7 days, a slow, controlled separation (about 0.5–1 mm/day) of the two bone fragments is undertaken to allow length augmentation by the sustained addition of new woven bone at the fracture site, formed under tension. When adequate length has been achieved, the two bone ends are immobilized for some weeks to allow the woven bone callus to be reinforced and ultimately replaced by mature, dense lamellar bone. For success, the original periosteum and blood supply must be retained. Although this technique was initially developed to increase the length of long bones, it has been adapted for use in craniofacial situations where there is marked bony underdevelopment, such as the small mandible of micrognathism. The mandible can be increased in length and height, depending on the orientation of the pre-planned osteotomies. When teeth have been extracted, the alveolar bone atrophies. In such cases, distraction osteogenesis may allow for an increased alveolar height to render the site suitable for implants.

Question 3

Unlike the other cells associated with bone (e.g. osteoblasts, osteocytes, bone-lining cells), osteoclasts are derived not from stromal cells, but from blood cells. The pluripotent stem cell is of the monocyte/macrophage lineage. Early important transcription factors indicative of its eventual fate are c-Fos and PU-1. Differentiation from the myeloid progenitor to the mononuclear osteoclast precursor involves the activity of many factors, two of the most important of which are macrophage-colony stimulating factor (M-CSF) and receptor activator of nuclear factor kappa B ligand (RANKL). These two factors are produced by osteoblast/stromal cells. As osteoclast progenitors have a receptor (c-Fms) for M-CSF and a receptor (RANK) for RANKL, close association between the two cell types drives the differentiation of the osteoclast precursors into mononuclear pre-osteoclasts. As a method of controlling the rate of formation of osteoclast precursors, the osteoblast also secretes osteoprotegerin (OPG), which acts as a soluble decoy molecule by binding with RANKL and thereby inhibiting osteoclast formation. The rate at which the osteoblast/stromal cells release these factors is influenced by parathormone, whose receptors lie on the osteoblast cell membrane. Indeed, pre-osteoclasts have fewer receptors than osteoblasts. However, one important receptor is for calcitonin. Interrelations of these factors is illustrated in Figure 16.8.

Fusion of mononuclear osteoclasts into multinucleated osteoclasts and their subsequent activation is also driven by the RANKL/RANK system. Many complex membrane interactions must occur when cells are undergoing fusion to become multinucleated. Initially, the cell is non-polarized and it is only on attaching to bone by cell–matrix interactions (involving transmembrane receptors such as integrins and matrix components such as collagen and osteopontin) that the osteoclast becomes polarized and develops the ruffled border, sealing zone and the systems to successfully demineralize bone and degrade its organic matrix. Following its resorptive phase, osteoclasts are thought to be removed by apoptosis.

Self-assessment: answers

Two additional important factors involved in the activation of osteoclasts are acidification and hypoxia:

- Acidification. In appropriate media, osteoclasts cultured on bone at pH 7.4 (physiological or blood pH) are virtually inactive. However, when the pH is lowered to 7.0, there is a large increase in resorption. This reduction in pH also acts synergistically with osteolytic agents such as RANKL. In this respect, it is worth noting that the activity of a number of cytokines and growth factors results in the release of hydrogen ions from the affected cells.
- Hypoxia. There is evidence to suggest that a reduction in oxygen levels in the microenvironment of bone tissue provides a stimulus for osteoclasis, although the mechanism is poorly understood. The hypoxia may be associated with acidification, or it may cause the release of factors such as prostaglandins and vascular endothelial growth factor (VEGF).

Factors that influence apoptosis of osteoclasts have recently been identified. Apoptosis can be inhibited by RANKL and PTH, while it can be stimulated by bisphosphonates. For this reason, the latter drugs have been used to combat osteoporosis.

The importance of factors listed above in association with the formation and activity of osteoclasts has been deduced from studies designed to produce deficiencies or over-expression of the factor. Thus, mice lacking the ability to produce either M-CSF, RANKL or RANK do not develop osteoclasts. They are therefore unable to resorb bone, and thick bone (osteopetrosis) results. Their teeth may be prevented from erupting (due to the inability to resorb bone overlying the erupting teeth), but this can be corrected by restoring the missing factor. In contrast, mice lacking the ability to produce OPG (the osteoclast inhibitor) have increased numbers of osteoclasts and develop osteoporosis.

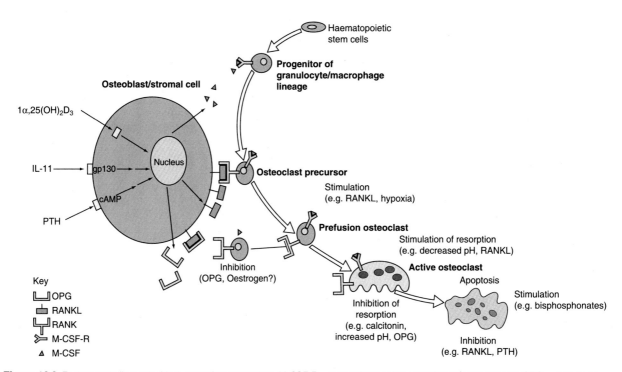

Figure 16.8 Factors controlling osteoblast–osteoclast interactions. M-CSF-R = macrophage colony-stimulating factor receptor; OPG = osteoprotegerin; PTH = parathyroid hormone; RANK = receptor activator of nuclear factor κ B; RANKL = receptor activator of nuclear factor κ B ligand. Courtesy of Drs A. Grigoriadis and T. Arnett.

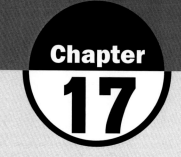
Oral mucosa and gingival crevicular fluid: structure and composition

Functions	**235**
Classification	**235**
Epithelium	**236**
Cytokeratins	**237**
Non-keratinocytes	**237**
Lamina propria	**237**
Regional variation	**237**
Self-assessment: questions	**241**
Self-assessment: answers	**245**

Overview

The oral mucosa shows regional variations relating to different functions in different regions. Masticatory mucosa is found in areas subjected to significant loading such as the hard palate and gingiva. Lining mucosa is subjected to far less stress and is found in regions such as the lip, cheek and floor of mouth. The anterior two-thirds of the dorsum of the tongue is lined by a specialized gustatory mucosa. Where the teeth are exposed in the mouth, the site is sealed and protected by the specialized junctional epithelium. Gingival crevicular fluid (GCF) is an exudate of the periodontal tissues and collects in the gingival sulcus. It is thought to have protective properties towards the tooth and gingival tissues, as it may flush away bacterial cells and host inflammatory molecules from the gingival sulcus, and may have antibacterial properties. The health of the oral mucosa (and teeth) is dependent on the quantity and quality of saliva produced by glands lying in the submucosa.

Learning objectives

You should:
- know the basic structure of the different types of oral mucosa
- understand the reasons for the regional variation of oral mucosa and its significance in different clinical situations; a full appreciation of the normal appearance of the oral mucosa is essential in obtaining a diagnosis for the many pathological conditions seen within the oral cavity
- have a detailed knowledge of the gingiva, as this is essential for an appreciation of periodontal disease
- know the composition, formation and function of GCF
- understand how inflammation influences GCF composition and production
- know that GCF contains proteins which may act as biomarkers of disease progression, and appreciate its usefulness as a possible diagnostic and prognostic fluid.

The oral mucosa lines the oral cavity. It consists of two basic layers separated by a basement membrane:

- An outer stratified squamous epithelium
- An underlying connective tissue layer, the lamina propria.

In many regions, a third layer (the submucosa) is found between the lamina propria and the underlying bone (palate) or muscle (cheeks and lips). The submucosa consists of a looser connective tissue containing the main nerves and blood vessels, as well as glands.

Functions

The oral mucosa has a number of important functions:

- It is protective mechanically against both compressive and shearing forces associated with mastication.
- It provides a barrier to microorganisms, toxins and various antigens.
- It has a role in immunological defence, both humoral and cell-mediated.
- Salivary glands within the oral mucosa secrete saliva which has many functions, including lubrication and buffering activity, as well as providing some antibodies.
- The viscoelastic mucous film also acts as a barrier, helping to retain water and electrolytes.
- The oral mucosa is richly innervated, providing sensory inputs associated with the modalities of touch, proprioception, pain and taste.

Classification

The oral mucosa may be classified into three types – masticatory, lining and specialized mucosa:

- Masticatory mucosa is found in regions where there is high compression and friction, and is characterized by

a keratinized epithelium and a thick lamina propria, which is usually bound down directly to underlying bone (mucoperiosteum).
- In lining mucosa, the epithelium is non-keratinized, as it is subjected to less stress.
- The tongue is regarded as a specialized mucosa, as it contains taste buds and is papillated. The vermilion (red) zone of the lip may also be classified as specialized.

Within the oral cavity about 60% of the mucosa is lining mucosa, about 25% of the mucosa is masticatory mucosa and the remaining 15% is specialized mucosa.

Epithelium

Oral epithelium is classified as a stratified squamous epithelium, as it has several layers of cells with distinct morphologies.

Masticatory epithelium

For masticatory epithelium, four layers are present:

Basal layer

The basal layer (stratum germinativum or stratum basale) is the single cell layer adjacent to the lamina propria and is demarcated from it by a basement membrane. It consists of low columnar/cuboidal cells, among which is a population of stem cells. On mitosis, stem cells give rise to two daughter cells, one of which remains a stem cell. Stem cells generate transit-amplifying cells that will undergo a number of further cell divisions, migrate from the basal cell layer and differentiate to give rise to replacement keratinocytes in the epithelial layers above. The cells of the basal layer are the least differentiated within the oral epithelium. Cell contacts in the form of desmosomes, hemidesmosomes, intermediate and gap junctions are present, allowing for adhesion and cell signalling.

Prickle cell layer

Above the basal layer lies the prickle cell layer (stratum spinosum). The cells of this region show the first stages of maturation, being larger and rounder than those in the basal layer. The transition from basal to prickle cell layer is characterized by the appearance of new cytokeratin types. They contribute to the formation of the tonofilaments, which become thicker and more conspicuous towards the surface. In the upper part of the prickle cell layer, small, intracellular membrane-coating granules appear. These granules are rich in phospholipids and, in the more superficial layers of the stratum spinosum, come to lie close to the cell membrane. Within the prickle cell layer, desmosomes increase in number and eventually occupy about 50% of the intercellular space. The term 'parabasal' is used to refer to the deepest layer of cells of the prickle cell layer that lie next to the basal layer. They may show features similar to that of the basal layer and may undergo cell proliferation.

Granular layer

Above the prickle cell layer lies the granular layer (stratum granulosum). The cells of the granular layer show a further increase in maturation compared with those of the basal and prickle cell layers. Many organelles are reduced or lost, such that the cytoplasm is predominantly occupied by the cytokeratin tonofilaments and tonofibrils. The cells are larger and flatter, and contain numerous small granules called keratohyaline granules. These contain profilaggrin, the precursor to the protein filaggrin that eventually binds the cytokeratin filaments together into a stable network. The membrane-coating granules first seen in the prickle cell layer move towards the superficial surface of the keratinocyte and discharge their lipid-rich contents into the extracellular space. This intercellular 'cement', together with the cell contacts (especially tight junctions in the upper region of the granular layer), helps limit the permeability of the layer and prevents water loss. Synthesis increases of the additional proteins, loricrin and involucrin, first apparent in the prickle cell layer. These proteins will help form a more resistant cell wall (envelope).

Keratinized layer

The most superficial layer in masticatory epithelium is the keratinized layer (cornified layer, stratum corneum). In this final stage in the maturation of the epithelial cells, there is loss of all organelles including the nucleus. The cells of the keratinized layer become filled entirely with closely packed tonofilaments surrounded by the matrix protein filaggrin. This mixture of proteins is collectively called keratin; it contributes to the mechanical and chemical resistance of the layer. In the cornified layer, involucrin becomes cross-linked (by the enzyme transglutaminase) to form a thin (10 nm), highly resistant, electron-dense, cornified envelope just beneath the plasma membrane. The cells of the keratinized layer are shed (squames), necessitating the constant turnover of epithelial cells. Desmosomes weaken and disappear to allow for this desquamation.

In some areas such as the gingiva, the nuclei may be retained in the cornified layer. These cells are described as parakeratinized (in contrast to the more usual orthokeratinized cells without nuclei).

Lining epithelium

In lining epithelium, the cells are non-keratinized at the surface. Like the cells in keratinized epithelia, cells from the basal layer enlarge and flatten as they shift towards the surface. The surface layers differ from the cells of keratinized epithelia in that they lack keratohyaline granules. This accounts for the less developed and dispersed tonofilaments present in lining epithelium. There are also more organelles in the surface layers compared with those in keratinized cells, although there are still considerably fewer than in the basal layer. Nuclei persist within the surface layers. Membrane-coating granules are smaller and lack the lipid-rich lamellar structure of those in keratinizing epithelia. This is thought to account for the greater permeability of lining epithelium compared to keratinized epithelium. Lining epithelium generally lacks the proteins filaggrin and loricrin, but contains involucrin.

Turnover time of the epithelium is fastest in the region of the junctional and sulcular epithelia (about 5 days), which are located immediately adjacent to the tooth surface. This is probably about twice as fast as that seen in lining mucosa, such as the cheek. Turnover time in masticatory mucosa is a little slower than that in non-masticatory (lining) mucosa.

Cytokeratins

Within epithelial cells, cytokeratin intermediate filaments function as components of the cytoskeleton and cell contacts (desmosomes and hemidesmosomes). The products of each cytokeratin gene family are divided into the neutral or basic type II cytokeratins (numbered 1–8) and the acidic type I cytokeratins (numbered 9–20). They occur in pairs; the type I cytokeratin is the smaller of each pair. There is a specific distribution of cytokeratins within epithelia:

- Cytokeratins 5 and 14 are usually restricted to the basal and parabasal layers (although cytokeratin 14 may also be expressed by suprabasal keratinocytes).
- Cytokeratins 1 and 10 (or CK 2 and 11) are characteristically found in the suprabasal layers of masticatory mucosa.
- In lining mucosa, the suprabasal keratinocytes stain primarily for cytokeratins 4 and 13.
- In the epithelium covering the soft palate, cytokeratins 7, 8 and 18 (normally associated with simple epithelia, such as ductal luminal cells) are present.

Non-keratinocytes

As many as 10% of the cells in the oral epithelium are non-keratinocytes, and include melanocytes, Langerhans cells and Merkel cells.

Melanocytes

Melanocytes are pigment-producing cells located in the basal layer. They are derived from the neural crest. They are dendritic cells, having long processes that extend in different directions and across several epithelial layers. Melanocytes characteristically contain pigment that is packaged in small granules termed melanosomes. The pigment is passed to adjacent keratinocytes when the tips of the dendrites are actively phagocytosed. In dark-skinned patients, patches of melanin pigment may be seen in the mouth, particularly in the gingiva.

Langerhans cells

Langerhans cells are dendritic cells situated in the layers above the basal layer. They are derived from bone marrow precursors. They act as antigen-presenting cells. Ultrastructurally, the Langerhans cell contains characteristic trilaminar, rod-shaped granules called Birbeck granules.

Merkel cells

Merkel cells are found in the basal layer, often closely apposed to nerve fibres. They are thought to act as receptors and are derived from the neural crest. Merkel cells can be identified using antibodies for cytokeratins 8/18 and 20. Merkel cells are common in masticatory epithelia but less frequently found in lining mucosa. Ultrastructurally, the nucleus of the Merkel cell is often deeply invaginated and may contain a characteristic rodlet. The cytoplasm contains a collection of electron-dense granules, which may liberate a transmitter towards the adjacent nerve terminal, giving the cell a sensory function. Desmosomes are associated with the cell membrane. Free nerve endings not associated with a Merkel cell are also found within the epithelium. These are nociceptors.

Inflammatory cells

Some inflammatory cells may also be found in the epithelium, having migrated through it from the underlying lamina propria. Lymphocytes are the most common type of inflammatory cell, though polymorphonuclear leukocytes and plasma cells may also be encountered. The greater degree of permeability of non-keratinized epithelium may account for the larger number of inflammatory cells said to occur there compared with masticatory epithelium.

Lamina propria

The lamina propria underlying the oral epithelium provides mechanical support for the epithelium, as well as nutrition. Its ridges, the dermal papillae, interdigitate with the epithelial folds or rete; the folding in masticatory mucosa is more pronounced than in lining mucosa. Its nerves have an important sensory function, while its blood cells and salivary glands have important defensive roles. The principal cells of the lamina propria are fibroblasts, responsible for the production and maintenance of extracellular matrix. The collagen fibres are mainly type I (about 90%), with about 8% type III. Elastin fibres are also present, their number varying according to site. As with all general connective tissues, the usual defence cells are present, such as macrophages, mast cells and lymphocytes. Inflammatory cells will increase dramatically in inflammation, such as following gingivitis.

Regional variation

There is regional variation in the structure of the oral mucosa related to different degrees and types of stress during mastication, speech and facial expression. As a consequence, the structure of the oral mucosa varies in terms of the thickness of the epithelium, the degree of keratinization, the complexity of the connective tissue-epithelium interface, the composition of the lamina propria, and the presence or absence of the submucosa.

Seventeen

Masticatory mucosa

Masticatory mucosa is found where there is high compression and friction, and is characterized by a keratinized epithelium and a thick lamina propria, with a highly folded interface. The mucosa of the gingiva and palate is masticatory, the bulk of which is firmly bound down to underlying bone by dense collagen bundles forming a mucoperiosteum. In the roof of the hard palate, however, a submucosa is present, within which is found the main neurovascular bundles. There are also minor mucous glands (predominantly posteriorly) that open on to the surface by ducts, and adipose tissue (predominantly anteriorly). The nasal surface of the hard palate is lined by a respiratory mucosa.

Gingiva

The majority of the gingiva surrounding the neck of the tooth is attached to the tooth and alveolar bone, with no submucosa. Its external surface (oral gingival epithelium) is a masticatory mucosa that may show orthokeratinization or parakeratinization. Its margin (1 mm) is the free gingiva, which may be demarcated from the attached gingiva by the free gingival groove. The gingival margin marks the floor of the gingival crevice or sulcus.

The internal surface of the gingiva adjacent to the tooth shows two zones of epithelium:

- The crevicular (sulcular) epithelium that faces the gingival crevice
- The junctional epithelium that is in direct contact with the enamel surface at the base of the crevice.

These two epithelia comprise the dentogingival junction; both are non-keratinized.

Crevicular (sulcular) epithelium

The crevicular epithelium has a more folded interface with the underlying connective tissue. In addition, the two epithelia can also be distinguished by their different cytokeratin profiles. The superficial layers of the crevicular epithelium stain positive for the cytokeratins typical of lining epithelium (e.g. cytokeratins 4 and 13). However, junctional epithelium not only lacks the cytokeratins typical of lining epithelium, but expresses the basal keratinocyte cytokeratins 5, 14 and 19 throughout all its layers, typical of the cytokeratin profile of the odontogenic epithelium from which it is derived.

Junctional epithelium

The junctional epithelium shows a number of additional specialized features that distinguish it from other oral epithelia:

- In addition to the normal (external) basal lamina at its junction with the adjacent lamina propria, it has a second (internal) basal lamina uniting it to the enamel surface.
- It has fewer desmosomes and this is correlated with larger intercellular spaces that may comprise up to 5% of the volume of the tissue. This can be correlated in turn with its increased permeability, which allows crevicular fluid and defence cells to pass into the crevicular space.

- It has the highest turnover rate.
- The peripheral cells adjacent to the enamel surface have organelles, such as Golgi material and roughened endoplasmic reticulum, related to the synthesis and secretion of the (internal) basal lamina.
- The composition of its integrins is different, implying a difference in the adhesive mechanisms within its cells.

The lamina propria associated with the junctional epithelium has a rich blood supply arranged as a complex anastomosing network. This crevicular plexus is the obvious source of gingival crevicular fluid. The vessels of the plexus are very sensitive to stimulation and are likely to vasodilate under the slightest of insults. In response to plaque, they may become more permeable, increasing the production of crevicular fluid.

Principal gingival collagen fibres

The dentogingival junction seals the underlying connective tissue of the periodontium from the oral environment. The strength of the seal is thought to be dependent not only upon the properties of the junctional epithelium, but also upon the groups of principal gingival collagen fibres. Among these groups are:

- dentogingival fibres (arising from the root surface above the alveolar crest and inserting into the lamina propria of the gingiva)
- longitudinal fibres (extending along the free gingiva, some possibly for the whole length of the dental arch)
- circular fibres (encircling each tooth within the marginal and interdental gingiva)
- alveologingival fibres (running from the crest of the alveolar bone and into the overlying lamina propria of the gingiva)
- dentoperiosteal fibres (passing from cementum over the alveolar crest to insert into the periosteum)
- trans-septal fibres (passing horizontally from the root of one tooth, above the alveolar crest, to be inserted into the root of the adjacent tooth).

Interdental gingiva

The interdental gingiva is the part of the gingiva lying between adjacent teeth. The shape and arrangement of the gingival tissues between the teeth depend on the shape of the contact between the teeth:

- From the buccal or lingual aspects, the interdental gingiva has a wedge-shaped appearance.
- Between the anterior teeth (which contact only at a small point), it would appear similarly 'pointed' when viewed in a buccolingual plane.
- In the posterior cheek teeth, which have a broader area of contact, the appearance from the buccal or lingual side would show the typical wedge shape but, across its buccolingual plane, there are two peaks on the buccal and lingual aspects with a curved depression between them (the interdental col), which fills the contour around the contact point.

The epithelium lining the col is non-keratinized and initially derived from the reduced enamel epithelium. Its epithelium is thin and, as the region is not easy to keep plaque-free, inflammatory cells may be seen infiltrating the underlying lamina propria. When teeth are spaced, the col does not exist and the gingiva here is covered by a keratinized epithelium.

Gingival crevicular fluid

Gingival crevicular fluid (GCF) may be regarded as a transudate (or exudate) of the periodontal tissues. It gathers in the gingival sulcus and may be sampled by non-invasive means at the gingival margin. GCF is thought to be protective towards the tooth and gingival tissues, as it washes away potentially harmful cells (bacterial and host) and molecules from the gingival sulcus. It also contains antibacterial substances along with high calcium and phosphate concentrations. The major constituents of GCF are derived from plasma, interstitial fluid, microbial sources, dental plaque matrix, host inflammatory cells and host tissues. Flow rate of the GCF can also be directly related to the degree of gingival inflammation. In healthy tissues, low levels of flow rates are observed (typically 0.05–0.2 μl/min) and the fluid has a composition similar to interstitial fluid.

Osmosis

The GCF reaches the sulcus by intercellular routes across the epithelial wall, and this passage of fluid into the sulcus is thought to be mediated by osmosis. In the healthy patient, small amounts of subgingival plaque give rise to macromolecular plaque, which is usually removed by desquamating epithelial cells or phagocytosis. However, macromolecules can diffuse intercellularly towards the basement membrane, which is a limiting barrier. This creates an osmotic gradient and interstitial fluid flows into junctional and sulcular epithelium and sulcus.

Flow of GCF is influenced by several factors, the major one being the passage of fluid from capillaries into the gingival tissues. Flow rate is also directly affected by:

- removal of the fluid by the lymphatic system of the gingival tissues
- the filtration coefficient of the junctional and sulcular epithelia
- differences in oncotic pressure of the interstitial fluid and sulcular fluid.

The basement membrane filters out large components.

Inflammation

Inflammation can have direct influences on GCF production. In inflamed periodontal and gingival tissues, GCF flow rate is increased due to a greater osmotic gradient being created and fluid flows across a weakened basement membrane. There is a loose organization of the junctional and sulcular epithelium, which serves to increase fluid flow from the capillaries into the connective tissues as a consequence of the host response. The production of an inflammatory exudate allows the passage of cells and large proteins into the

fluid, and pressure sources such as mastication and tooth brushing may cause an increase in GCF flow. These forces are thought to produce transient elevations in the pressure of interstitial fluids and increased GCF flow.

Biochemical composition

Biochemically, GCF contains both inorganic and organic components. Its composition is similar to plasma; however, it may be modified by the local environment and ecosystem.

Inorganic constituents include sodium, potassium, calcium and magnesium. Calcium levels within the GCF are higher than those in saliva, which has important implications for pellicle protein interaction, enhancing salivary protein precipitation, attachment of bacteria and calculus formation.

In health, the concentration of organic components of GCF are similar to those of plasma. In disease, there is an increase in components relating to the degradation of the underlying connective tissues and host response to invading pathogenic bacteria. The presence of such constituents highlights the potential of GCF for diagnostic/prognostic use. The serum-derived proteins found in the GCF include:

- Serum albumin, important in protein transport and as an antioxidant
- Immunoglobulins IgA, IgG and IgM
- Fibrinogen, essential for blood clot formation
- Complement components of both the classical and alternative pathways, which can cause release of lysosomal enzymes from leucocytes mediating cell lysis
- Protease inhibitors α_1-antitrypsin, α_2-macroglobulin and α_1-antichymotrypsin.

In addition to the above, GCF also contains components of bacterial origin, including urea, lactic acid, hydrogen sulphide, lipopolysaccharides and bacterial enzymes (acid phosphatase, lysozyme, hyaluronidase). These bacterial enzymes can be accompanied by the presence of enzymes derived from the host inflammatory cells and resident connective tissues. Such enzymes, with roles in the inflammatory response to periodontitis and inflammatory-mediated tissue destruction, include cathepsin D, cathepsin G, alkaline phosphatase, elastase and collagenases.

Lining mucosa

Lining mucosa is not subject to high levels of friction but must be mobile and distensible. It is thus non-keratinized and has a loose lamina propria. Within the lamina propria, the collagen fibres are arranged as a network to allow free movement, and the elastin fibres allow recoil to prevent the mucosa being chewed. Commonly, lining mucosa also has a submucosa. The lips, cheeks, alveolus, floor of the mouth, ventral surface of the tongue and soft palate have a lining mucosa.

Lip

The lip has skin on its outer surface and labial mucosa on its inner surface. Between these two tissues lies the vermilion

Seventeen

zone (also known as the red or transitional zone) of the lip. The lips have striated muscles in their core that are part of the muscles of facial expression. Substantial amounts of minor mucous salivary glands are present in the sub-mucosa beneath the oral mucosa. The epithelial thickness gradually increases from the skin to the mucosal aspect.

Vermilion zone

The vermilion zone lacks the appendages of skin. Its epithelium is keratinized, but thin and translucent. The connective tissue papillae of the lamina propria are rela-tively long and narrow, and contain capillary loops. The proximity of these vessels to the surface, combined with the translucency of the epithelium, gives the surface a red appearance — hence its name. The junctional region between the vermilion zone and the oral mucosa is known as the intermediate zone. It lacks a granular layer and tends to have a thick parakeratinized layer. In infants, this becomes thickened and forms the suckling pad. The vermilion zone has a unique transitional phenotype with features of both epidermal and oral mucosal epithelium.

Ventral surface of the tongue

The ventral surface of the tongue and the floor of the mouth are covered by typical lining mucosa. The epithe-lium is thin and non-keratinized, and shows short papil-lae. The submucosa is extensive on the floor of the mouth but indistinct (if not absent) on the ventral surface of the tongue, where the mucosa binds down to the tongue mus-cles. The thinness of the epithelium and the vascularity of the connective tissue make this a route by which some drugs can rapidly reach the bloodstream.

Specialized mucosa

The anterior two-thirds of the dorsum of the tongue may be considered a specialized gustatory mucosa due to the presence of taste buds and papillae.

Dorsal surface of the tongue

An indistinct groove, the sulcus terminalis, divides the dorsal surface of the tongue into an anterior two-thirds (palatal surface) and a posterior third (pharyngeal sur-face). The anterior two-thirds of the tongue is covered with numerous papillae, namely filiform, fungiform, foliate and circumvallate.

Filiform papillae

Filiform papillae are the most numerous papillae and each consists of an overlying stratified squamous epithelium that is keratinized and forms hair-like tufts (although the

regions between the papillae are non-keratinized). The central core of lamina propria has smaller, secondary papillae branching from it. The filiform papillae have an abrasive function during mastication when the bolus is compressed against the palate.

Fungiform papillae

Fungiform papillae are found as isolated, mushroom-shaped papillae scattered between the filiform papillae. They are covered by a relatively thin epithelium that may or may not be keratinized, and have a vascular core of lam-ina propria. Taste buds are found on their surface.

Foliate papillae

Foliate papillae may be present as one or two longitudinal clefts at the side of the posterior part of the tongue. Taste buds are found within the non-keratinized epithelium of these papillae.

Circumvallate papillae

Circumvallate papillae are the largest papillae and are sur-rounded by a trench-like feature. They number between about 8 and 15, and lie in front of the sulcus terminalis; they do not project beyond the normal surface level of the tongue. Each circumvallate papilla is generally covered by a non-keratinized epithelium. Taste buds predominate on the internal wall of the trench in the epithelium. Small serous glands (of von Ebner) empty into the base of the trench. Groups of mucous glands are also seen within the muscle of the tongue, particularly in the posterior part.

Taste buds

Taste buds are located within the epithelium around the walls of the circumvallate papillae, but are also found in small numbers on the fungiform and foliate papillae, on the soft palate and on the epiglottis. Two types of cell are present in the taste bud: the supporting cell and the taste cell. A small pore opens from the surface into the taste bud. Simple cytokeratins are expressed by taste buds. See Chap-ter 5 for more information on the sense of taste.

Lingual tonsil

A collection of lymphoid follicles lies on the posterior third of the tongue, which is covered by a lining mucosa. These are collectively known as the lingual tonsil and form a component of Waldeyer's ring, which protects the opening into the pharynx (together with the palatine tonsil, and the tubal and pharyngeal tonsils within the nasopharynx). The follicles are deep crypts lined with epithelium and containing a mass of lymphoid material. The follicles usually open onto the surface of the tongue. The mucosa in this region also contains many mucous glands.

Self-assessment: questions

True/false statements

Which of the following statements are true and which are false?

a. Sebaceous glands are found in the oral mucosa of the lips and cheeks.
b. Parakeratosis refers to the incomplete loss of nuclei during keratinization.
c. Approximately 10% of cells in the oral epithelium are non-keratinocytes.
d. Langerhans cells, like melanocytes, are derived from ectomesenchyme (neural crest) cells.
e. The gingiva forms a characteristic interdental col between teeth which are spaced.
f. The sulcular epithelium is unique in having both an internal and an external basement membrane (basal lamina).
g. The junctional epithelium possesses a granular layer.
h. The junctional epithelium can completely regenerate following surgical removal.
i. The attached gingiva has a narrow submucosa.
j. The alveolar mucosa has well-developed dermal papillae.
k. Like skin, keratinized masticatory epithelium contains a stratum lucidum.
l. Fungiform papillae on the anterior two-thirds of the tongue are keratinized.
m. The vermilion (red) zone on the lip is keratinized, with pronounced dermal papillae.
n. Like other lining epithelium, junctional epithelium contains cytokeratins 4 and 13.
o. Trans-septal fibres pass from the cementum of adjacent teeth above the alveolar crest.
p. Cytokeratins 1 and 10 are characteristic of masticatory epithelium.
q. The free gingiva is stippled when healthy.
r. The turnover time of masticatory epithelium is generally quicker than that for lining epithelium.
s. Unlike the melanocyte, the Merkel cell exhibits some desmosomes.
t. Turnover time for collagen in the gingiva is similar to that in the periodontal ligament.
u. Gingival crevicular fluid (GCF) represents plasma solely derived from blood vessels in the underlying periodontal tissues.
v. Flow rate of the GCF can be directly related to the degree of gingival inflammation.
w. GCF contains organic components alone.
x. Bacterial and host enzymes can be identified in GCF.

Extended matching questions

Theme: Oral mucosa

Lead-in

Select the most appropriate option to answer items 1–5. Each option can be used once, more than once or not at all.

Item list

1. Junctional epithelium
2. Merkel cell
3. Vermilion (red) zone of the lip
4. Circumvallate papilla
5. Granular layer

Option list

A. It has both an internal and an external basal lamina
B. It is characterized by cytokeratins 4 and 13
C. It lies just above the stratum lucidum in the hard palate
D. Serous glands drain into it
E. It is derived from neural crest and contains cytokeratin
F. It is keratinized
G. It contains the precursor to filaggrin
H. It is a dendritic cell
I. It contains sweat glands
J. It is derived from blood cell precursors

Picture questions

Figure 17.1 (Courtesy of Professor H. E. Schroeder)

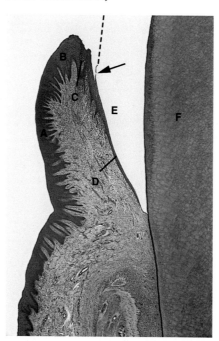

In this demineralized section where the broken vertical line (arrowed) represents the acquired pellicle:

a. Identify this region of the oral cavity.
b. Identify the structures labelled A–F.
c. Classify A–D according to whether they are masticatory or lining mucosa.
d. Which of the layers A–D has the highest turnover rate?
e. List four differences between C and D.

Self-assessment: questions

Figure 17.2 (Courtesy Mr Karyawasam)

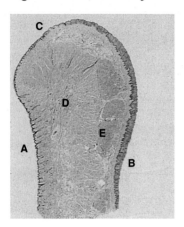

a. Identify the region illustrated.
b. Identify the regions/structures labelled A–D.
c. What glands are represented by label E?
d. What cytokeratin pair characterizes the epithelium at B?

Figure 17.3

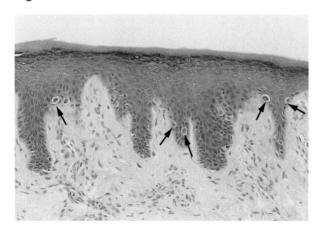

a. Which of zones A–C in Figure 17.2 is represented by this micrograph?
b. What is the significance of the clear cells arrowed?

Figure 17.4 (Courtesy of Professor C. A. Squier)

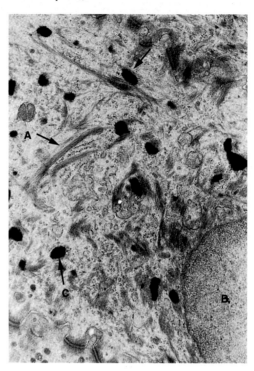

a. Identify the structures labelled A–C in this electron micrograph of a keratinocyte from one of the layers of the oral epithelium.
b. What layer does it come from?
c. What does C contain?
d. Does skin have similar cells?

Self-assessment: questions

Figure 17.5 (Courtesy of Dr A. W. Barrett)

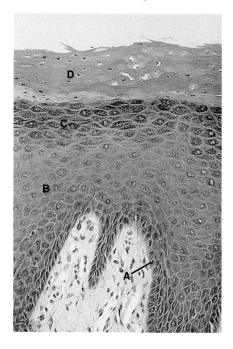

a. Identify the layers labelled A–D.
b. What region of the oral cavity may this represent?
c. Is there any added feature worth noting in layer D?
d. What are the essential differences between the epithelium illustrated here and the epidermis in skin?

Figure 17.6 (Figure B Courtesy of Dr M. E. Atkinson)

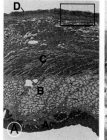 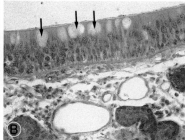

Figure 17.6B represents a higher power view of the window shown in the upper layer of Figure 17.6A

a. What region of the oral cavity is illustrated in the micrograph (Figure 17.6A)? Indicate your reasons.
b. What type of epithelium is found on surface A?
c. What type of epithelium is found on surface D and shown at higher magnification in Figure 17.6B? What are the pale structures arrowed?
d. What type of tissue is C in Figure 17.6A and what is its probable innervation?

e. What is the sensory innervation of the structures arrowed in Figure 14.6B?

Figure 17.7

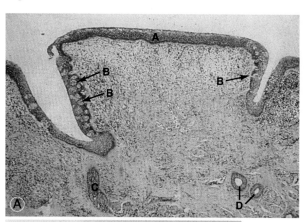

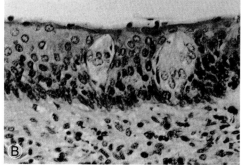

a. Identify the structure shown in Figure 17.7A.
b. What type of epithelium occurs at A?
c. Identify the pale structures (B) which are shown at higher magnification in Figure 17.7B.
d. Identify C.
e. Identify D.

Figure 17.8 (Courtesy of Professor C. A Squier)

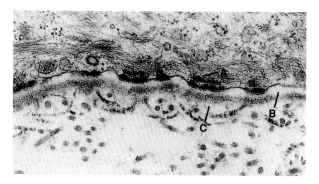

a. Identify the structures labelled A–C.

Self-assessment: questions

b. What is the principal component of B?
c. What is the principal component of C?
d. What cell produces B and C?

Figure 17.9

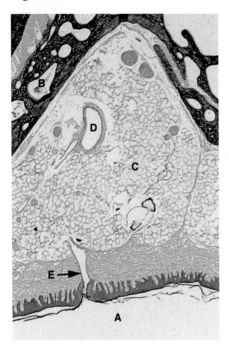

a. Identify this region of the oral cavity.
b. Classify the type of epithelium at A.
c. Identify B–E.
d. What is the innervation of C?

Figure 17.10 (Courtesy of Dr D. Adams)

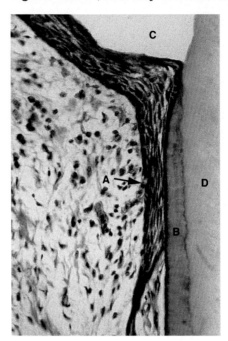

a. Identify the structures labelled A–D.
b. What is the means of attachment of A and B?
c. Is this from a young or old patient?
d. Is this normal, healthy tissue?

Essay questions

1. Is the junctional epithelium a typical lining epithelium?
2. Name the non-keratinocytes present within the oral cavity, describing their origin, morphology and function.
3. Discuss the synthesis of gingival crevicular fluid (GCF) and its biological function. How might GCF be informative clinically?
4. How is the function of the oral surface of the hard palate related to its function?

Self-assessment: answers

True/false answers

a. **True.** These ectopic glands appear as yellowish patches known as Fordyce spots.

b. **True.** Parakeratosis is normally present in the masticatory mucosa of the gingival and palate.

c. **True.** These cells include melanocytes, Langerhans cells and Merkel cells.

d. **False.** Langerhans cells are derived from blood cells.

e. **False.** An interdental col only occurs between cheek teeth that are in contact and will be lined by a non-keratinized epithelium. When teeth are spaced, the col will disappear and be replaced by a keratinized epithelium.

f. **False.** The sulcular epithelium only has one basement membrane (basal lamina). The junctional epithelium possesses two basal laminae; the internal basal lamina is found at the interface with the tooth surface, the external basal lamina at the interface with the underlying connective tissue.

g. **False.** The junctional epithelium is non-keratinized and lacks a granular layer.

h. **True.** Regeneration occurs from the adjacent oral epithelium. If this were not true, much periodontal surgery would be unsuccessful.

i. **False.** No submucosa exists beneath the attached gingiva.

j. **False.** The alveolar mucosa is a lining mucosa.

k. **False.** A stratum lucidum is absent from the oral epithelium. Unlike skin, the oral mucosa also lacks hair follicles and sweat glands.

l. **False.** Fungiform papillae are covered with a non-keratinized epithelium.

m. **True.** Together with the underlying blood vessels, this gives the vermilion zone its red coloration. The vermilion zone also lacks mucous glands found in labial mucosa.

n. **False.** Junctional epithelium contains simpler cytokeratins, such as cytokeratin 19, perhaps reflecting its derivation from odontogenic epithelium.

o. **True.** These fibres provide an anatomical basis whereby all the teeth in the arch are linked together.

p. **True.** Cytokeratins 4 and 13 are characteristic of lining epithelium.

q. **False.** The free gingiva is smooth.

r. **False.** Turnover time for the hard palate is of the order of about 3–4 weeks, whereas that for buccal mucosa is nearer 2 weeks.

s. **True.** The non-dendritic Merkel cell also contains some tonofibrils.

t. **False.** The turnover time of gingival collagen is about three times slower than that of the periodontal ligament.

u. **False.** The major constituents of GCF are derived not only from plasma, but also from interstitial fluid, microbial sources, dental plaque matrix, host inflammatory cells and host tissues.

v. **True.** GCF flow rate is increased due to a greater osmotic gradient being created and fluid flows across a weakened basement membrane.

w. **False.** GCF contains both organic and inorganic components, as it is modified by the surrounding environment and ecosystem.

x. **True.** GCF contains a range of enzymes of both bacterial and host origin. These may include alkaline phosphatase and cathepsins.

Extended matching answers

Item 1 = Option A. The presence of a basal lamina on its external and internal surfaces makes this epithelium unique.

Item 2 = Option E. Due to the presence of cytokeratins, Merkel cells can be identified by immunohistochemical techniques using antibodies for cytokeratins 8/18 and 20.

Item 3 = Option F. This keratin layer is thin and translucent and, as underlying blood capillaries lie close to its surface, the vermilion assumes a red coloration.

Item 4 = Option D. The serous glands (of von Ebner), by draining into the trenches surrounding the circumvallate papillae, bring ingested material into solution for tasting.

Item 5 = Option G. The precursor of filaggrin is profilaggrin. The protein filaggrin eventually binds keratin filaments together into a stable network.

Picture questions

Figure 17.1

a. Dentogingival junction.

b. A = attached gingival epithelium. B = free gingival epithelium. C = sulcular (crevicular) epithelium. D = junctional epithelium. E = enamel space. F = dentine.

c. A and B = masticatory (keratinized) epithelium. C and D = lining (non-keratinized) epithelium.

d. The junctional epithelium (D) has the highest turnover rate.

e. The junctional epithelium has fewer desmosomes, larger intercellular spaces, two basal lamina, a higher turnover rate, is more permeable, contains more organelles associated with the synthesis and extracellular secretion of protein and has a different cytokeratin profile.

Figure 17.2

a. Lip.

b. A = skin of lip. B = labial mucosa of lip. C = vermilion zone. D = orbicularis oris muscle.

c. E = mucous glands of lip.

d. Being a lining epithelium, it is characterized by cytokeratins 4 and 13.

245

Self-assessment: answers

Figure 17.3

a. The thin, keratinized layer, the absence of skin appendages, the pronounced dermal papillae and the absence of minor salivary glands indicate that this is the vermilion zone of the lip.
b. The clear cells in the basal layer represent non-keratinocytes (melanocytes and Merkel cells). They generally lack the tonofilaments and the many desmosomes of typical keratinocytes, and do not stain as readily as them when visualized in routine haematoxylin and eosin preparations.

Figure 17.4

a. A = tonofibril. B = nucleus. C = keratohyalin granule.
b. Granular layer.
c. Keratohyalin granules contain profilaggrin, the precursor to filaggrin.
d. Yes.

Figure 17.5

a. A = basal layer. B = prickle cell layer. C = granular layer. D = keratinized layer.
b. Because of the keratinized layer and the prominent epithelial rete, it is likely to come from the masticatory mucosa of the hard palate or gingiva.
c. Nuclei have been retained in the keratinized layer. The term for this is parakeratinized.
d. Skin would show sweat glands and hair follicles, and may contain an extra layer near the surface, the stratum lucidum.

Figure 17.6

a. Because of the presence of muscle and glandular tissue, and because of the absence of bone, skin and masticatory mucosa, this section is probably from the soft palate.
b. A = stratified squamous (lining) epithelium.
c. D = respiratory (ciliated) epithelium lining the nasal surface of the soft palate. The arrows indicate goblet cells.
d. B = mucous glands. They probably derive their parasympathetic nerve supply from the facial nerve (via the pterygopalatine ganglion), which is distributed in branches emanating from this ganglion (e.g. lesser palatine nerve).
e. The muscles of the palate (C) are innervated by the cranial accessory nerve (via the pharyngeal plexus), except for the tensor veli palatine muscle, which is supplied by the mandibular branch of the trigeminal nerve.

Figure 17.7

a. Circumvallate papilla of tongue.
b. Lining (non-keratinized) epithelium.
c. B = taste bud, innervated by the glossopharyngeal nerve.
d. C = serous glands (of von Ebner).
e. D = salivary ducts.

Figure 17.8

a. A = hemidesmosome. B = lamina lucida. C = lamina densa.
b. Lining (non-keratinized) epithelium.
c. The lamina densa contains type IV collagen.
d. The lamina lucida and lamina densa are products of the basal cells (stratum germinativum) of the epithelium.

Figure 17.9

a. Hard palate.
b. Masticatory (keratinized/parakeratinized) epithelium.
c. B = bone of hard palate. C = mucous glands in submucosa. D = greater palatine artery. E = duct of mucous gland.
d. The parasympathetic innervation of minor mucous glands is the greater petrosal branch of the facial nerve via the pterygopalatine ganglion and greater palatine nerve.

Figure 17.10

a. A = junctional epithelium. B = cementum. C = enamel space. D = dentine.
b. A basal lamina-like structure.
c. As the attachment has migrated on to the cementum, this must represent an older patient.
d. The apical migration of the junctional epithelium on to cementum, together with an obvious infiltration of inflammatory cells, indicates this to be diseased tissue.

Outline essay answers

Question 1

The junctional epithelium is the epithelial collar that surrounds the tooth and extends from the region of the cement–enamel junction to the bottom of the gingival crevice. In its basic histological appearance, the junctional epithelium is a lining epithelium in that it is a stratified squamous epithelium comprising two main layers: a single basal layer, above which are a variable number of layers comprising what may be termed the prickle cell layer. Unlike other lining mucosa, junctional

Self-assessment: answers

epithelium shows more variation in thickness. Cervically, where it is continuous with the crevicular epithelium, it may be 15–30 cells thick (up to 100 μm), whilst apically it narrows to only 1–3 cells thick. Unlike masticatory epithelium, lining epithelium lacks the granular and keratinized layers.

Like all epithelium, the junctional epithelium is separated from the underlying lamina propria by a basal lamina. Unlike other types of lining mucosa, where this interface shows some degree of folding, that associated with the junctional epithelium is remarkably flat.

Like other lining epithelia, junctional epithelium contains stem cells situated in the basal layer that give rise to daughter cells that pass to the superficial layers and are eventually shed into the gingival crevice. However, the rate of proliferation and turnover within the junctional epithelium is the highest within oral epithelium, the complete cycle being in the order of days rather than weeks.

Like other lining epithelia, junctional epithelial cells contain cytokeratins. Whereas those that characterize lining epithelia are cytokeratins 4 and 13, those found in junctional epithelium are the cytokeratins found in odontogenic tissue, such as cytokeratin 19, reflecting its origin from the reduced enamel epithelium.

The basal layer of the junctional epithelium is separated by a basal lamina (external basal lamina) from the underlying lamina propria. However, uniquely, the junctional epithelium is also joined to the enamel at its free surface by a second basal lamina (internal basal lamina). The internal basal lamina also differs from the external basal lamina in lacking type IV collagen and anchoring fibrils. As the internal basal lamina can only be produced by the superficial cells of the prickle cell layer, this is reflected in the morphology of the cell which, unusually, contains numerous free ribosomes, cisternae of rough endoplasmic reticulum and prominent Golgi material.

As with the prickle cell layer in lining epithelium, desmosomes link the same cells in the junctional epithelium. However, they are fewer in number and this is correlated with larger intercellular spaces that may comprise up to 5% of the volume of the tissue in the junctional epithelium. This renders the junctional epithelium permeable to tissue fluid derived from underlying capillaries in the lamina propria, known as gingival crevicular fluid. In addition, defence cells can cross the junctional epithelium. Indeed, even healthy gingival tissue may exhibit neutrophils in the intercellular spaces, indicative of its protective role. The lack of membrane-coating granules may also assist the permeability of the cell layer. In this context, cells of the junctional epithelium, together with underlying fibroblasts and endothelial cells, express intercellular adhesion molecule 1 (ICAM-1), which helps in the transmigration of neutrophils from the adjacent capillaries and through the junctional epithelium.

Question 2

As many as 10% of the cells in the oral epithelium are non-keratinocytes. The three main non-keratinocytes are melanocytes, Langerhans cells and Merkel cells. In addition, inflammatory cells migrate through the epithelium. All (except for the Merkel cells) lack the tonofilaments and desmosomes characteristic of keratinocytes. Non-keratinocytes may appear as clear cells in sections stained routinely with haematoxylin and eosin. Lacking the typical cytokeratins associated with normal keratinocytes, they remain unstained in sections of epithelium stained for cytokeratins.

Melanocytes are pigment-producing cells located in the basal layer. They are derived from the neural crest and are present in the skin by about 8 weeks of intrauterine life. Once located in the epithelium, they are assumed to be long-lived, but with some powers of self-replication, and are seen to divide in vitro. Melanocytes have long processes that extend in several directions and across several epithelial layers. As suggested by their name, melanocytes produce the pigment melanin, using the enzyme tyrosinase. Their presence in the oral mucosa would appear to have little obvious functional significance.

The long processes of the melanocyte extend between adjacent keratinocytes and each melanocyte establishes contact with about 30–40 keratinocytes. Keratinocytes release numerous mediators that are essential for normal melanocyte function. Ultrastructurally, the cytoplasm of melanocytes characteristically contains pigment that is packaged in small, dark granules termed melanosomes. As the melanosomes mature under the activity of tyrosinase, their melanin content increases. The pigment is passed to adjacent keratinocytes as the tips of the dendrites are actively phagocytosed by the keratinocytes. Melanin pigmentation is usually not pronounced in the buccal mucosa, tongue or hard palate.

The number of melanocytes varies in different regions, but the difference in the degree of pigmentation between populations is the result of a combination of the size and degree of branching of the cells (rather than the absolute number), the size of the melanosomes, the number and degree of dispersion of the melanosomes, the degree of melanization of the melanosomes, and the rate of degradation of the pigment.

Langerhans cells are dendritic cells situated in the layers of epithelium above the basal layer. They are derived from bone marrow precursors that are probably related to the monocyte lineage and leave the blood stream to enter the lamina propria, before penetrating the basal lamina to reach the epithelium. Such migration may relate to certain chemokines released by keratinocytes, with surface receptors on the Langerhans cells. Langerhans cells act as part of the immune system as antigen-presenting cells. They express class II molecules of the major histocompatibility complex and Fc receptors, and move back and forth

Self-assessment: answers

from the epithelium via dermal lymphatics to local lymph nodes, presenting antigenic material to T lymphocytes. Indeed, lymphocytes present within the oral epithelium are commonly associated with Langerhans cells. Langerhans cells play an important role in skin in producing contact hypersensitivity reactions, in anti-tumour immunity and in graft rejection; they also react as propagators of human immunodeficiency virus (HIV)-1 transmission to T cells. The cells may be localized due to the presence of ATPase on the cell membrane. Ultrastructurally, the Langerhans cell contains characteristic trilaminar, rod-shaped granules called Birbeck granules. These may be up to 50 nm long and 4 nm wide, and have a vesicular swelling at one end, resembling a tennis racquet.

The Merkel cell is found in the basal layer, often closely apposed to nerve fibres. It is thought to act as a receptor and is derived from the neural crest. As the Merkel cells contain cytokeratin, they can be identified by immunohistochemical techniques using antibodies for cytokeratin 8 and 18. They are common in masticatory epithelia such as gingiva, but less frequent in lining mucosa such as the buccal mucosa.

Ultrastructurally, the nucleus of the Merkel cell is often deeply invaginated and may contain a characteristic rodlet. The cytoplasm contains numerous mitochondria, abundant free ribosomes and a collection of electron-dense granules (80–180 nm in diameter), adjacent to the nerve terminal, and these may liberate a transmitter towards the terminal, giving the cell a sensory function. Desmosomes are associated with the cell membrane.

D cells associated with the inflammatory response are present within the epithelium.

Cells associated with the inflammatory response are present within the epithelium. Lymphocytes are the most common type of inflammatory cell, although polymorphonuclear leukocytes and plasma cells are also seen. Lymphocytes are retained within the epithelial layer by binding to integrins (that may increase in disease). The greater degree of permeability of non-keratinized epithelium may account for the larger number of inflammatory cells said to occur there compared with masticatory epithelium.

Question 3

GCF may be regarded as a transudate (or exudate) of the periodontal tissues. It gathers in the gingival sulcus and may be collected by non-invasive means at the gingival margin. The constituents of GCF are derived from plasma, interstitial fluid, microbial dental plaque, host inflammatory cells and host tissues, and its flow rate relates to the degree of gingival inflammation. In healthy tissues, small amounts of subgingival plaque give rise to macromolecular plaque and this is usually removed by desquamating epithelial cells or phagocytosis. Macromolecules diffuse intercellularly to basement membrane (limiting barrier)

and an osmotic gradient is created; interstitial fluid flows into junctional and sulcular epithelium and into the gingival sulcus. In inflamed tissues, the fluid flow rate increases, leading to a greater osmotic gradient. Fluid flows across a weakened basement membrane, as there is loose organization of the junctional and sulcular epithelium. There is also increased fluid flow from capillaries into connective tissues as a consequence of the host response.

Functions of GCF include protection of the tooth and gingival tissues. It washes away potentially harmful cells and molecules from the gingival sulcus and may contain antibacterial substances. It also contains high calcium and phosphate concentrations important for remineralization. Its value as a biomarker may be as an indicator of current disease metabolic activity, involving both soft and mineralized periodontal tissue, as it is non-invasive and site-specific. It may be used as a prognostic or diagnostic indicator of disease progression or future disease activity, or as an indicator of response to therapy. It may also provide information regarding the mechanisms of periodontal tissue destruction. Examples of such biomarkers include markers of microbial origin (lipopolysaccharides (LPS) and trypsin-like protease and bacterial collagenases), markers from the host response (polymorphonuclear leukocyte (PMN) enzymes MMP-8 and elastase, cytokines, cathepsin D and IgG-specific antigens, interleukin (IL)-1 and prostaglandin E2), and markers resulting from the degradation of the connective tissues, such as collagen cross-links, proteoglycans and osteocalcin.

Question 4

The oral surface of the hard palate is exposed to significant forces during mastication. It is therefore adapted to resist these loads. It also has important sensory functions and is a source for the secretion of saliva from minor salivary glands. In its capacity to resist masticatory loads, the oral surface of the hard palate is covered by a keratinized, masticatory mucosa, whose structure shows the relevant adaptations. Its epithelium consists of keratinized (or parakeratinized), stratified, squamous epithelium. Cells are generated from stem cells in the proliferative basal layer and, over a period of about 3 weeks, these migrate to the surface where they are shed. Normal desquamation of the epithelial cells will be accompanied by the loss of bacteria adhering to the cells on the surface. In their passage from the basal layer, the cells increase in size and undergo differentiation, acquiring cytokeratin microfilaments. Initially they become prickle cells that contact via numerous desmosomes, providing a system of mechanical support within the epithelial layer (eventually coming to occupy about 50% of the intercellular space). Prickle cells also produce small, intracellular membrane-coating granules. These granules are rich in phospholipids. In the more superficial layers of the stratum spinosum, the granules come to lie close to the cell membrane.

Self-assessment: answers

Prickle cells move upwards into the granular layer. The cells of the granular layer show a further increase in maturation. Many organelles are reduced or lost, such that the cytoplasm is predominantly occupied by the cytokeratin tonofilaments and tonofibrils. The membrane-coating granules first seen in the prickle cell layer move towards the superficial surface of the keratinocyte and discharge their lipid-rich contents into the extracellular space. This intercellular 'cement', together with the cell contacts (especially tight junctions in the upper region of the granular layer), helps limit the permeability of the layer and prevents water loss. The cells are larger and flatter, but most significantly now contain large numbers of small granules (0.5–1.0 µm in length) called keratohyaline granules. These contain profilaggrin, the precursor to the protein filaggrin that eventually binds the keratin filaments together into a stable network. Synthesis of additional proteins, loricrin and involucrin, which will help form a more resistant cell wall (envelope), is evident in the granular layer.

In the superficial layer of the epithelium, the continued maturation of the epithelial cells results in the loss of all organelles (including nuclei and keratohyaline granules). The cells of the keratinized layer become filled entirely with closely packed tonofilaments surrounded by the matrix protein filaggrin. This mixture of proteins is collectively called keratin. The keratin is also strongly cross-linked by disulphide bonds, contributing to the mechanical and chemical resistance of the layer. In the cornified layer, involucrin becomes cross-linked (by the enzyme transglutaminase) to form a thin (10 nm), highly resistant, electron-dense, cornified envelope just beneath the plasma membrane. Approximately 75% of the cornified envelope is loricrin. Although only constituting 5% of the cell envelope, involucrin is an important component on the internal aspect, acting as a binding site for lipids that are extruded to form a water-insoluble barrier.

The cells of the keratinized layer may be termed epithelial squames; it is these cells that are shed (the process of desquamation), necessitating the constant turnover of epithelial cells. Desmosomes weaken and disappear to allow for this desquamation. In the oral surface of the hard palate, there are areas where nuclei are retained in the otherwise keratinized layer. These cells are described as being parakeratinized, in contrast to the more normal orthokeratinized condition.

In addition to the keratinocytes mentioned above, as many as 10% of the cells in the oral epithelium are non-keratinocytes. The structure and function of these cells has been described in the answer to Essay 2.

To increase the mechanical bonding between the masticatory epithelium and the underlying lamina propria, the interface is markedly folded, deep epithelial rete interdigitating with dermal papillae. The underlying connective tissue of the lamina propria consists of cells, principally fibroblasts, embedded in an extracellular matrix consisting of fibres and ground substance to provide support and nutrition for the overlying epithelial cells. To limit mobility of the hard palate, the lamina propria consists of numerous bundles of collagen fibres that are bound down in the midline (median palatine raphe) and laterally (gingiva) to underlying bone, forming a mucoperiosteum. Few elastin fibres are present. Between these two regions, in the roof of the hard palate adjacent to the cheek teeth, a submucosa is present in which is situated the main neurovascular bundles. Together with nerves passing through the incisive fossa anteriorly, myelinated and unmyelinated sensory nerve fibres are distributed throughout the hard palate to subserve the sensory modalities of pain, pressure and temperature. The sensory endings appropriate to these functions can therefore be visualized within the lamina propria. Autonomic fibres mainly controlling the vascular system will also be evident in the lamina propria.

Minor salivary glands of the mucous type will be present in the submucosa. Ducts pass from the glands to penetrate the overlying keratinized epithelium and drain into the mouth, contributing saliva to the oral cavity. Saliva has many important functions, particularly those related to lubrication.

As for all soft connective tissues, the lamina propria will also contain defence cells. Such cells may be adapted to phagocytose and digest material inside the cell, or to release molecules extracellularly to help combat foreign material, including immunological reactions. These include macrophages, mast cells and lymphocytes. A population of stem cells will ensure that precursors are present to replace any cells that are turning over.

Revision summary charts

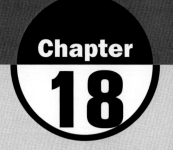

Chapter 18

1. The oral cavity   251
2. The jaws   252
3. Temporomandibular joint   253
4. Incisors of the human dentition   254
5. Canines of the human dentition   255
6. Premolars of the human dentition   256
7. Molars of the human dentition   257
8. The alignment and occlusion of the human permanent dentition   258
9. Anatomy of the orofacial musculature   259
10. Mastication   260
11. Swallowing   261
12. The tongue   262
13. Flavour   263
14. Vasculature and innervation of orodental structures   264
15. Major salivary glands   265
16. Salivary gland structure   266
17. Saliva biochemistry   267
18. Physiology of salivary secretion   268

19. Craniofacial development   269
20. Enamel integuments   270
21. Early tooth development   271
22. Root development   272
23. Tooth eruption   273
24. Mineralization   274
25. Enamel   275
26. Enamel biochemistry   276
27. Enamel formation   277
28. Dentine structure   278
29. Zones in dentine   279
30. Dental pulp   280
31. Oral nociception   281
32. Cementum   282
33. The periodontal ligament   283
34. Tooth support mechanism   284
35. Periodontal ligament mechanoreceptors   285
36. Bone   286
37. Oral mucosa   287
38. Gingival crevicular fluid   288

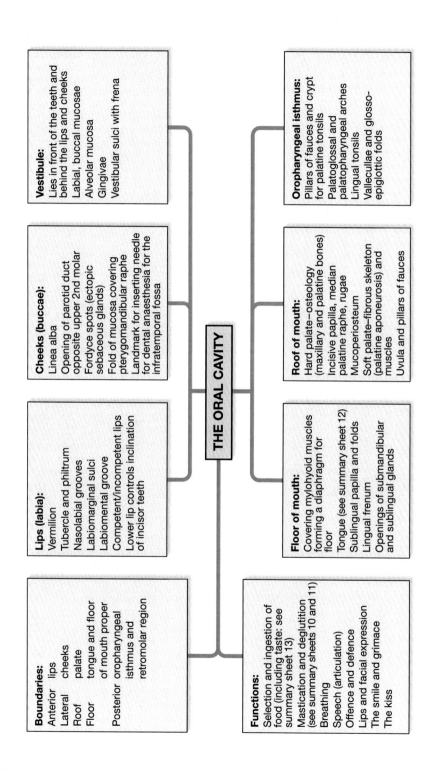

THE ORAL CAVITY

Boundaries:
Anterior lips
Lateral cheeks
Roof palate
Floor tongue and floor
       of mouth proper
Posterior oropharyngeal
       isthmus and
       retromolar region

Functions:
Selection and ingestion of
food (including taste: see
summary sheet 13)
Mastication and deglutition
(see summary sheets 10 and 11)
Breathing
Speech (articulation)
Offence and defence
Lips and facial expression
The smile and grimace
The kiss

Lips (labia):
Vermilion
Tubercle and philtrum
Nasolabial grooves
Labiomarginal sulci
Labiomental groove
Competent/incompetent lips
Lower lip controls inclination
of incisor teeth

Cheeks (buccae):
Linea alba
Opening of parotid duct
opposite upper 2nd molar
Fordyce spots (ectopic
sebaceous glands)
Fold of mucosa covering
pterygomandibular raphe
Landmark for inserting needle
for dental anaesthesia for the
infratemporal fossa

Vestibule:
Lies in front of the teeth and
behind the lips and cheeks
Labial, buccal mucosae
Alveolar mucosa
Gingivae
Vestibular sulci with frena

Floor of mouth:
Covering mylohyoid muscles
forming a diaphragm for
floor
Tongue (see summary sheet 12)
Sublingual papilla and folds
Lingual frenum
Openings of submandibular
and sublingual glands

Roof of mouth:
Hard palate—osteology
(maxillary and palatine bones)
Incisive papilla, median
palatine raphe, rugae
Mucoperiosteum
Soft palate—fibrous skeleton
(palatine aponeurosis) and
muscles
Uvula and pillars of fauces

Oropharyngeal isthmus:
Pillars of fauces and crypt
for palatine tonsils
Palatoglossal and
palatopharyngeal arches
Lingual tonsils
Valleculae and glosso-
epiglottic folds

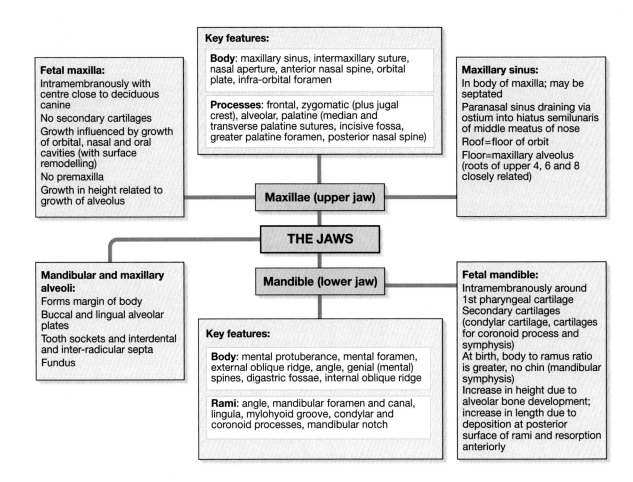

Key features:

Body: maxillary sinus, intermaxillary suture, nasal aperture, anterior nasal spine, orbital plate, infra-orbital foramen

Processes: frontal, zygomatic (plus jugal crest), alveolar, palatine (median and transverse palatine sutures, incisive fossa, greater palatine foramen, posterior nasal spine)

Fetal maxilla:
Intramembranously with centre close to deciduous canine
No secondary cartilages
Growth influenced by growth of orbital, nasal and oral cavities (with surface remodelling)
No premaxilla
Growth in height related to growth of alveolus

Maxillary sinus:
In body of maxilla; may be septated
Paranasal sinus draining via ostium into hiatus semilunaris of middle meatus of nose
Roof=floor of orbit
Floor=maxillary alveolus (roots of upper 4, 6 and 8 closely related)

Maxillae (upper jaw)

THE JAWS

Mandible (lower jaw)

Mandibular and maxillary alveoli:
Forms margin of body
Buccal and lingual alveolar plates
Tooth sockets and interdental and inter-radicular septa
Fundus

Fetal mandible:
Intramembranously around 1st pharyngeal cartilage
Secondary cartilages (condylar cartilage, cartilages for coronoid process and symphysis)
At birth, body to ramus ratio is greater, no chin (mandibular symphysis)
Increase in height due to alveolar bone development; increase in length due to deposition at posterior surface of rami and resorption anteriorly

Key features:

Body: mental protuberance, mental foramen, external oblique ridge, angle, genial (mental) spines, digastric fossae, internal oblique ridge

Rami: angle, mandibular foramen and canal, lingula, mylohyoid groove, condylar and coronoid processes, mandibular notch

Eighteen

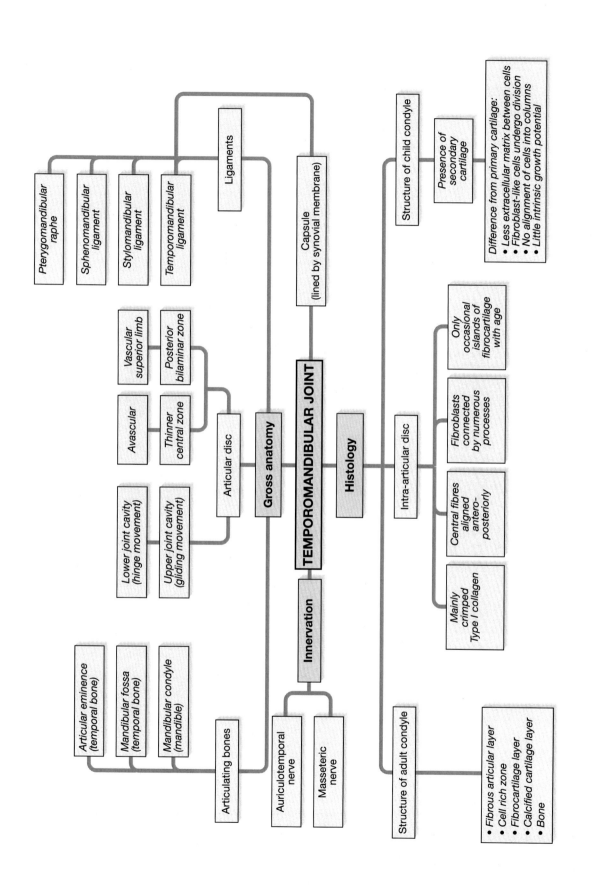

THE INCISORS OF THE HUMAN DENTITION

Deciduous incisors

Maxillary incisors

1st (central) incisor

Key features:
Similar to the permanent incisor but appears 'plumper'
No mamelons/labial lobe grooves
Prominent cingulum palatally but poorly defined marginal ridges
An addition cingulum at cervical margin of labial surface

2nd (lateral) incisor

Key features:
Similar to the permanent incisor but mesio-incisal angle is more acute and disto-incisal angle more rounded
Cingulum present both palatally and labially

Mandibular incisors

1st (central) incisor

Key features:
Similar to the permanent incisor but with low labial cingulum
Palatal cingulum and marginal ridges are indistinct

2nd (lateral) incisor

Key features:
Similar to the permanent incisor but is more bulbous and the incisal margin slopes downwards distally

Permanent incisors

Maxillary incisors

1st (central) incisor

Key features:
Widest incisor mesiodistally
Wedge-shaped
3 mamelons; labial lobe grooves; palatal cingulum
Mesial surface of crown less angulated from root surface
Crown length=root length
Disto-incisal corner rounded
Well defined marginal ridges

2nd (lateral) incisor

Key features:
Less wide mesiodistally
Wedge-shaped
Longer root relative to crown length
Mesial surface of crown less angulated from root surface
Foramen caecum near cingulum
Disto-incisal corner rounded
Well defined marginal ridges

Mandibular incisors

1st (central) incisor

Key features:
Symmetrical crown
Wedge-shaped
Crown lingually tilted
Less distinct cingulum
Root more flattened mesiodistally

2nd (lateral) incisor

Key features:
Compared with lower 1st incisor:
Less symmetrical with incisal edge having oblique orientation and distal surface diverging from tooth's long axis (fan-shaped incisor)

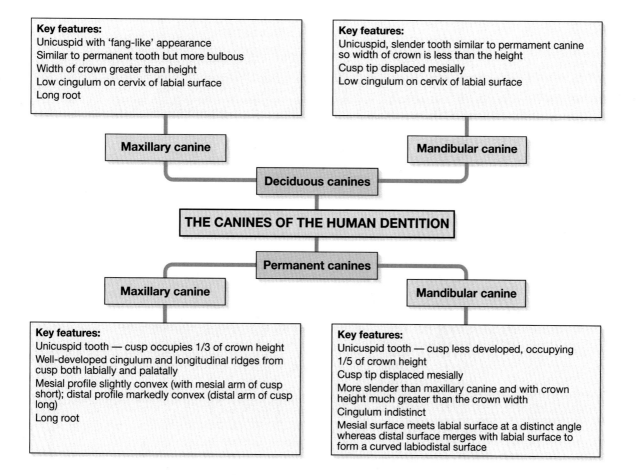

Key features:
Unicuspid with 'fang-like' appearance
Similar to permanent tooth but more bulbous
Width of crown greater than height
Low cingulum on cervix of labial surface
Long root

Key features:
Unicuspid, slender tooth similar to permanent canine so width of crown is less than the height
Cusp tip displaced mesially
Low cingulum on cervix of labial surface

Maxillary canine

Mandibular canine

Deciduous canines

THE CANINES OF THE HUMAN DENTITION

Permanent canines

Maxillary canine

Mandibular canine

Key features:
Unicuspid tooth — cusp occupies 1/3 of crown height
Well-developed cingulum and longitudinal ridges from cusp both labially and palatally
Mesial profile slightly convex (with mesial arm of cusp short); distal profile markedly convex (distal arm of cusp long)
Long root

Key features:
Unicuspid tooth — cusp less developed, occupying 1/5 of crown height
Cusp tip displaced mesially
More slender than maxillary canine and with crown height much greater than the crown width
Cingulum indistinct
Mesial surface meets labial surface at a distinct angle whereas distal surface merges with labial surface to form a curved labiodistal surface

Eighteen

THE PREMOLARS OF THE HUMAN DENTITION

Premolars absent in deciduous dentition

Maxillary premolars

1st Premolar

Key features:
Bicuspid with buccal and palatal cusps nearly equal in size with buccal cusp slightly larger. Oval occlusal outline
Two roots (buccal and palatal)
Canine fossa on mesial surface of crown and root with the occlusal fissure crossing the mesial marginal ridge

2nd Premolar

Key features:
Bicuspid with buccal and palatal cusps equal in size. Oval occlusal outline
Single root
No canine fossa; occlusal fissure confined to occlusal surface
Palatal cusp seen from the palatal aspect of the tooth inclines mesially, the mesial shoulder of the cusp being shorter than the distal shoulder

Mandibular premolars

1st Premolar

Key features:
Bicuspid with buccal cusp large and lingual cusp very small. Thus, the occlusal surface slopes obliquely and is not transverse as for the other premolars. Circular occlusal outline
Single root
A longitudinal ridge links the buccal and lingual cusps, creating mesial and distal fossae on either side (the distal fossa is more pronounced)

2nd Premolar

Key features:
Bicuspid with buccal and lingual cusps more equal in size. Tip of lingual cusp displaced mesial.
Lingual cusp often bicuspid. Square occlusal outline
Single root
No longitudinal ridge linking the buccal and the lingual cusps and there is a mesiodistal occlusal fissure

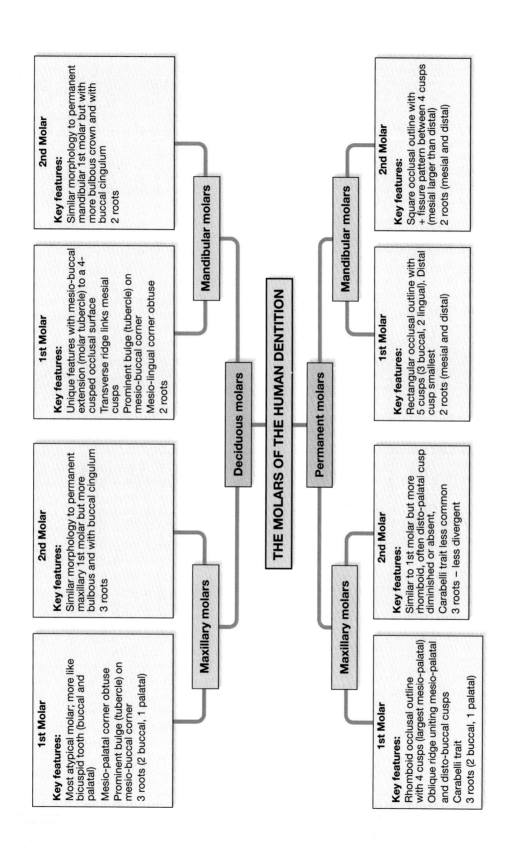

THE MOLARS OF THE HUMAN DENTITION

Deciduous molars

Mandibular molars

2nd Molar

Key features:
Similar morphology to permanent mandibular 1st molar but with more bulbous crown and with buccal cingulum
2 roots

1st Molar

Key features:
Unique features with mesio-buccal extension (molar tubercle) to a 4-cusped occlusal surface
Transverse ridge links mesial cusps
Prominent bulge (tubercle) on mesio-buccal corner
Mesio-lingual corner obtuse
2 roots

Maxillary molars

2nd Molar

Key features:
Similar morphology to permanent maxillary 1st molar but more bulbous and with buccal cingulum
3 roots

1st Molar

Key features:
Most atypical molar; more like bicuspid tooth (buccal and palatal)
Mesio-palatal corner obtuse
Prominent bulge (tubercle) on mesio-buccal corner
3 roots (2 buccal, 1 palatal)

Permanent molars

Mandibular molars

2nd Molar

Key features:
Square occlusal outline with + fissure pattern between 4 cusps (mesial larger than distal)
2 roots (mesial and distal)

1st Molar

Key features:
Rectangular occlusal outline with 5 cusps (3 buccal, 2 lingual). Distal cusp smallest
2 roots (mesial and distal)

Maxillary molars

2nd Molar

Key features:
Similar to 1st molar but more rhomboid, often disto-palatal cusp diminished or absent,
Carabelli trait less common
3 roots – less divergent

1st Molar

Key features:
Rhomboid occlusal outline with 4 cusps (largest mesio-palatal)
Oblique ridge uniting mesio-palatal and disto-buccal cusps
Carabelli trait
3 roots (2 buccal, 1 palatal)

Eighteen

257

THE ALIGNMENT AND OCCLUSION OF THE HUMAN PERMANENT DENTITION

Alignment

Maxillary teeth

Incisors proclined and aligned slightly distally

Canine slightly proclined with slight mesial angulation

Premolars are only slightly buccally and mesially inclined

Molars are buccally inclined and show distal alignments

Alignment

Mandibular teeth

Incisors proclined and not mesially or distally aligned

Canine slightly proclined with slight mesial angulation

Premolars show slight mesial and lingual angulations

Molars are lingually inclined and show mesial alignments

Alignment

Curvatures of arches

Occlusal planes are not flat (though become so with wear and age)

Anteroposterior curve of Spee

Transverse curves of Wilson (buccal inclinations of maxillary molars with lingual inclinations of mandibular molars)

Occlusion

Centric occlusion

Terminal position of jaw movements with mandibular condyles centrally positioned in mandibular fossae of temporomandibular joint

Each maxillary tooth contacts its corresponding mandibular antagonist and its distal neighbour (except third molar)

Centric stops

Occlusion

Overbite and overjet

Maxillary arch slightly larger than mandibular — horizontal overlap of the mandibular teeth by maxillary teeth is termed 'overjet'

In addition, for the incisors and canines, vertical overlapping of mandibular teeth by maxillary teeth is termed 'overbite'

Malocclusion
(Angle's classification)

Class I – normal molar relationship (malalignment elsewhere in arches)

Class II – prenormal maxillary arch relationship (maxillary incisors proclined (division 1); incisors retroclined (division 2))

Class III – postnormal maxillary arch relationship (incisors can be edge-to-edge or with reverse overjet)

Malocclusion
(incisor classification)

Class I – no malposition of incisors

Class II – incisal margins of mandibular incisors behind cingulum plateau of maxillary incisors (division 1 = proclined incisors; division 2 = retroclined incisors)

Class III – incisal margins of mandibular incisors are in front of cingulum plateau

Eighteen

ANATOMY OF THE OROFACIAL MUSCULATURE

Muscles of mastication
(innervated by mandibular division of trigeminal)

Masseter – elevator of mandible; puts power into the bite; attached from zygomatic arch to the entire lateral surface of mandibular ramus

Temporalis – elevator (anterior and vertical fibres); retractor (posterior and horizontal fibres); attached from floor of temporal fossa and temporal fascia to internal aspect of mandibular coronoid process

Lateral pterygoid – protrudes and depresses mandible; side-to-side movements; superior head attached to roof of infratemporal fossa; inferior head from lateral side of lateral pterygoid plate. Inserts onto neck of condyle and intra-articular disc of temporomandibular joint

Medial pterygoid – protrudes and elevates mandible; side-to-side movements; attached mainly from medial side of lateral pterygoid plate to inner aspect of angle of mandible

Muscles of the floor of the mouth
(innervations variable)

Mylohoid – forms diaphragm for floor of mouth; attached to mylohyoid line of mandible and to the hyoid bone (innervated by mandibular nerve)

Digastric – 2 bellies with intermediate tendon; depresses and retracts mandible; attached to digastric groove of temporal bone and to digastric fossa at chin (posterior belly innervated by facial; anterior belly by mandibular nerve)

Geniohyoid – from mandibular inferior genial spine to body of hyoid (C1 innervation)

Genioglossus – from superior genial spine into tongue (protrudes and depresses tongue) (innervated by hypoglossal nerve)

Hypoglossus – from greater horn of hyoid to lateral margins of tongue (depresses tongue) (innervated by hypoglossal)

Muscles of facial expression (oral group)
(innervated by facial)

Orbicularis oris – changes shape of lips

Levator labii superioris – elevates upper lip

Zygomaticus major and minor – elevate and laterally extend upper lip

Levator anguli oris – elevates corner of lips when smiling

Depressor labii inferioris – depresses lower lip

Depressor anguli oris – depresses corner of lips when grimacing

Mentalis – protrudes lower lip when expressing doubt or disdain

Risorius – the grinning muscle

Buccinator – holds food between teeth; expels air between lips

Muscles of the soft palate
(mainly innervated from pharyngeal plexus)

Musculus uvulae – intrinsic muscles changing shape of soft palate

Tensor veli palatini – forms palatine aponeurosis (the 'skeleton' of the soft palate) and tenses palate for elevation (innervated by mandibular nerve)

Levator veli palatini – raises the tense soft palate during swallowing to protect nasopharynx

Palatoglossus – anterior pillar of fauces; raises back of tongue

Palatopharyngeus – posterior pillar of fauces; longitudinal muscle of pharynx that raises pharynx and larynx during swallowing

Co-ordination of teeth, jaw elevator and depressor muscles, temporomandibular joint, tongue, lips, palate and salivary glands (the so-called **masticatory apparatus**)

Control of mastication

Primarily a voluntary process, involving the cerebral cortex and motor neurones in the trigeminal motor nucleus.

Controlled by **central pattern generator** and modulated by inputs from sensory feedback from the mouth and reflexes of mastication

MASTICATION

Teeth are the main organ of mastication and adapted for the main functional requirement of the diet

Masticatory forces:
• Maximum forces:
  500 – 700 N between the molar teeth
• During mastication, forces between
  70 – 150 N are achieved

Involves both vertical and lateral movements of the jaws in human beings in so-called chewing cycle

Chewing cycle involves:
• Opening phase
• Closing phase
• Occlusal or intercuspal phase

Eighteen

Regarded as a complex process comprising a subset of a continuous series of automatic events that transport food from the incisor teeth to the stomach
Swallowing fluid is traditional three-stage process but swallowing solids or solids mixed with liquids is more complex

Control of swallowing
Like mastication, swallowing is driven by a **central pattern generator** within the brain stem, located in two parts of the medulla (**dorsal and ventral**)

SWALLOWING

Swallowing can also be initiated by a series of reflexes brought about by stimulation of mechanoreceptors and chemoreceptors at the back of the mouth
Receptors innervated by Vth, IXth and Xth cranial nerves

Dorsal pattern generator receives inputs which trigger the swallowing process and lead to contraction and relaxation of the muscles involved in swallowing

Ventral pattern generator receives inputs from the dorsal part and then relays them to the appropriate motor neurones involved in swallowing (of the Vth, VIIth, IXth, Xth, XIth and XIIth cranial nerves and the first 3 cervical segments of the spinal cord)

Surface features (Anterior 2/3 of dorsum)
Sulcus terminalis
Gustatory (partially keratinized) mucosa
Circumvallate papillae
Filiform and fungiform papillae

Surface features (Posterior 1/3 of dorsum)
Sulcus terminalis
Non-keratinized mucosa
Lingual follicles – lingual tonsil
Foramen caecum
Foliate papillae
Lateral and median glossoepiglottic folds and valleculae
Anterior pillar of fauces (palatoglossal fold)

Surface features (Ventral surface)
Non-keratinized mucosa
Lingual frenum
Deep lingual veins
Fimbriated folds
Sublingual papilla
Sublingual folds

THE TONGUE

Sensory innervation
Anterior 2/3 of dorsum – general sensation lingual nerve; taste chorda tympani of facial nerve
Posterior 1/3 of dorsum – general sensation and taste glossopharyngeal nerve (near epiglottis vagus nerve)
Ventral surface – lingual nerve

Musculature
Intrinsic ms (change shape) – superior and inferior longitudinal, transverse and vertical fibres
Extrinsic ms (change position) – genioglossus, hyoglossus, styloglossus and palatoglossus muscles
Innervated by hypoglossal nerve (excepting palatoglossus by pharyngeal plexus)

Functions
Mastication
Taste and food selection; common chemical sense
Swallowing
Speech
Thermosensation

Eighteen

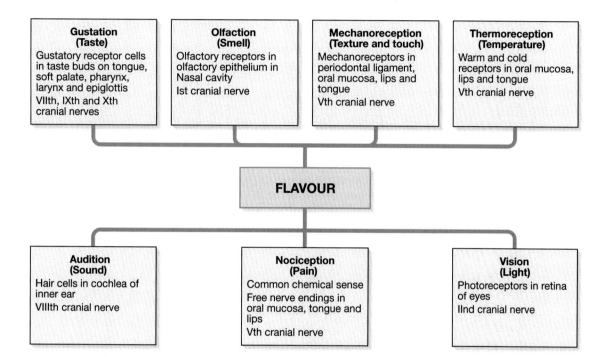

**Gustation
(Taste)**

Gustatory receptor cells in taste buds on tongue, soft palate, pharynx, larynx and epiglottis

VIIth, IXth and Xth cranial nerves

**Olfaction
(Smell)**

Olfactory receptors in olfactory epithelium in Nasal cavity

Ist cranial nerve

**Mechanoreception
(Texture and touch)**

Mechanoreceptors in periodontal ligament, oral mucosa, lips and tongue

Vth cranial nerve

**Thermoreception
(Temperature)**

Warm and cold receptors in oral mucosa, lips and tongue

Vth cranial nerve

FLAVOUR

**Audition
(Sound)**

Hair cells in cochlea of inner ear

VIIIth cranial nerve

**Nociception
(Pain)**

Common chemical sense

Free nerve endings in oral mucosa, tongue and lips

Vth cranial nerve

**Vision
(Light)**

Photoreceptors in retina of eyes

IInd cranial nerve

VASCULATURE AND INNERVATION OF ORODENTAL STRUCTURES

Innervation

Motor innervation
Tongue muscles – hypoglossal
Lips and cheeks – facial
Floor of mouth (mylohyoid) – mandibular
Soft palate and oropharyngeal isthmus – mainly pharyngeal plexus

Innervation of salivary glands
Parotid – lesser petrosal branch of glossopharyngeal via otic ganglion (postganglioic fibres with auriculotemporal nerve)
Submandibular and sublingual – chorda tympani branch of facial (travelling with lingual nerve) via submandibular ganglion

Innervation of oral cavity
Inferior alveolar nerve (mandibular nerve) for mandibular teeth and posterior, middle, anterior superior alveolar nerves (maxillary nerve) for maxillary teeth
Tongue (see summary sheet 12)
Nasopalatine and greater and lesser palatine nerves (maxillary nerve) for palate
Buccal nerve (mandibular nerve) for cheeks and glossopharyngeal nerve at oropharyngeal isthmus. Lips infra-orbital and mental nerves

Cutaneous innervation (relating only to nerves supplying orodental tissues)
Infra-orbital branch of maxillary nerve
Buccal branch of mandibular nerve
Mental branch of inferior alveolar nerve (mandibular nerve)

Vasculature

Lymphatics (extremely variable)
Submental nodes – tip of tongue, lower lip, anterior mandibular teeth
Submandibular nodes – most of dorsum of tongue (ipsilateral and contralateral), posterior mandibular teeth, most of upper jaw/maxillary teeth
Juguloidigastric nodes – posterior tongue (ipsilateral and contralateral), palate (posterior part into pharyngeal nodes), floor of mouth
Buccal (facial) lymph node
Waldeyer's tonsillar ring

Veins (very variable)
Facial vein (to internal jugular vein)
From teeth to pterygoid venous plexus and/or facial vein (note inferior alveolar vein)
From palate to pterygoid venous plexus and/or pharyngeal venous plexus
From tongue to lingual and deep lingual veins and to jugular vein

Arteries
Facial artery and superior and inferior labial branches
Inferior alveolar artery (from maxillary artery); superior alveolar arteries (from maxillary artery/infra-orbital arteries
Greater and lesser palatine arteries and nasopalatine (from maxillary artery)
Buccal artery (from maxillary artery)
Lingual artery

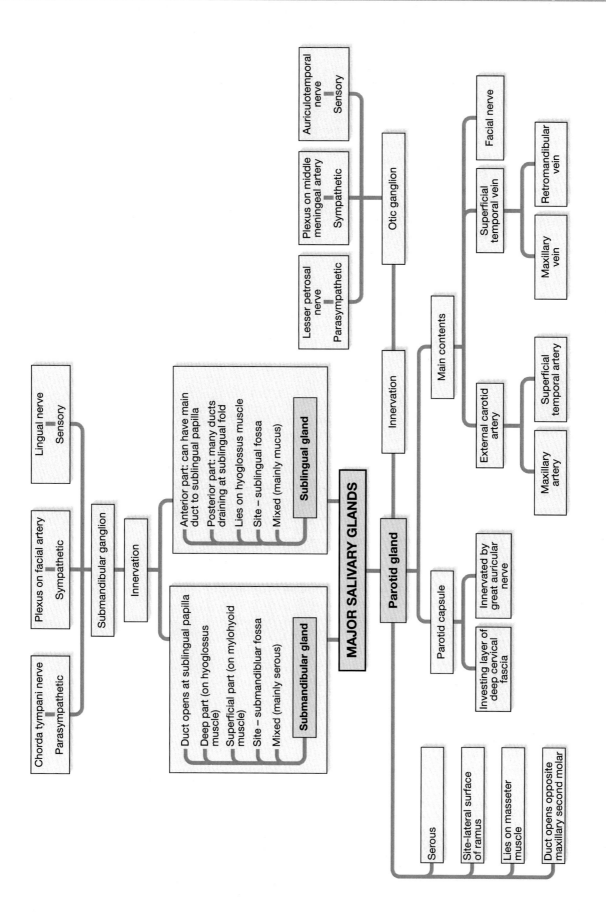

Eighteen

MAJOR SALIVARY GLANDS

Submandibular gland

Innervation
- Chorda tympani nerve — Parasympathetic
- Plexus on facial artery — Sympathetic
- Lingual nerve — Sensory
- Submandibular ganglion

- Duct opens at sublingual papilla
- Deep part (on hyoglossus muscle)
- Superficial part (on mylohyoid muscle)
- Site – submandibluar fossa
- Mixed (mainly serous)

Sublingual gland
- Anterior part: can have main duct to sublingual papilla
- Posterior part: many ducts draining at sublingual fold
- Lies on hyoglossus muscle
- Site – sublingual fossa
- Mixed (mainly mucus)

Parotid gland

Innervation
- Lesser petrosal nerve — Parasympathetic
- Plexus on middle meningeal artery — Sympathetic
- Auriculotemporal nerve — Sensory
- Otic ganglion

Main contents
- External carotid artery
  - Maxillary artery
  - Superficial temporal artery
- Superficial temporal vein
  - Maxillary vein
  - Retromandibular vein
- Facial nerve

Parotid capsule
- Investing layer of deep cervical fascia
- Innervated by great auricular nerve

- Serous
- Site-lateral surface of ramus
- Lies on masseter muscle
- Duct opens opposite maxillary second molar

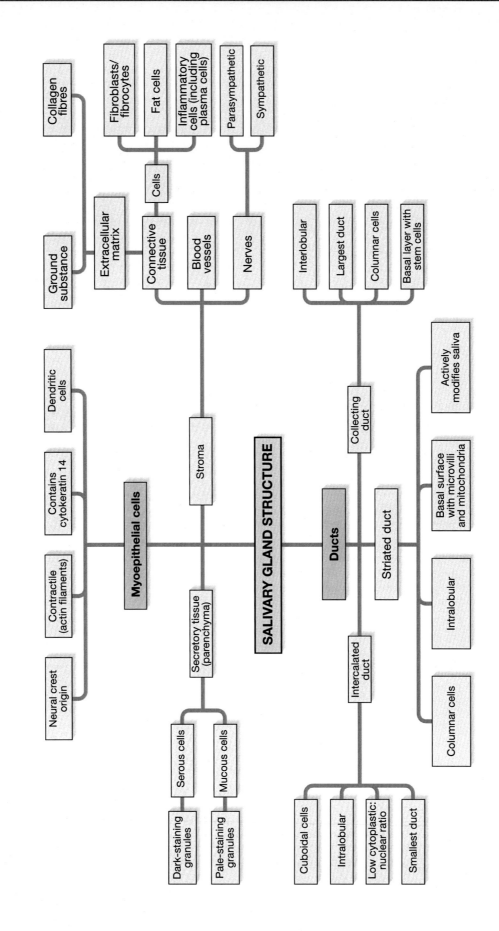

SALIVARY GLAND STRUCTURE

Stroma
- Connective tissue
  - Extracellular matrix
    - Collagen fibres
    - Ground substance
  - Cells
    - Fibroblasts/fibrocytes
    - Fat cells
    - Inflammatory cells (including plasma cells)
- Blood vessels
- Nerves
  - Parasympathetic
  - Sympathetic

Secretory tissue (parenchyma)
- Serous cells
  - Dark-staining granules
- Mucous cells
  - Pale-staining granules

Myoepithelial cells
- Neural crest origin
- Contractile (actin filaments)
- Contains cytokeratin 14
- Dendritic cells

Ducts
- Intercalated duct
  - Cuboidal cells
  - Intralobular
  - Low cytoplastic: nuclear ratio
  - Smallest duct
- Striated duct
  - Columnar cells
  - Intralobular
  - Basal surface with microvilli and mitochondria
  - Actively modifies saliva
- Collecting duct
  - Interlobular
  - Largest duct
  - Columnar cells
  - Basal layer with stem cells

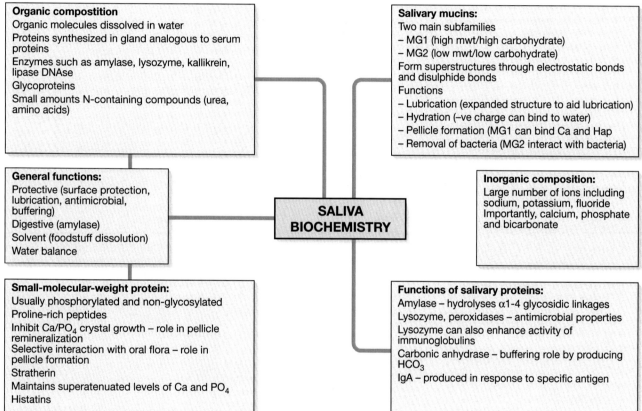

Organic compostition
Organic molecules dissolved in water
Proteins synthesized in gland analogous to serum proteins
Enzymes such as amylase, lysozyme, kallikrein, lipase DNAse
Glycoproteins
Small amounts N-containing compounds (urea, amino acids)

Salivary mucins:
Two main subfamilies
– MG1 (high mwt/high carbohydrate)
– MG2 (low mwt/low carbohydrate)
Form superstructures through electrostatic bonds and disulphide bonds
Functions
– Lubrication (expanded structure to aid lubrication)
– Hydration (–ve charge can bind to water)
– Pellicle formation (MG1 can bind Ca and Hap
– Removal of bacteria (MG2 interact with bacteria)

General functions:
Protective (surface protection, lubrication, antimicrobial, buffering)
Digestive (amylase)
Solvent (foodstuff dissolution)
Water balance

SALIVA BIOCHEMISTRY

Inorganic composition:
Large number of ions including sodium, potassium, fluoride
Importantly, calcium, phosphate and bicarbonate

Small-molecular-weight protein:
Usually phosphorylated and non-glycosylated
Proline-rich peptides
Inhibit Ca/PO_4 crystal growth – role in pellicle remineralization
Selective interaction with oral flora – role in pellicle formation
Stratherin
Maintains superatenuated levels of Ca and PO_4
Histatins

Functions of salivary proteins:
Amylase – hydrolyses α1-4 glycosidic linkages
Lysozyme, peroxidases – antimicrobial properties
Lysozyme can also enhance activity of immunoglobulins
Carbonic anhydrase – buffering role by producing HCO_3
IgA – produced in response to specific antigen

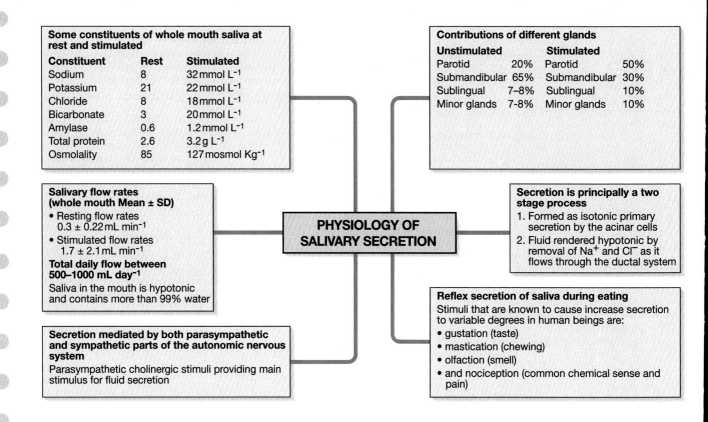

Some constituents of whole mouth saliva at rest and stimulated

Constituent	Rest	Stimulated
Sodium	8	32 mmol L^{-1}
Potassium	21	22 mmol L^{-1}
Chloride	8	18 mmol L^{-1}
Bicarbonate	3	20 mmol L^{-1}
Amylase	0.6	1.2 mmol L^{-1}
Total protein	2.6	3.2 g L^{-1}
Osmolality	85	127 mosmol Kg^{-1}

Contributions of different glands

Unstimulated		Stimulated	
Parotid	20%	Parotid	50%
Submandibular	65%	Submandibular	30%
Sublingual	7–8%	Sublingual	10%
Minor glands	7–8%	Minor glands	10%

Salivary flow rates (whole mouth Mean ± SD)
- Resting flow rates
  0.3 ± 0.22 mL min^{-1}
- Stimulated flow rates
  1.7 ± 2.1 mL min^{-1}

Total daily flow between 500–1000 mL day^{-1}

Saliva in the mouth is hypotonic and contains more than 99% water

PHYSIOLOGY OF SALIVARY SECRETION

Secretion is principally a two stage process
1. Formed as isotonic primary secretion by the acinar cells
2. Fluid rendered hypotonic by removal of Na$^+$ and Cl$^-$ as it flows through the ductal system

Secretion mediated by both parasympathetic and sympathetic parts of the autonomic nervous system

Parasympathetic cholinergic stimuli providing main stimulus for fluid secretion

Reflex secretion of saliva during eating

Stimuli that are known to cause increase secretion to variable degrees in human beings are:
- gustation (taste)
- mastication (chewing)
- olfaction (smell)
- and nociception (common chemical sense and pain)

CRANIOFACIAL DEVELOPMENT

Facial development

Key features:

5 facial processes appear around primitive mouth (stomodeum): frontonasal process over prosencephalon, 2 mandibular processes from 1st pharyngeal arch (below stomodeum) and extending from these 2 maxillary processes

Ectodermal placodes – nasal, lens and optic placodes

Frontonasal process around nasal pits (from invaginating nasal placodes) – medial and lateral nasal processes centrally with the 2 maxillary processes laterally. Note that the upper lip seems to be eventually formed entirely by the maxillary processes that merge in the midline where the medial nasal processes initially are located

Jaw development

Key features:

Mandible – develops intramembranously around (not in) the cartilage of the 1st pharyngeal arch (Meckel's cartilage). Development of the ramus of the mandible is associated with the appearance of secondary cartilages (condylar and coronoid cartilages). There is also a secondary cartilage at the midline – mandibular symphysis

Maxilla – develops intramembranously from centres of ossification located near the developing deciduous canine teeth. No secondary cartilages

Growth of mandible by surface remodelling, with little contribution from condylar cartilage. Growth of maxilla by surface deposition plus sutural growth

Palate development

Key features:

Initially there is a primary palate (rostral aspect of frontonasal process) and a common oronasal chamber. Subsequently, palatal shelves appear from maxillary processes. These processes are vertical and have to elevate to the horizontal position before fusing

Elevation of the palatal shelves is thought to occur because of rapid hydration of the mesenchymal extracellular matrix to produce a turgor pressure

Hyaluronan is involved in this process

Fusion involves the initial formation of a midline epithelial seam which subsequently breaks down (with loss of the basement membrane) as a result of apoptosis and redifferentiation of the epithelial cells

Tongue development

Key features:

Anterior 2/3 of tongue formed by lateral lingual swellings and a midline tuberculum impar (median lingual swelling) beneath the endoderm of the 1st pharyngeal arch. Thus, the sensory innervation is derived from the mandibular division of the trigeminal (with taste from the facial nerve – the nerve of the 2nd pharyngeal arch)

Posterior 1/3 formed by copula primarily from the 3rd and 4th pharyngeal arches. Thus, the sensory innervation is derived from the glossopharyngeal (and vagus) nerves

The tongue musculature is derived from occipital myotomes that are therefore innerved by the hypoglossal nerves

Note the origin of the thyroid gland from the developing tongue (remaining as the foramen caecum on the fully formed tongue)

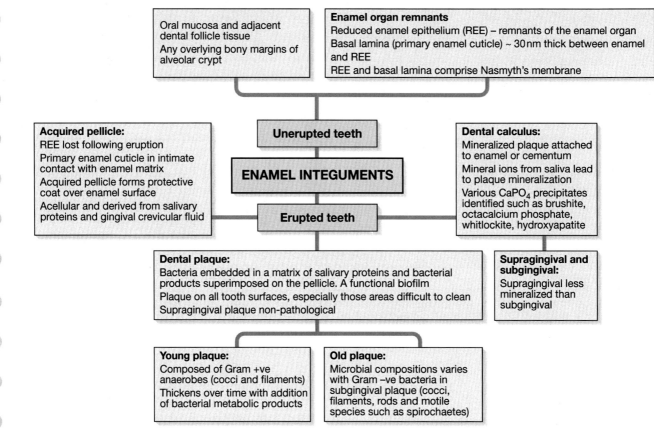

Oral mucosa and adjacent dental follicle tissue
Any overlying bony margins of alveolar crypt

Enamel organ remnants
Reduced enamel epithelium (REE) – remnants of the enamel organ
Basal lamina (primary enamel cuticle) ~ 30 nm thick between enamel and REE
REE and basal lamina comprise Nasmyth's membrane

Acquired pellicle:
REE lost following eruption
Primary enamel cuticle in intimate contact with enamel matrix
Acquired pellicle forms protective coat over enamel surface
Acellular and derived from salivary proteins and gingival crevicular fluid

Unerupted teeth

ENAMEL INTEGUMENTS

Erupted teeth

Dental calculus:
Mineralized plaque attached to enamel or cementum
Mineral ions from saliva lead to plaque mineralization
Various $CaPO_4$ precipitates identified such as brushite, octacalcium phosphate, whitlockite, hydroxyapatite

Dental plaque:
Bacteria embedded in a matrix of salivary proteins and bacterial products superimposed on the pellicle. A functional biofilm
Plaque on all tooth surfaces, especially those areas difficult to clean
Supragingival plaque non-pathological

Supragingival and subgingival:
Supragingival less mineralized than subgingival

Young plaque:
Composed of Gram +ve anaerobes (cocci and filaments)
Thickens over time with addition of bacterial metabolic products

Old plaque:
Microbial compositions varies with Gram –ve bacteria in subgingival plaque (cocci, filaments, rods and motile species such as spirochaetes)

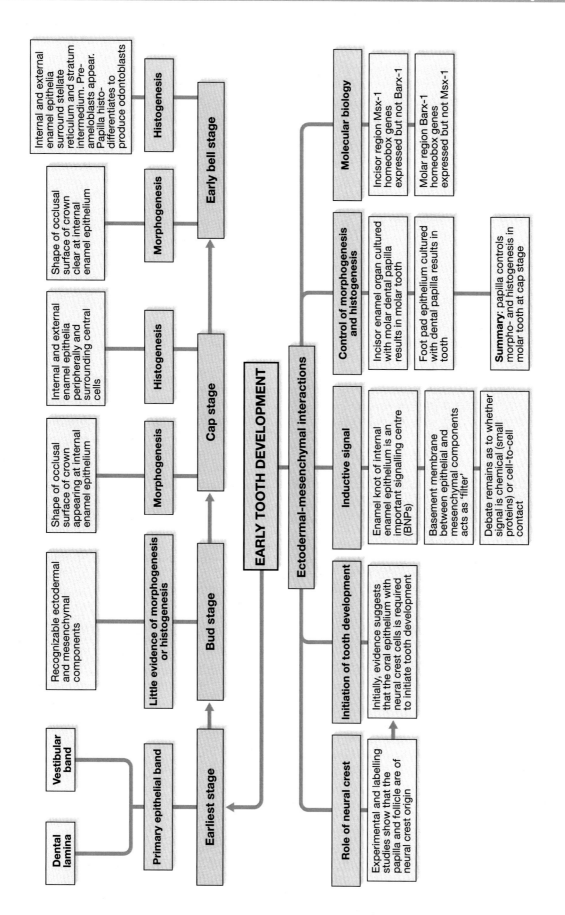

EARLY TOOTH DEVELOPMENT

Dental lamina

Vestibular band

Primary epithelial band

Earliest stage

Bud stage
- Recognizable ectodermal and mesenchymal components
- Little evidence of morphogenesis or histogenesis

Cap stage
- Shape of occlusal surface of crown appearing at internal enamel epithelium — **Morphogenesis**
- Internal and external enamel epithelia peripherally and surrounding central cells — **Histogenesis**

Early bell stage
- Shape of occlusal surface of crown clear at internal enamel epithelium — **Morphogenesis**
- Internal and external enamel epithelia surround stellate reticulum and stratum intermedium. Pre-ameloblasts appear. Papilla histo-differentiates to produce odontoblasts — **Histogenesis**

Ectodermal–mesenchymal interactions

Role of neural crest
- Experimental and labelling studies show that the papilla and follicle are of neural crest origin

Initiation of tooth development
- Initially, evidence suggests that the oral epithelium with neural crest cells is required to initiate tooth development

Inductive signal
- Enamel knot of internal enamel epithelium is an important signalling centre (BNPs)
- Basement membrane between epithelial and mesenchymal components acts as 'filter'
- Debate remains as to whether signal is chemical (small proteins) or cell-to-cell contact

Control of morphogenesis and histogenesis
- Incisor enamel organ cultured with molar dental papilla results in molar tooth
- Foot pad epithelium cultured with dental papilla results in tooth
- **Summary:** papilla controls morpho- and histogenesis in molar tooth at cap stage

Molecular biology
- Incisor region Msx-1 homeobox genes expressed but not Barx-1
- Molar region Barx-1 homeobox genes expressed but not Msx-1

Eighteen

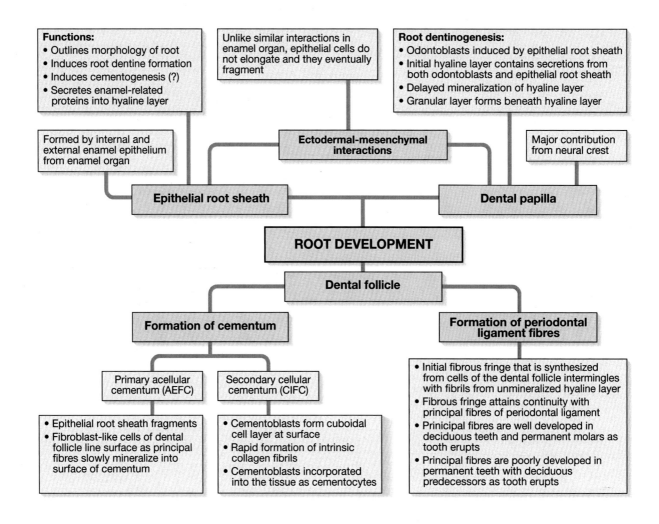

Functions:
- Outlines morphology of root
- Induces root dentine formation
- Induces cementogenesis (?)
- Secretes enamel-related proteins into hyaline layer

Unlike similar interactions in enamel organ, epithelial cells do not elongate and they eventually fragment

Root dentinogenesis:
- Odontoblasts induced by epithelial root sheath
- Initial hyaline layer contains secretions from both odontoblasts and epithelial root sheath
- Delayed mineralization of hyaline layer
- Granular layer forms beneath hyaline layer

Formed by internal and external enamel epithelium from enamel organ

Ectodermal-mesenchymal interactions

Major contribution from neural crest

Epithelial root sheath

Dental papilla

ROOT DEVELOPMENT

Dental follicle

Formation of cementum

Formation of periodontal ligament fibres

Primary acellular cementum (AEFC)

Secondary cellular cementum (CIFC)

- Epithelial root sheath fragments
- Fibroblast-like cells of dental follicle line surface as principal fibres slowly mineralize into surface of cementum

- Cementoblasts form cuboidal cell layer at surface
- Rapid formation of intrinsic collagen fibrils
- Cementoblasts incorporated into the tissue as cementocytes

- Initial fibrous fringe that is synthesized from cells of the dental follicle intermingles with fibrils from unmineralized hyaline layer
- Fibrous fringe attains continuity with principal fibres of periodontal ligament
- Prinicipal fibres are well developed in deciduous teeth and permanent molars as tooth erupts
- Principal fibres are poorly developed in permanent teeth with deciduous predecessors as tooth erupts

Eighteen

The role of the periodontal ligament and dental follicle:
Root resection and transection experiments for teeth of continuous growth indicate that the source of eruptive forces resides in the periodontal ligament (PDL) and transplantation experiments for teeth of limited growth suggests that the forces are generated in the PDL's precursor, the dental follicle

Evidence against a 'tractional' eruptive force pulling the tooth via the collagen network:
From studies using lathyrogens
From tooth transplantation experiments
From studies of the development of the PDL
Eruption of rootless teeth

The fibroblast contraction/migration hypothesis
Evidence is available indicating that PDL fibroblasts migrate according tp eruptive behaviour (passive migration or active migration to effect eruption?)
Fibroblasts in vitro have features of migratory or contractile cells but, in vivo, lack these myofibroblast-like features, resembling cells rapidly turning over collagen

The vascular/tissue hydrostatic pressure hypothesis
Supported by evidence from changes in tooth position with arterial pulse, events at death, effects of vasoactive drugs, effects of cutting or stimulating the vasomotor innervation, measurements of tissue hydrostatic pressure, the biochemistry of the extracellular matrix of the PDL, and the morphology of the PDL vasculature (incl fenestrations)

Eruptive mechanism generating eruptive forces

TOOTH ERUPTION

Interproximal drift

Key features:
Usually mesial drift for human dentition (although distal drift possible)
Mesial drift can help provide space for eruption of third molars
Hypotheses for force generation:
mesial inclination of teeth and direction of biting forces
muscular activity (particularly buccinator)
bone deposition on distal surfaces of tooth sockets
contaction of trans-septal collagen fibres in gingiva
vascular/tissue fluid hydrostatic pressures

Eruptive process

Key features:
Pre-eruptive, eruptive/prefunctional and functional phrases. Eruption commences once tooth root starts to form. Continues throughout life
As tooth erupts, bony crypt remodels and, as tooth approaches oral cavity, resorption of the connective tissues of the oral mucosa occurs with the formation of an epithelial eruptive pathway on fusion of the reduced enamel epithelium and the oral epithelium (note formation of junctional epithelium
Note resorption of deciduous predecessor by 'odontoclasts' (phasic, with some attempts at repair)
Presence of gubernaculum for erupting permanent teeth

273

Matrix vesicles

Controls mineralization of mantle dentine

Controlled micro-environment to concentrate Ca and PO_4 with enzymes

Mineral crystals form within the vesicle

Bud off from the odontoblast process

Approx 30–200nm in size

Thought to have initiating role in mineralization

Heterogenous nucleation

Crystal growth induced by provision of a second solid phase on which a crystal lattice can be formed

Promoted on crystalline material with similar spacings – epitaxy

Seeding of small amounts of hydroxyapatite (Hap) on matrix – grows at expense of Ca PO_4 surrounding it

Controls mineralization of dentine and enamel

Limiting factors

Pyrophosphates present in pre-dentine and bone

In dentine and bone, pyrophosphatases degrade pyrophosphates removing inhibition of mineralization

MINERALIZATION

Enamel mineralization

Size, morphology, stability of crystals determined by supersaturation of Ca PO_4

Influenced by numerous regulators

Initial crystals grow by fusion

Once prismatic structure present, grow in length, not width, controlled by amelogenin nanospheres

Nanospheres act as spacers preventing fusion

Nanospheres degraded as enamel matures

Circumpaulpal dentine

Odontoblasts actively transport Ca to dentine

Deposition occurs within gap zone of collagen type I

Chondroitin sulphate (CS) proteoglycans secreted at the mineralization front

Associated with the gap zones, CS proteoglycans guide mineral deposition

Dentine phosphoprotein (DPP) highly acidic with high affinity for Hap and control of levels of DPP controls rate of mineralization

Dermatan sulphate (DS) proteoglycans in pre-dentine inhibit mineral deposition

Osteopontin promotes mineralization and osteonectin inhibits Hap crystal growth

Bone

Strong similarities to dentine Initial process governed by matrix vesicles followed by heterogenous nucleation

Osteoid contains DS proteoglycans (inhibit)

Mineralization front contains CS proteoglycans

Other acidic proteins (osteopontin, osteonectin, bone sialoprotein control mineralization)

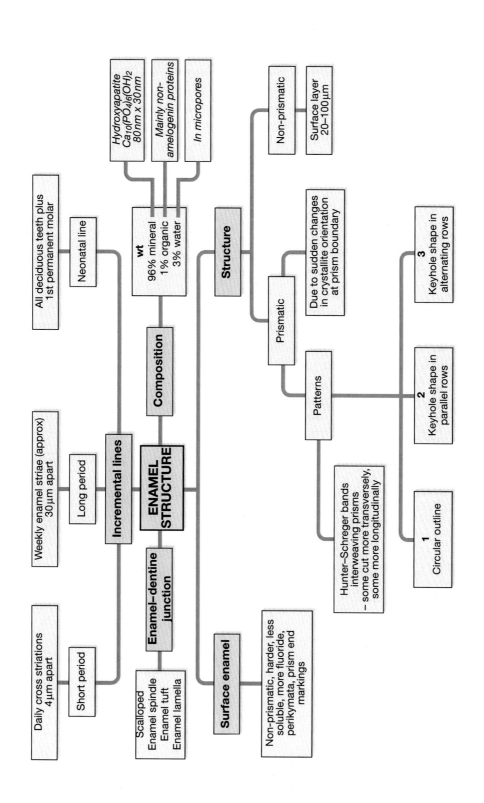

ENAMEL STRUCTURE

Incremental lines

Weekly enamel striae (approx) 30 µm apart — Long period

Daily cross striations 4 µm apart — Short period

All deciduous teeth plus 1st permanent molar — Neonatal line

Composition

wt
96% mineral
1% organic
3% water

Hydroxyapatite $Ca_{10}(PO_4)_6(OH)_2$ 80nm x 30nm

Mainly non-amelogenin proteins

In micropores

Enamel–dentine junction

Scalloped
Enamel spindle
Enamel tuft
Enamel lamella

Surface enamel

Non-prismatic, harder, less soluble, more fluoride, perikymata, prism end markings

Structure

Non-prismatic — Surface layer 20–100 µm

Prismatic — Due to sudden changes in crystallite orientation at prism boundary

Patterns

1 Circular outline

2 Keyhole shape in parallel rows

3 Keyhole shape in alternating rows

Hunter–Schreger bands interweaving prisms – some cut more transversely, some more longitudinally

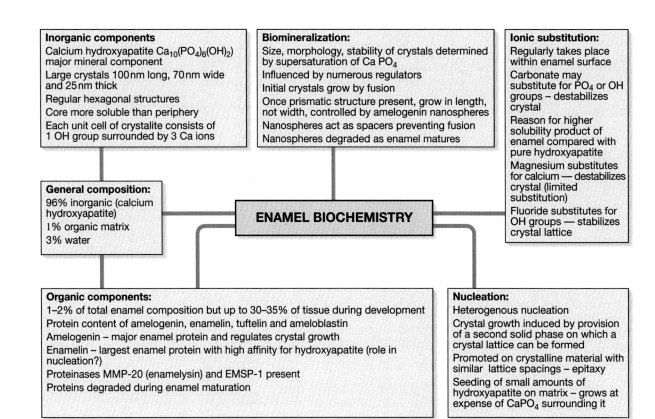

Inorganic components
Calcium hydroxyapatite $Ca_{10}(PO_4)_6(OH)_2$ major mineral component
Large crystals 100 nm long, 70 nm wide and 25 nm thick
Regular hexagonal structures
Core more soluble than periphery
Each unit cell of crystalite consists of 1 OH group surrounded by 3 Ca ions

Biomineralization:
Size, morphology, stability of crystals determined by supersaturation of Ca PO_4
Influenced by numerous regulators
Initial crystals grow by fusion
Once prismatic structure present, grow in length, not width, controlled by amelogenin nanospheres
Nanospheres act as spacers preventing fusion
Nanospheres degraded as enamel matures

Ionic substitution:
Regularly takes place within enamel surface
Carbonate may substitute for PO_4 or OH groups – destabilizes crystal
Reason for higher solubility product of enamel compared with pure hydroxyapatite
Magnesium substitutes for calcium — destabilizes crystal (limited substitution)
Fluoride substitutes for OH groups — stabilizes crystal lattice

General composition:
96% inorganic (calcium hydroxyapatite)
1% organic matrix
3% water

ENAMEL BIOCHEMISTRY

Organic components:
1–2% of total enamel composition but up to 30–35% of tissue during development
Protein content of amelogenin, enamelin, tuftelin and ameloblastin
Amelogenin – major enamel protein and regulates crystal growth
Enamelin – largest enamel protein with high affinity for hydroxyapatite (role in nucleation?)
Proteinases MMP-20 (enamelysin) and EMSP-1 present
Proteins degraded during enamel maturation

Nucleation:
Heterogenous nucleation
Crystal growth induced by provision of a second solid phase on which a crystal lattice can be formed
Promoted on crystalline material with similar lattice spacings – epitaxy
Seeding of small amounts of hydroxyapatite on matrix – grows at expense of $CaPO_4$ surrounding it

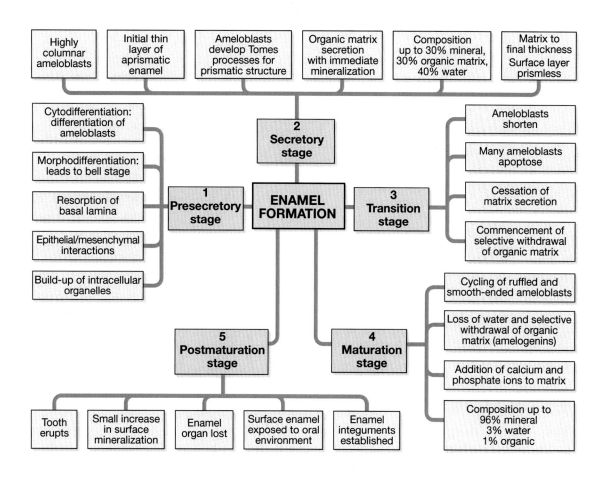

| Highly columnar ameloblasts | Initial thin layer of aprismatic enamel | Ameloblasts develop Tomes processes for prismatic structure | Organic matrix secretion with immediate mineralization | Composition up to 30% mineral, 30% organic matrix, 40% water | Matrix to final thickness Surface layer prismless |

2 Secretory stage

| Ameloblasts shorten |
| Many ameloblasts apoptose |
| Cessation of matrix secretion |
| Commencement of selective withdrawal of organic matrix |

| Cytodifferentiation: differentiation of ameloblasts |
| Morphodifferentiation: leads to bell stage |
| Resorption of basal lamina |
| Epithelial/mesenchymal interactions |
| Build-up of intracellular organelles |

1 Presecretory stage

ENAMEL FORMATION

3 Transition stage

5 Postmaturation stage

4 Maturation stage

| Cycling of ruffled and smooth-ended ameloblasts |
| Loss of water and selective withdrawal of organic matrix (amelogenins) |
| Addition of calcium and phosphate ions to matrix |
| Composition up to 96% mineral 3% water 1% organic |

| Tooth erupts | Small increase in surface mineralization | Enamel organ lost | Surface enamel exposed to oral environment | Enamel integuments established |

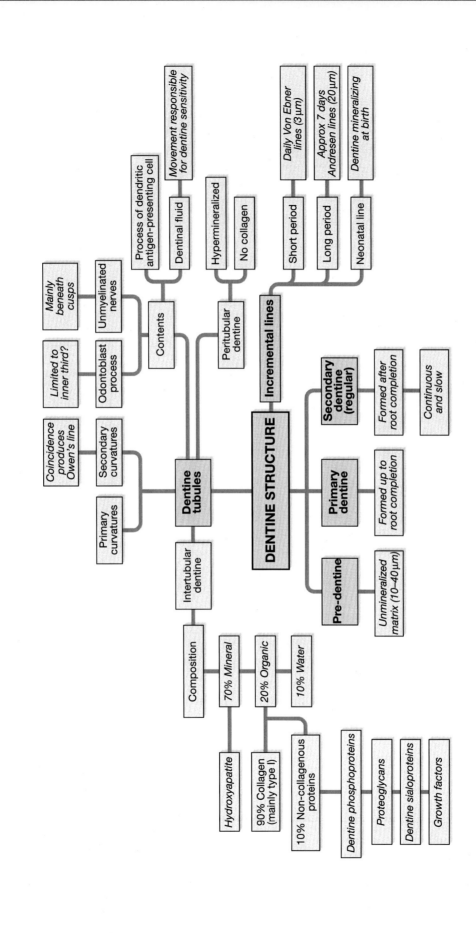

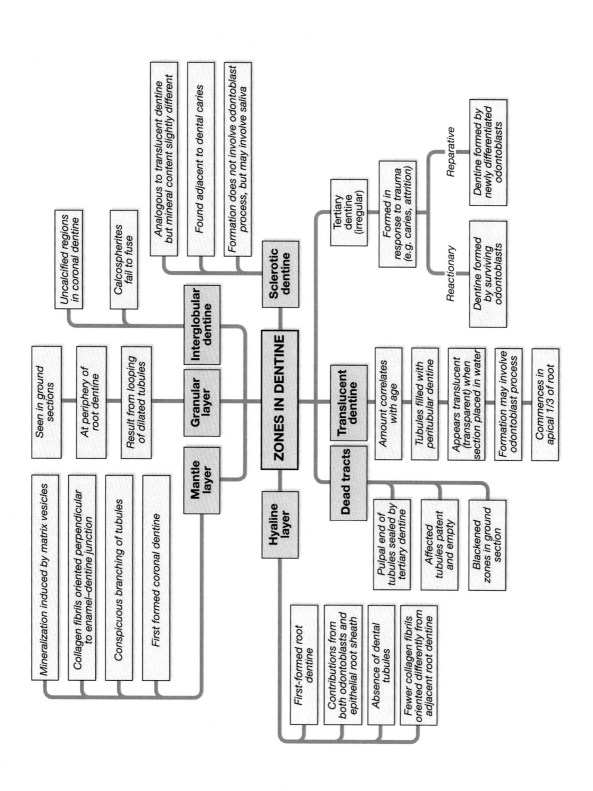

ZONES IN DENTINE

Mantle layer
- Mineralization induced by matrix vesicles
- Collagen fibrils oriented perpendicular to enamel–dentine junction
- Conspicuous branching of tubules
- First formed coronal dentine

Granular layer
- Seen in ground sections
- At periphery of root dentine
- Result from looping of dilated tubules

Interglobular dentine
- Uncalcified regions in coronal dentine
- Calcospherites fail to fuse

Sclerotic dentine
- Analogous to translucent dentine but mineral content slightly different
- Found adjacent to dental caries
- Formation does not involve odontoblast process, but may involve saliva

Tertiary dentine (irregular)
- Formed in response to trauma (e.g. caries, attrition)
  - Reparative — Dentine formed by newly differentiated odontoblasts
  - Reactionary — Dentine formed by surviving odontoblasts

Translucent dentine
- Amount correlates with age
- Tubules filled with peritubular dentine
- Appears translucent (transparent) when section placed in water
- Formation may involve odontoblast process
- Commences in apical 1/3 of root

Dead tracts
- Pulpal end of tubules sealed by tertiary dentine
- Affected tubules patent and empty
- Blackened zones in ground section

Hyaline layer
- First-formed root dentine
- Contributions from both odontoblasts and epithelial root sheath
- Absence of dental tubules
- Fewer collagen fibrils oriented differently from adjacent root dentine

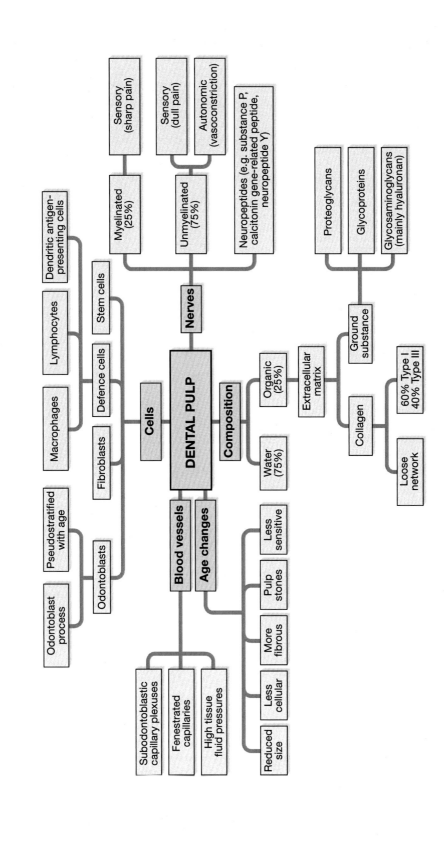

DENTAL PULP

Nerves

Myelinated (25%)
- Sensory (sharp pain)

Unmyelinated (75%)
- Sensory (dull pain)
- Autonomic (vasoconstriction)

Neuropeptides (e.g. substance P, calcitonin gene-related peptide, neuropeptide Y)

Cells

- Dendritic antigen-presenting cells
- Lymphocytes
- Stem cells
- Macrophages
- Defence cells
- Fibroblasts
- Odontoblast process
- Pseudostratified with age
- Odontoblasts

Composition

Organic (25%)
- Extracellular matrix
  - Ground substance
    - Proteoglycans
    - Glycoproteins
    - Glycosaminoglycans (mainly hyaluronan)
  - Collagen
    - 60% Type I 40% Type III
    - Loose network

Water (75%)

Blood vessels
- Subodontoblastic capillary plexuses
- Fenestrated capillaries
- High tissue fluid pressures

Age changes
- Less sensitive
- Pulp stones
- More fibrous
- Less cellular
- Reduced size

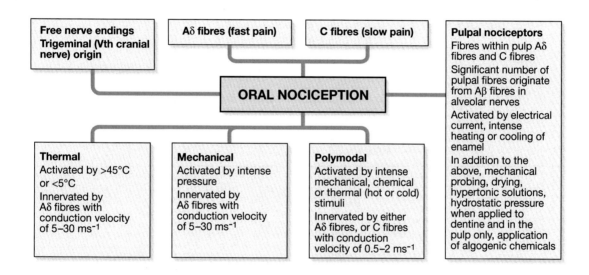

Free nerve endings
Trigeminal (Vth cranial nerve) origin

Aδ fibres (fast pain)

C fibres (slow pain)

ORAL NOCICEPTION

Pulpal nociceptors
Fibres within pulp Aδ fibres and C fibres
Significant number of pulpal fibres originate from Aβ fibres in alveolar nerves
Activated by electrical current, intense heating or cooling of enamel
In addition to the above, mechanical probing, drying, hypertonic solutions, hydrostatic pressure when applied to dentine and in the pulp only, application of algogenic chemicals

Thermal
Activated by >45°C or <5°C
Innervated by Aδ fibres with conduction velocity of 5–30 ms^{-1}

Mechanical
Activated by intense pressure
Innervated by Aδ fibres with conduction velocity of 5–30 ms^{-1}

Polymodal
Activated by intense mechanical, chemical or thermal (hot or cold) stimuli
Innervated by either Aδ fibres, or C fibres with conduction velocity of 0.5–2 ms^{-1}

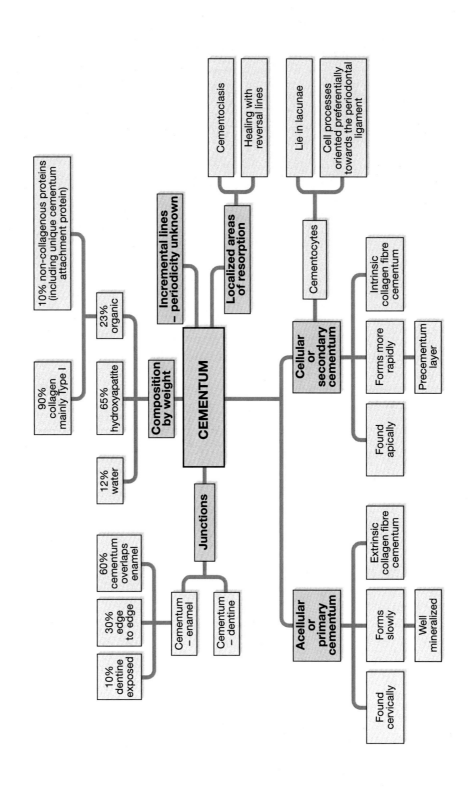

CEMENTUM

Composition by weight
- 90% collagen mainly Type I
  - 10% non-collagenous proteins (including unique cementum attachment protein)
  - 23% organic
- 65% hydroxyapatite
- 12% water

Incremental lines – periodicity unknown

Localized areas of resorption
- Cementoclasis
- Healing with reversal lines

Cementocytes
- Lie in lacunae
- Cell processes oriented preferentially towards the periodontal ligament

Junctions
- Cementum – enamel
  - 60% cementum overlaps enamel
  - 30% edge to edge
  - 10% dentine exposed
- Cementum – dentine

Cellular or secondary cementum
- Intrinsic collagen fibre cementum
- Forms more rapidly
- Precementum layer
- Found apically

Acellular or primary cementum
- Extrinsic collagen fibre cementum
- Forms slowly
- Well mineralized
- Found cervically

282

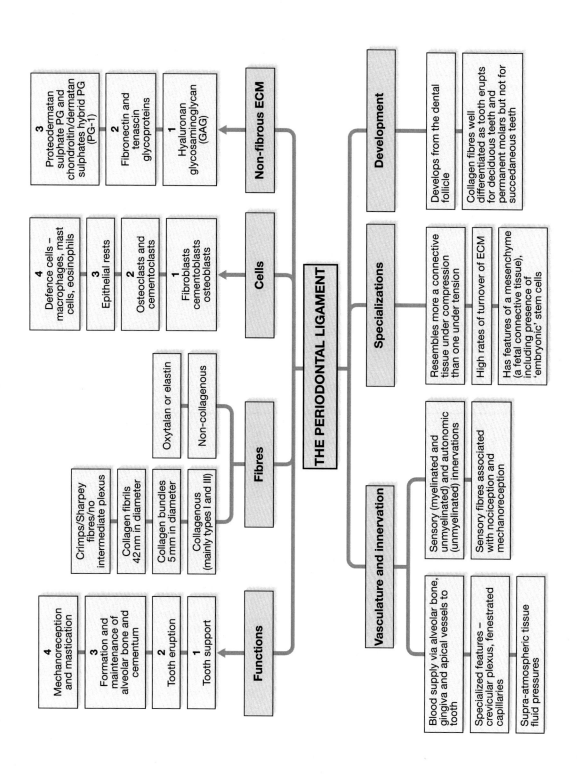

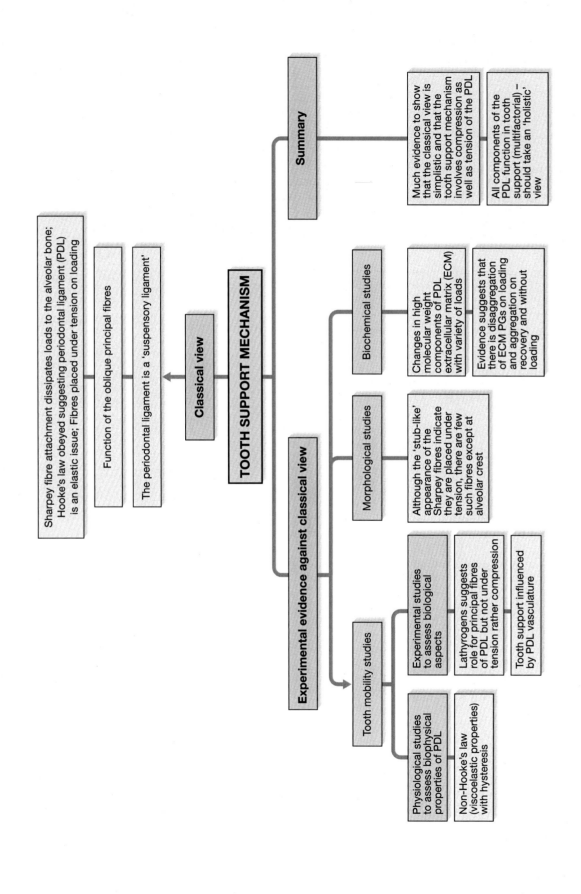

TOOTH SUPPORT MECHANISM

Classical view

Sharpey fibre attachment dissipates loads to the alveolar bone; Hooke's law obeyed suggesting periodontal ligament (PDL) is an elastic issue; Fibres placed under tension on loading

Function of the oblique principal fibres

The periodontal ligament is a 'suspensory ligament'

Experimental evidence against classical view

Tooth mobility studies

Physiological studies to assess biophysical properties of PDL

Non-Hooke's law (viscoelastic properties) with hysteresis

Experimental studies to assess biological aspects

Lathyrogens suggests role for principal fibres of PDL but not under tension rather compression

Tooth support influenced by PDL vasculature

Morphological studies

Although the 'stub-like' appearance of the Sharpey fibres indicate they are placed under tension, there are few such fibres except at alveolar crest

Biochemical studies

Changes in high molecular weight components of PDL extracellular matrix (ECM) with variety of loads

Evidence suggests that there is disaggregation of ECM PGs on loading and aggregation on recovery and without loading

Summary

Much evidence to show that the classical view is simplistic and that the tooth support mechanism involves compression as well as tension of the PDL

All components of the PDL function in tooth support (multifactorial) – should take an 'holistic' view

Slowly adapting Ruffini-type stretch receptors
Adaptation dependent on position within the ligament and force applied

Stimulated when force applied to crown of tooth and when ligament in which they lie is stretched
Thresholds between 10 mN and 200 mN

Innervated by Vth cranial nerve
Aβ fibres with conduction velocities of 25–90 ms^{-1}

PERIODONTAL LIGAMENT MECHANORECEPTORS

Cell bodies in trigeminal ganglion or mesencephalic nucleus of Vth cranial nerve

Involved in reflex control of salivary secretion
When stimulated they cause a reflex secretion of saliva and contribute to the so-called masticatory-salivary reflex

Involved in reflex control of mastication
When stimulated they cause short latency inhibition of jaw closing muscles and contribute to the so-called jaw opening reflexes

Involved in sensory perception of movement of the teeth
They contribute to the sensation of forces applied to the teeth during eating and also inform when something is wedged between the teeth

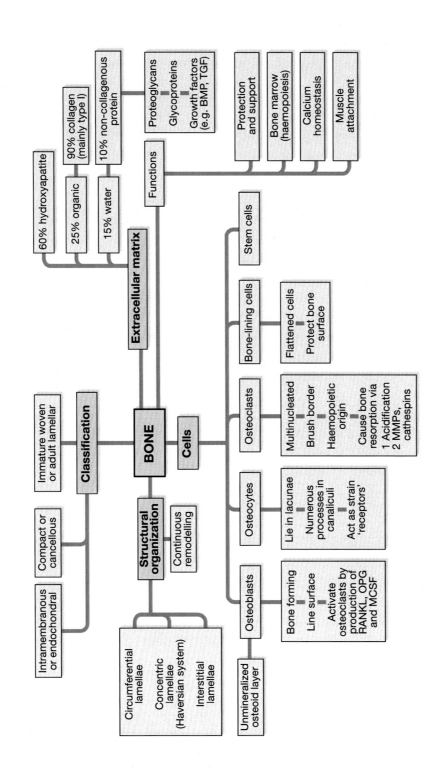

BONE

Extracellular matrix

- 60% hydroxyapatite
- 25% organic
  - 90% collagen (mainly type I)
  - 10% non-collagenous protein
    - Proteoglycans
    - Glycoproteins
    - Growth factors (e.g. BMP, TGF)
- 15% water

Functions
- Protection and support
- Bone marrow (haemopoiesis)
- Calcium homeostasis
- Muscle attachment

Classification
- Immature woven or adult lamellar
- Compact or cancellous
- Intramembranous or endochondral

Structural organization
- Circumferential lamellae
- Concentric lamellae (Haversian system)
- Interstitial lamellae
- Continuous remodelling

Cells
- Osteoblasts
  - Bone forming
  - Line surface
  - Activate osteoclasts by production of RANKL, OPG and MCSF
  - Unmineralized osteoid layer
- Osteocytes
  - Lie in lacunae
  - Numerous processes in canaliculi
  - Act as strain 'receptors'
- Osteoclasts
  - Multinucleated
  - Brush border
  - Haemopoietic origin
  - Cause bone resorption via
    1 Acidification
    2 MMPs, cathespins
- Bone-lining cells
  - Flattened cells
  - Protect bone surface
- Stem cells

Eighteen

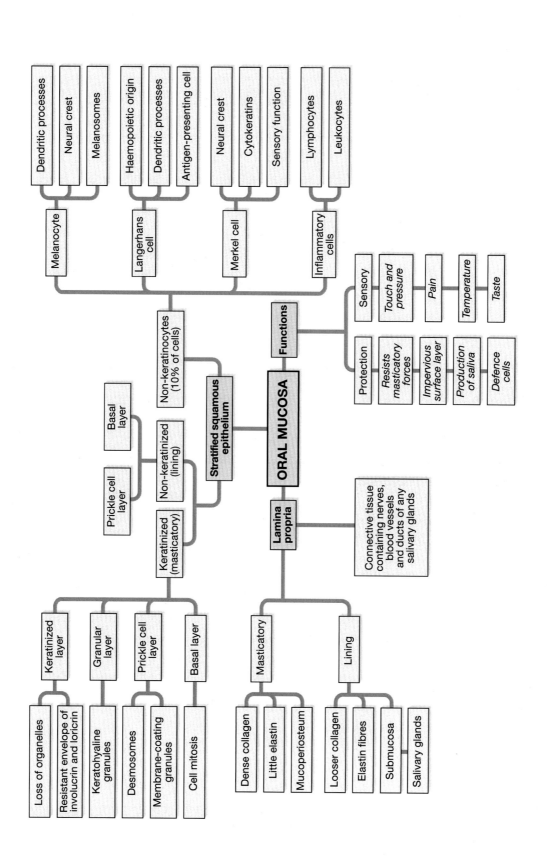

GCF flow
Flow rate directly linked to degree of inflammation
In health 0.05–0.2 μl/min
Reaches the sulcus by intercellular routes across epithelial wall
Mediated by osmosis
Affected by: passage of fluid from capillaries to gingival tissues
removal of fluid by lymphatic system
filtration coefficient of junctional and sulcular epithelia

Inflammation and GCF
Flow rate increased due to increased osmotic gradient and fluid flows across weakened basement membrane
Loose organization of junctional and sulcular epithelium increases fluid flow from capillaries into connective tissue
Inflammatory exudate allows passage of cells/large proteins into fluid

General composition
Transudate (exudate) of periodontal tissues
Collects in gingival sulcus
Major constituents from: plasma, interstitial fluid, plaque matrix, host inflammatory cells and tissue, microbial sources

GINGIVAL CREVICULAR FLUID (GCF)

Biochemical composition
Inorganic and organic components and modified by local environment
Inorganic components, Ca, Na, K, Mg
Ca levels higher in GCF than saliva – implications for pellicle protein interaction and bacterial attachment
In health concentration of organic components similar to plasma
Contains serum-derived proteins including albumin, IgA, IgG, IgM, fibrinogen, complement components and protease inhibitors
Bacterial components including bacterial enzymes, lipopolysaccharides (LPS), urea, lactic acid

Biomarkers
Components of bacterial and host origin as indicators of disease progression
Information regarding periodontal tissue destruction
Markers of bone resorption and pro/anti-inflammatory cytokines
Presence of active disease

Further reading

Oral anatomy, histology and embryology

Students will find more detailed information on all aspects of these topics, including reference lists of up-to-date original scientific articles, in the following textbook:

Berkovitz BKB, Holland RG, Moxham BJ. A colour atlas and textbook of oral anatomy, histology and embryology. 4th edn. Edinburgh: Mosby, 2009.

Oral biochemistry

The following list provides some original scientific articles that may be consulted as additional reading to complement the text of this book:

Bartlett JD, Ganss B, Goldberg M et al. (2006) Protein-protein interactions of the developing enamel matrix. Current Topics in Developmental Biology, 74: 57–115

Bartold PM, Narayanan AS (2006) Molecular and cell biology of healthy and diseased periodontal tissues. Periodontology 2000, 40: 29–49

Beertsen W, McCulloch CA, Sodek J (1997) The periodontal ligament: a unique, multifunctional connective tissue. Periodontology 2000, 13: 20–40

Bosshardt DD (2005) Are cementoblasts a subpopulation of osteoblasts or a unique phenotype? Journal of Dental Research, 84: 390–406

Butler WT (1998) Dentin matrix proteins. European Journal of Oral Science, 106: 204–210

Delima AJ, Van Dyke TE (2003) Origin and function of the cellular components in gingival crevice fluid. Periodontology 2000, 31: 55–76

Diekwisch TG, Thomas GH (2001) The developmental biology of cementum. International Journal of Developmental Biology, 45: 695–706

Embery G, Waddington RJ et al. (2000) Connective tissue elements as diagnostic aids in periodontology. Periodontology 2000, 24: 193–214

Giannobile WV, Al-Shammari KF, Sarment DP (2003) Matrix molecules and growth factors as indicators of periodontal disease activity. Periodontology 2000, 31: 125–134

Goodson JM (2003) Gingival crevice fluid flow. Periodontology 2000, 31: 43–54

Gorski JP (1998) Is all bone the same? Distinctive distributions and properties of non-collagenous matrix proteins in lamellar vs woven bone imply the existence of different underlying osteogenic mechanisms. Critical Reviews in Oral Biology and Medicine, 9: 201–223

Graham L, Cooper PR, Cassidy N et al. (2006) The effect of calcium hydroxide on solubilisation of bioactive dentine matrix components. Biomaterials, 27: 2865–2873

Kaufman E, Lamster IB (2002) The diagnostic applications of saliva: a review. Critical Reviews in Oral Biology and Medicine, 13: 197–212

Loos BG, Tjoa S (2005) Host-derived diagnostic markers for periodontitis: do they exist in gingival crevice fluid? Periodontology 2000, 39: 53–72

Margolis HC, Beniash E, Fowler CE (2006) Role of macromolecular assembly of enamel matrix proteins in enamel formation. Journal of Dental Research, 85: 775–793

Simmer J, Hu JC (2001) Dental enamel formation and its impact on clinical dentistry. Journal of Dental Education, 65: 896–905

Sloan AJ, Perry H, Matthews JB et al. (2000) Transforming growth factor-beta isoform expression in mature human healthy and carious molar teeth. Histochemical Journal, 32: 247–252

Sloan AJ, Waddington RJ (2009) Dental pulp stem cells: what, where, how? International Journal of Paediatric Dentistry, 19: 61–70

Smith AJ (2002) Pulp responses to caries and dental repair. Caries Research, 36: 223–232

Zhao S, Sloan AJ, Murray PE et al. (2000) Ultrastructural localisation of TGF-beta exposure in dentine by chemical treatment. Histochemical Journal, 32: 489–494

Oral physiology

The following list provides some original scientific articles that may be consulted as additional reading to complement the text of this book:

Cadden SW, Orchardson R (2001) The neural mechanisms of oral and facial pain. Dental Update, 28, 359–367

Cadden SW, Orchardson R (2009) Mastication and swallowing: 2. Control. Dental Update, 36, 390–398

Hector MP, Linden RWA (1999) Reflexes of salivary secretion. In: Garrett JP, Ekström J, Anderson LC (eds). Frontiers of Oral Biology, vol. 11. Neural Mechanisms of Salivary Gland Secretion. Basel: Karger, 196–217

Linden RWA (ed.) (1998) The scientific basis of eating, taste and smell, salivation, mastication and swallowing and their dysfunctions. Frontiers of Oral Biology, vol. 9. Basel: Karger

Linden RWA, Millar BJ, Scott BJJ (1995) The innervation of the periodontal ligament. In: Berkovitz BKB, Moxham BJ, Newman HN (eds). The Periodontal Ligament in Health and Disease, 2nd edn. London: Mosby-Wolfe, 133–159

Orchardson R, Cadden SW (2001) An update on the physiology of the dentine-pulp complex. Dental Update, 28, 200–209

Orchardson R, Cadden SW (2009) Mastication and Swallowing: 1. Functions, Performance and Mechanisms. Dental Update, 36, 327–337

Index

Aβ fibres, 172–173, 207
Abrasion, 153
Accessory ligaments, temporomandibular joint, 11
Accessory nerve, 39, 53, 69
Accessory parotid gland, 79
Acetylcholine, 81
Acid phosphatases, 80–81, 239
Acidic proteins, dentine matrix, 162, 167
Acinus, 83–84
    cells, 81–84
Aδ fibres, 164, 170–173
Adenoid tissue (pharyngeal tonsils), 69
Adhesins, 95
Age-related changes
    dentine, 163–165
    enamel, 147
    pulp, 173, 193
    salivary glands, 85, 92
Albumin, 239
Alcohol, free nerve endings stimulation, 55
Algogenic substances, 171
Alkaline phosphatase, 114, 114–115, 135–136, 166, 223, 239
Allodynia, 171
Alveolar bone, 221
    biochemical composition, 221
    cell types, 223–224
    development, 104
    gross morphology, 222
    histology, 222
    organic matrix, 221
    remodelling during tooth eruption, 104, 210
    self-assessment
        answers, 229–234
        questions, 226–228
    structural lines, 224
Alveolar nerve, 2
Alveolar plates, 222
Alveolar processes
    mandible, 2–3
        development, 102–103
    maxilla, 2, 103
Ameloblastin, 116–117, 136–137, 146
Ameloblasts, 115, 135, 145–146
    maturation stage, 145–146
        ruffle-ended morphology, 146
        smooth-ended morphology, 146
    post-maturation stage, 147

Amelogenesis, 115, 143–144
    maturation stage, 146–147
    post-maturation stage, 147
    presecretory stage, 144–145
    revision summary chart, 277f
    secretory stage, 145
    self-assessment
        answers, 157–160
        questions, 155–156
    transition stage, 145
Amelogenin, 116–117, 137, 143, 146
    nanospheres, 137, 146
        hydroxyapatite crystal growth regulation, 146–147
Amylase, 80–81
Andresen lines, 164, 168
Angle of mandible, 2–3
Angle's classification of malocclusion, 25
    class I, 25
    class II, 25
        division 1, 25
        division 2, 25
    class III, 25
Ankyloglossa, 51
Ankylosis, 119
Anterior nasal spine, 2, 70
Anterior olfactory nucleus, 56
Anterior superior alveolar artery, 68
Anterior superior alveolar nerve, 70–71
Antigen-presenting cells, 170, 237
Antimicrobial salivary constituents, 80–81
Antrum See Maxillary sinus
Apical foramen, 24, 170
    development, 116
Apoptosis, 117
    ameloblasts, 145
Articular eminence, 10–11
Articular tubercle, 11
Articulation, 58
Artificial sweeteners, 54–55
Ascending pharyngeal artery, 39
Attrition, 153
Auriculotemporal nerve, 11, 70–71, 79–80
Autonomic nerve fibres, periodontal ligament, 206

Bacterial products, gingival crevicular fluid, 239

Bell stage, 114, 144, 165–166, 168
    early, 114–115
    late, 115
    layers, 144
Bennett movement, 41
Bicarbonate ions, saliva, 82
Biglycan, 118, 136–137, 162, 164, 166, 195, 221–222
Bilabial consonant sounds, 58
Bioactive signalling molecules, odontogenesis, 115–116
Biofilms, 94–95
Birbeck granules, 237
Bitter taste, 54–55
    reflex salivary secretion, 82–83
Blood supply, 67–68, 67b
    cheek, 67–68
    digastric muscles, 37–38
    face, 67
    floor of mouth, 68
    gingiva, 67–68
        buccal, 67–68
        labial, 67–68
        lingual, 67
        palatal, 68
    lips, 68
    mandibular teeth/periodontium, 67
    masseter, 37
    maxillary sinus, 67–68
    mylohyoid muscle, 38
    palate, 39, 68
    pterygoids, 37
    pulp, 170
    revision summary chart, 264f
    self-assessment
        answers, 75–78
        questions, 73–74
    tongue, 53, 68
Body of mandible, 2–3
Body of maxilla, 2
Body temperature maintenance, 57
Bone
    biochemical composition, 221
    cell types, 223–224
    classification, 222
    histology, 222
    mechanosensors, 223
    mineralization, 136–137
    organization, 222

Page numbers followed by f, t, or b indicate figures, tables, or boxes, respectively.

Bone (*Continued*)
  resorption/deposition (remodelling), 224–225, 231–234
    formation phase, 224
    resorption phase, 224
    resting phase, 224
    reversl phase, 224
  revision summary chart, 286f
  stem cells, 223
  structural lines, 224
Bone marrow, 222
Bone morphogenetic proteins, 115, 162, 167, 170, 224
Bone sialoprotein, 117, 136–137, 162, 195–196, 221
Bone-lining cells, 223
Branchial arches *See* Pharyngeal arches
Broca's area, 59
Brushite, 96, 135–136
Buccae *See* Cheeks
Buccal artery, 67–68
Buccal, definition, 19t
Buccal gingiva
  blood supply, 67–68
  lymphatic drainage, 68
Buccal glands, 79, 85
Buccal lymph nodes, 68
Buccal nerve, 71
  anaesthetization, 69
Buccal veins, 68
Buccinator, 1, 38, 41
Bud stage, 114
Buffering capacity of saliva, 80
Bundle bone, 104, 222, 224

C fibres, 170–173
c-Fos, 225
Calcitonin, 224
Calcitonin gene-related peptide, 171, 171–172, 210
Calculus, 96–97
  classification, 96–97
  composition, 96
  formation, 96
  removal, 97
  subgingival, 96–97
  supragingival, 96–97
Canaliculi, 195, 223
Cancellous (spongy) bone, 222
  trabeculae, 222
Candida albicans, 81
Caniform teeth, 18
Canine groove, 21–22
Canines, 18, 21
  angulation/inclination, 24
  deciduous
    mandibular, 21
    maxillary, 21
    resorption/shedding, 118–119
  innervation
    mandibular, 70
    maxillary, 70
  permanent
    mandibular, 21
    maxillary, 21
  revision summary chart, 255f

Cap stage, 114–115, 168
Capsaicin, 55, 83
Carbohydrate, dietary, plaque matrix relationship, 95–96
Carbonic anhydrase, 80–81
Caries, plaque matrix relationship, 95–96
Cathepsin D, 239
Cathepsin G, 239
Cbfa-1 (runx2), 223, 225
Cementoblasts, 116–118, 138, 195
  periodontal ligament, 205–206
Cementoclasts, 205–206
Cementocytes, 117–118, 195
Cementogenesis, 116–118
Cementoid, 138
Cementum, 194
  acellular extrinsic fibre, 117, 137–138, 195
  acellular (primary), 116–117, 195, 202
  afibrillar, 196
  cellular intrinsic fibre, 138, 195–196
  cellular mixed stratified, 196
  cellular (secondary), 116–118, 195, 202
  chemical composition, 194–195
    inorganic, 194
    organic matrix, 195
  classification, 195–196
  extrinsic fibre, 195
  incremental lines, 195, 117–118
  intermediate, 196
  intrinsic fibre, 195
  junction with enamel, 194
  mineralization, 117–118, 137–138
  mixed fibre, 195
  periodontal ligament fibre attachment, 117
  physical properties, 194
  regeneration, 196
  resorption, 196
  revision summary charts, 282f
  self-assessment
    answers, 200–202
    questions, 197–199
Cementum-attachment protein, 117, 195
Central pattern generators, 41–43, 49–50
Central septum of nasal passage, 55
Centric occlusal position, 24–25
Centric stops, 25
Cervical loop, 114, 116
Cervical lymph nodes, 53, 68–69
Cervical margins, 19t
  deciduous/permanent dentition comparison, 19
Cheek
  anatomy, 1
  blood supply, 67–68
  muscle innervation, 71t
  venous drainage, 68
Chemoreceptors, 43
Chewing cycle, 40–41
  closing phase, 40
  jaw reflex activity, 42
  muscles of mastication, 41
  occlusal (intercuspal) phase, 40
  opening phase, 40
Chin
  anatomy, 2–3
  development, 103

Chondroitin sulphate, 12, 136, 162, 166, 169, 204, 221
Chorda tympani nerve, 53–54, 70–71, 80, 104
Chronology of tooth development, 119–120
  deciduous dentition, 119t
  permanent dentition, 120t
Cingulum, 19t
Circumferential lamellae, 222
Circumvallate papillae, 51–54, 85, 240
Cold receptors, 57
Cold sensitivity, 57
Collagen
  bone matrix, 221, 223
  cementum, 194, 195
  dental pulp, 169
  dentine, 162
  dentinogenesis, 166
    mineralization, 166
  gingival fibres, 238
  intra-articular disc, 12
  lamina propria, 237
  osteoid, 222
  periodontal ligament, 203–204
    crimps, 204, 211
    degradation, 205
    development, 210
    fuctional roles, 204
    principal fibres, 204
    response to mechanical loading, 204, 211
    turnover rate, 204
  predentine, 164
  type I, 162, 164, 166, 203–204
  type III, 204
  type V, 204
  type VI, 204
  type XII, 204
Collagenase, 205, 239
Collecting ducts, 83–84
Colony-stimulating factor, 114
Common chemical sense, 53, 55, 66
  oral nociceptor-salivary reflexes, 83
Common facial vein, 68
Compact (cortical) bone, 222
  organization of lamellae, 222
Complement components, 239
Compound glands, 79
Conditioned reflex salivation, 83
Condylar cartilage, 103
Condylar process, 2–3, 10
Connexin 43, 12
Consonant sounds, 58
  classification, 58–59
Constitutive secretion, 82
Contour line (of Owen), 162–164
Copula, 104
Coronoid process, 2–3, 36–37, 103
Cortical areas
  gustation, 55
  nociception, 172
  olfaction, 56
  speech, 59
  thermoreception, 57–58

Cortical bone *See* Compact bone
Cranial nerves
    reflexes, 72
    swallowing, 43
Craniofacial complex development, 101
    revision summary chart, 269f
    self-assessment
        answers, 109–112
        questions, 105–108
Craniomandibular joint *See* Temporomandibular joint
Crevicular plexus, 206, 238
Crevicular/sulcular epithelium, 238
Cribriform plate, 55–56, 222, 224
Cross-striations, enamel, 145
Crowns, 19t
    deciduous/permanent dentition comparison, 19
    formation, 104
Curves of Spee, 24
Curves of Wilson, 24
Cusps, 19t, 40
    deciduous/permanent dentition comparison, 19
Cutaneous sensory innervation of face, 69, 71
Cyclic adenosine monophosphate (cAMP), 54–56
Cytokeratin 1, 237
Cytokeratin 4, 237–238
Cytokeratin 5, 237–238
Cytokeratin 7, 237
Cytokeratin 8, 237
Cytokeratin 10, 237
Cytokeratin 13, 237–238
Cytokeratin 14, 237–238
Cytokeratin 18, 237
Cytokeratin 19, 238
Cytokeratins, 236–237
    crevicular/sulcular epithelium, 238
    type I, 237
    type II, 237
Cytokines, bone remodelling, 224

Deciduous (primary) dentition, 18
    canines, 21
    chronology of development, 119t
    dental formula, 18
    differences from permanent dentition, 19
    enamel striae, 143
    incisors, 18, 20
    molars, 23–24
        root canals, 24
    pulp chamber, 24
    resorption/shedding, 118–119
Decorin, 118, 136–137, 162, 164, 166, 169, 195, 221–222
Deep cervical lymph nodes, 53, 68–69
Deep temporal nerve, 11
Defence cells
    dental pulp, 170
    periodontal ligament, 206
Dendritic antigen-presenting cells, 170
Dental arches, 24

Dental follicle, 94, 104, 114, 167, 194, 203
    cementogenesis, 116, 118
    layers, 114, 116
    root development, 116
Dental formulae, 18
Dental lamina, 113–114
Dental notation, 18
Dental papilla, 114–116, 144–145, 165–167
    dental pulp development, 168
    epithelial-mesenchymal interactions, 115
    pulp formation, 169
Dental pulp *See* Pulp
Dentinal fluid, 163
Dentinal tubules, 162–163
    contents, 163
    fluid movement, dentine sensitivity, 165
Dentine, 161, 169
    age-related changes, 163–165
    chemical composition, 162
        collagen, 162
        non-collagenous proteins, 162
    circumpulpal, 136, 162–163
    dead tracts, 165
    development *See* Dentinogenesis
    incremental lines, 167, 168
        long-period (Andresen lines), 164, 168
        short-period (von Ebner lines), 164, 168
    interglobular, 163–164, 166
    intertubular, 162–163
    mantle, 135–136, 144–145, 163, 166–167
    mineralization, 135–136, 140–141, 162–163, 166–167
        biochemical aspects, 166–167
        root, 136
    peritubular (intratubular), 163, 165, 167–168
    physical properties, 161–162
    posteruptive changes, 164–165
    regional variations (zones), 163–164
    revision summary charts
        structure, 278f
        zones, 279f
    sclerotic, 165
    secondary, 164, 167–169
    sensory nerve terminals, 163
    structure, 153–154
    structure/composition
        self-assessment answers, 177–180
        self-assessment questions, 174–176
    tertiary, 164, 168–170, 190–191
        reactionary, 164, 168
        reparative, 164, 168
    translucent, 163, 168
Dentine matrix proteins, 162, 167
Dentine phosphoprotein (DPP), 136, 162, 167
Dentine phosphoproteins, 162, 167
Dentine sensitivity, 163, 165, 179
Dentine sialophosphoprotein gene, 162, 167
Dentine sialoprotein, 196, 118, 162, 167, 196

Dentinogenesis, 115, 165, 169
    odontoblasts
        differentiation, 165–166
        organic matrix secretion, 166
    primary/secondary curvatures, 162–163
    root, 167
    self-assessment, 181–182
Dentogingival junction, 238
    development, 113
Depressor anguli oris, 38
Depressor labii inferioris, 38
Dermal papillae, 237
Dermatan sulphate, 12, 136–137, 166, 169, 204, 222
Development
    craniofacial complex, 101
    dentine (dentinogenesis), 165
    dentogingival junction, 118
    face, 101
    jaws, 101
    palate, 102
    periodontal ligament, 210
    root, 210
    thyroid gland, 104
    tongue, 102, 104
    tooth (odontogenesis)
        early, 113–114
        initiation, 115–116
Diacylglycerol, 54–55
Digastric fossa, 2–3, 37
Digastric muscle, 2–3, 36–38, 41
    blood supply, 37–38
    innervation, 37–38, 71
Digastric nerve, 37
Digastric tendon, 37
Digestive enzymes, saliva, 80
Diphyodonty, 18
Distal, definition, 19t
Dryopithecus cusp pattern, 23–24
Dynorphins, 172

Ear ossicles, 102–103
Elastase, 239
Elastin, 203–204, 237
Electrolytes, saliva, 80
    concentration variation with flow rate, 81–82
    modification, 84
Enamel, 142–160
    aprismatic (non-prismatic), 145
    composition, 142–143
    deciduous/permanent dentition comparison, 19
    development *See* Amelogenesis
    hydroxyapatite, 142–143
    incremental lines, 143–145
        cross-striations, 143
        enamel striae, 143–144
    investing organic layers *See* Enamel integuments
    ionic substitution, 143
        fluoride, 143
    junction with cementum, 194
    maturation, 145–146
    mineralization, 137, 147

Enamel *(Continued)*
  non-prismatic, 143
  organic matrix, 143, 146–147, 159–160
    degradation, 146
    proteinases, 146–147
    proteins, 146–147
    synthesis, 145
  physical properties, 142
  revision summary charts, 275f
    biochemistry, 276f
  self-assessment
    answers, 151–154
    questions, 148–150
  structure, 142, 152–154
    age changes, 147
    See also Enamel prisms (rods)
  surface, 142, 144
  water content, 143
Enamel cord, 115
Enamel integuments, 94
  revision summary chart, 270f
  self-assessment
    answers, 100
    questions, 98–99
Enamel knot, 115
Enamel lamellae, 144, 146
Enamel matrix serine proteinase-1
    (EMSP-1), 146–147
Enamel niche, 115
Enamel organ, 94
  bell stage, 114–115, 144
    layers, 144
  bud stage, 114
  cap stage, 114
Enamel prisms (rods), 143
  formation, 145
Enamel spindles, 144–145, 163
Enamel striae (of Retzius), 143–145
  neonatal line, 143–144
  perikymata grooves, 143
Enamel tufts, 144, 146
Enamel–dentine junction, 144–145
Enamel-related proteins, 116–117
Enamelin, 137, 143, 146
Enamelysin (MMP-20), 146
Encephalins, 172
Endochondral bone, 222
Endogenous opioid peptides, 172
Endorphins, 172
Entorhinal cortex, 56
Eosinophils, 206
Epiglottis, 51–52
  swallowing, 43
  taste buds, 53–54, 240
Epitaxy, 136–137, 147, 223
Epithelial cell rests, periodontal ligament,
    206
Epithelial folds (rete), 237
Epithelial root sheath (of Hertwig),
    116–117, 165, 167, 206
  fenestration, 116–117
Epithelial–mesenchymal interactions,
    133–134
  amelogenesis, 144–145
  cementogenesis, 116–117
  dental papilla, 168

Epithelial–mesenchymal interactions
    (Continued)
  odontoblast differentiation, 165–166
  odontogenesis, 115
    bioactive signalling molecules,
        115–116
  root development, 116
    dentinogenesis, 167
Erosion, 153
Erupted tooth, investing organic layers, 94
Erupting tooth, soft tissues covering, 94
Exernal oblique ridge, 2–3
Exocrine glands, 79
Exocytosis, 82
External auditory meatus, 79
External carotid artery, 67, 79–80
External enamel epithelium, 114, 116–117,
    144

Face
  blood supply, 67
  cutaneous innervation, 69, 71
  development, 101
  lymphatic drainage, 68
Facial artery, 37–38, 67–68
  ascending palatine branch, 39
  submental branch, 38
Facial expression muscles, 38
  innervation, 38
Facial nerve, 38, 53, 69–70, 79–80
  chorda tympani branch, 53–54, 70–71,
      80, 104
  digastric branch, 37–38
Facial veins, 68
Feeding process, 40
  posterior oral seal, 40–41
  role of mechanoreceptors, 207
  salivary flow, 82
  transport of food in mouth
    Stage I, 40
    Stage II, 40–41
Fenestrated capillaries, 206
Fibrinogen, 239
Fibroblasts
  dental pulp, 170
  lamina propria, 237
  periodontal ligament, 204–205
    role in tissue remodelling, 205
Fibronectin, 118, 169, 195–196,
    221–222
  periodontal ligament, 204–205
Filaggrin, 236
Filiform papillae, 52, 240
Fimbriae, 95
Fimbriated folds, 51
Fissure, 19t
Flavour sensation, 55–56
  revision summary chart, 263f
Floor of mouth, 38
  anatomy, 2
  blood supply, 68
  innervation
    of muscles, 71t
    sensory, 70–71
  lining mucosa, 240
  lymphatic drainage, 68

Fluoride
  cementum, 194
  ionic substitution in enamel, 143
Foliate papillae, 52–54, 240
Foramen caecum, 20, 51–52, 104
Foramen ovale, 70–71
Foramen rotundum, 71
Foramen spinosum, 71
Fossa, 19t
Free nerve endings, 55
  cold/warm thermoreceptors, 57
  nociceptors, 171
  periodontal ligament, 206–207, 210
  temporomandibular joint capsule, 11
Frena, 1
Frontal processes, 2, 103
Frontonasal process, 101–102
Fructosyltransferases, 96
Fungiform papillae, 52–54, 207, 240

G-proteins, 54–56
Gag reflex, 70
Gamma-aminobutyric acid (GABA), 172
Ganglionic nerve, 71
Gastro-oesphageal reflux, 83
Gate control theory of pain, 172
Genial spines, 2–3
Genial tubercle, 52
Genioglossus, 2–3, 38, 52
Geniohyoid, 2–3, 38, 41
  innervation, 38
Gingiva, 238–239
  blood supply, 67–68
  collagen fibres, 238
  epithelium
    crevicular/sulcular, 238
    external surface, 238
    internal surface, 238
    junctional, 237–238
  free, 238
  innervation, 69t
  interdental, 238–239
  lymphatic drainage, 68
  oral mucosa, 238
  venous drainage, 68
Gingival crevice (sulcus), 118, 238
  epithelium, 238
Gingival crevicular fluid, 235–249
  biochemical composition, 239
    serum-derived proteins, 239
  flow rate, 239
    influence of inflammation, 239
  formation
    crevicular plexus, 238
    osmosis, 239
  functions, 239
  revision summary chart, 288f
  self-assessment
    answers, 245–249
    questions, 241–244
Gla-proteins, 162, 167
Glenoid fossa *See* Mandibular fossa
Glomeruli of olfactory bulb, 56
Glosso-epiglottic folds, 51–52
Glossopharyngeal nerve, 70, 53–54, 69–70, 104
  lesser petrosal branch, 70, 80

Glottal consonant sounds, 59
Glottis, in swallowing, 43
Glucosyltransferases, 96
Glutamate, 54–55, 172
Glycine, 172
Glycoproteins
    bone, 221
    dental pulp, 169
    osteoid, 222
    periodontal ligament, 204–205
    saliva, 80–81
Glycosaminoglycans
    bone, 221
    dental pulp, 169
    tooth development, 114–115
Golgi tendon organs, 11
Granular layer (of Tomes), 162–164, 167
Granular layer (stratum granulosum), 236
Greater palatine artery, 68
Greater palatine foramen, 2, 70
Greater palatine nerve, 1–2, 70–71
Greater palatine veins, 68
Greater palatine vessels, 1–2
Ground substance
    intra-articular disc, 12
    periodontal ligament, 204–205
Growth factors
    bone matrix, 221
    bone remodelling, 224
    dentine, 162, 167
    odontoblast differentiation, 165–166
    osteoid, 222
    saliva, 81
Growth, postnatal of mandible, 103
Gubernacular canal, 119
Gubernacular cord, 119
Gustation See Taste
Gustatory afferent neurones, 55
Gustatory pathway, 55
Gustatory-salivary reflex, 82–83

Hard palate, 1–2, 9t
    bones, 2
    mechanoreceptors, 207–208
    oral mucosa, 238, 248–249
    ossification, 102
        maxillary centre, 102
        palatine centres, 102
    sensory innervation, 70
    venous drainage, 68
Haversian system, 222
Heparan sulphate, 221
Heterodont dentition, 40
Heterogenous nucleation, 137
    enamel mineralization, 147
    osteoid mineralization, 223
Histatins, 81
Holding contacts (centric stops), 25
Homeobox genes, 115
Hooke's law, 210
Howship's lacunae (resorption lacunae), 103–104, 118, 223–224
Hunger, 55
Hunter–Schreger bands, 143, 145
Hyaline layer, 116–117, 136, 164, 167
Hyaluronan, 169

Hyaluronidase, 239
Hydrokinetic secretion, 82
Hydroxyapatite, 96, 135–137, 145–146, 153
    bone, 221
    cementum, 194
    crystal formation, 142
    dentine, 162–164, 166
    enamel, 142–143
    ionic substitution, 143
Hyoglossus, 38, 52, 70–71, 80
Hyoid bone, 37–38, 40–41, 51–52
    role in speech articulation, 58
Hypoglossal nerve, 52–53, 69, 104
Hypopharynx, in swallowing, 42–43
Hypothalamus, 57
Hysteresis, periodontal ligament, 210

Immunoglobulin A (IgA), 80–81
Immunoglobulins, gingival crevicular fluid, 239
Incisal margin, 19t
Incisiform teeth, 18
Incisive artery, 67
Incisive canal, 2–3, 70
Incisive foramen, 1–2, 68, 70
Incisive fossa, 2–3
Incisive nerve, 69–70
Incisive papilla, 1–2
    mechanoreceptors, 207–208
Incisor plexus, 69
Incisor relationships, classification of malocclusion, 25–26
    Class I, 26
    Class II, 26
        Division 1, 26
        Division 2, 26
    Class III, 26
Incisors, 18–20
    angulation/inclination, 24
    deciduous
        mandibular first (central), 20
        mandibular second (lateral), 20
        maxillary first (central), 20
        maxillary second (lateral), 20
        resorption/shedding, 118–119
    dental notation, 18
    development (odontogenesis), 115
    innervation
        mandibular, 70
        maxillary, 70
    permanent
        eruption rates, 119
        mandibular first (central), 20
        mandibular second (lateral), 20
        maxillary first (central), 19
        maxillary second (lateral), 20
    revision summary chart, 254f
Incremental lines
    cementum, 194, 117–118
    dentine, 167, 168
        long-period (Andresen lines), 164, 168
        short-period (von Ebner lines), 164, 168
    enamel, 143–145
Inferior alveolar artery, 2–3, 67, 206

Inferior alveolar nerve, 2–3, 69–71
    anaesthetization, 69
        complications, 77–78
    dental branches, 69
    incisive branch, 69–70
    mental branch, 2–3, 69
    mylohyoid branch, 38
Inferior alveolar veins, 68
Inferior genial tubercle (mental spine), 38
Inferior labial artery, 68
Inferior labial vein, 68
Inferior salivatory nucleus, 70
Inflammation, 171
    influence on gingival crevicular fluid, 239
Inflammatory cells, oral epithelium, 237
Infrahyoid, 41
Infraorbital artery, 68
Infraorbital canal, 70
Infraorbital foramen, 2
Infraorbital nerve, 2, 70–71
    anaesthetization, 69
Infratemporal fossa, 36, 53, 67–68, 70–71
Innervation, 67b, 69–70
    canines, 70
    cheek muscles, 71t
    cutaneous of face, 69, 71
    digastric muscle, 37–38, 71
    facial expression muscles, 38
    floor of mouth, 70–71, 71t
    geniohyoid, 38
    gingiva, 69t
    incisors, 70
    jaw elevator/depressor muscles, 69
    lateral pterygoid, 71
    lips, 69–71, 71t
    masseter, 37, 71
    medial pterygoid, 71
    molars, 69–70
    muscles of mastication, 36, 71
    mylohyoid muscle, 38, 71
    oral cavity
        muscles, 69, 71, 71t
        sensory, 70
    oral mucosa, 70
    palate, 70–71, 71t
        hard, 70
        soft, 39, 70
    parotid gland, 70, 80
    pillars of fauces (oropharyngeal isthmus), 70
    premolars, 69–70
    pterygoids, 37
    pulp, 168, 170–171
    revision summary chart, 264f
    salivary glands, 70–71
    self-assessment
        answers, 75–78
        questions, 73–74
    sublingual gland, 70–71, 80
    submandibular gland, 70–71, 80
    taste buds, 53–54
    teeth, 69–71, 69t
    temporalis, 37, 71
    temporomandibular joint, 11

Innervation (Continued)
 tensor tympani, 71
 tongue, 53, 65, 71, 71t, 104
 uvula, 70
Inositol trisphosphate, 54–55, 81
Insulin-like growth factor, 162, 167, 224
Intercalated duct, 83–85
Interdental col, 238–239
Interdental gingiva, 238–239
Interdental septa, 222
 development, 103–104
Interleukins, 224
Intermaxillary segment, 101
 development, 111
Intermaxillary suture, 2
Intermediate zone, 240
Internal enamel epithelium, 114–117, 144,
 167
 enamel formation, 144
 presecretory stage, 144–145
 secretory stage, 145
 transition stage, 145
 enamel knot, 115
Internal jugular veins, 68
Internal oblique ridge, 2–3
Interneurones, 172
 olfactory bulb, 56
Inter-radicular septa, 222
Intra-alveolar venous networks, 206
Intra-articular disc (meniscus), 10–12,
 16–17, 37
 blood vessels, 12
 cells, 12
 ground substance, 12
Intracellular collagen profiles, 205
Intragemmal cells, 54
Intragemmal nerve fibres, 54
Intramembranous bone, 222
Involucrin, 236–237
Ion channels, 54–55
 salivary ducts, 81–82

Jaw elevator/depressor muscles
 jaw reflexes, 42
 masticatory apparatus, 39–41
 motor innervation, 69
Jaw jerk reflex, 42
Jaw opening reflexes, 42
Jaw reflexes, 42
Jaw unloading reflex, 42
Jaws
 anatomy, 1–9
 development, 101–104
 alveolar bone, 104
 mandible, 102–103
 maxilla, 103–104
 revision summary chart, 252f
Jugulodigastric lymph nodes, 53,
 68–69
Jugulo-omohyoid lymph nodes, 68–69
Junctional epithelium, 238, 118, 147, 238,
 246–247

Kallikrein, 80
Keratin, 236
Keratinized layer (stratum corneum), 236

Keratinocytes, 236
Keratohyaline, 236

Labia See Lips
Labial commissures, 1
Labial, definition, 19t
Labial gingiva
 blood supply, 67–68
 lymphatic drainage, 68
Labial glands, 79, 85
Labiodental consonant sounds, 58
Lactoferrin, 80–81
Lacunae, 195
Lamellar bone, 104, 222
Lamina dura, 222
Lamina limitans, 163
Lamina propria, 235, 237
 filiform papillae, 240
 junctional epithelium, 238
 lining mucosa, 239
 masticatory mucosa, 238
Langerhans cells, 237
Laryngeal inlet, in swallowing, 42–43
Laryngopharyngeal transit time, 43
Laryngopharynx, in swallowing,
 42–43
Larynx
 taste buds, 53
 vocal folds, 58
 voice box function, 58
Lateral pterygoid, 10
 innervation, 71
Lesser palatine foramen, 70
Lesser palatine nerve, 70–71
Lesser petrosal nerve, 70, 80
Levator anguli oris, 38
Levator labii superioris, 38
Levator labii superioris alaeque nasi,
 38
Levator veli palatini, 39
Limbic system, 57
Linea alba, 1
Lingual artery, 52–53, 67–68
 sublingual branch, 38
Lingual, definition, 19t
Lingual follicles, 51–52
Lingual frenum, 2, 51, 53
Lingual gingiva
 blood supply, 67
 lymphatic drainage, 68
Lingual glands, 79, 85
Lingual nerve, 53, 70–71, 80, 104
Lingual septum, 52
Lingual swellings, 104
Lingual tonsils, 51–52, 69, 240
Lingual veins, 51, 53, 68
Lingula, 2–3, 102–103
Linguodental consonant sounds, 58
Linguopalatal consonant sounds, 59
Lining mucosa, 236, 239–240
Lips, 49
 anatomy, 1
 blood supply, 68
 competent/incompetent, 1
 development, 101, 111
 facial expression muscles, 38

Lips (Continued)
 innervation, 69, 71
 muscles, 71t
 sensory of mucosa, 70
 lining mucosa, 239–240
 lymphatic drainage, 68
 masticatory apparatus, 40
 anterior oral seal, 40
 mechanoreceptors, 208
 speech articulation, 58
 thermal sensitivity, 57
 venous drainage, 68
Loricrin, 236
Lubrication, oral cavity, 80–81
Lymphatic drainage, 67b, 68–69
 pulp, 170
 self-assessment
 answers, 75–78
 questions, 73–74
Lymphocytes, 237
Lysozyme, 80–81, 239
 antimicrobial activity, 80–81

Macrophage colony stimulating factor,
 224–225
Macrophages, 206
Major salivary glands, 79
 revision summary chart, 265f
Malocclusions, 25–26
 classification, 25
 Angle's, 25
 incisor relationships, 25–26
 jaw skeletal morphology variation, 25
 malposition of teeth, 25
 malrelationship of dental arches, 25
Mammelons, 19–20
Mandible
 anatomy, 2–3
 development, 102–103
 functional matrices, 103
 postnatal, 103
 secondary cartilages, 103
 muscle attachments, 9t
 processes, 101
 speech articulation, 58
Mandibular canal, 2–3, 67, 69
Mandibular condyle, 10–11, 37, 41
 articular surfaces, 11–12
 of child, 12
 secondary condylar cartilage, 12
 neck, 10–11
Mandibular foramen, 2–3, 67–69
Mandibular (glenoid) fossa, 10–11, 41
 articular surface, 12
Mandibular nerve, 11, 36–38,
 70–71, 77–78
 anterior trunk, 71
 motor fibres, 71
 posterior trunk, 71
 sensory fibres, 71
Mandibular symphysis, 102–103
Marginal ridge, 19t
Masseter, 2–3, 36–37, 41, 79
 blood supply, 37
 innervation, 37, 71
Masseteric nerve, 11

Mast cells, 206
Mastication, 36b, 39–40, 51, 80, 207
  chewing cycle, 40–41
  control, 41–42, 49–50
    pathways, 72
  forces generated between teeth, 41
  jaw movements, 40–41
  muscles *See* Muscles of mastication
  reflex salivary secretion, 83
  reflexes, 42
  relationship to swallowing, 42–43
  revision summary chart, 260f
  self-assessment
    answers, 47–50
    questions, 44–46
  working/non-working side, 40–41
Masticatory apparatus, 40
Masticatory mucosa, 235–236, 238–239
  gingiva, 238
Masticatory-salivary reflex, 83
Mastoid notch, 37
Matrix metalloproteinase-1, 205
Matrix metalloproteinases, 136–137, 164
  bone remodelling, 224
  osteoid, 222–223
Matrix vesicles
  mineralization, 135–136
    bone, 136–137
    mantle dentine, 166
  osteoid, 223
Maxilla
  anatomy, 2
  development, 103–104
  processes, 101–102
Maxillary air sinus, 70–71
Maxillary artery, 11, 37, 67–68
  mylohyoid branch, 38
  palatine branches, 39
Maxillary nerve, 70–71
Maxillary sinus, 2, 70
  air sinus, 2
  blood supply, 67–68
  development, 103–104
  ostium, 2
Maxillary tuberosity, 2, 37, 70
Mechanoreceptors, 41–43, 66
  central pathways, 209–210
  classification, 207
  masticatory-salivary reflex, 83
  periodontal ligament, 206–210
    revision summary chart, 285f
  rapidly adapting, 207
    type I (RAI), 207–208
    type II (RAII), 207–208
  slowly adapting, 207
    type I (SAI), 207
    type II (SAII), 207–208
Meckel's cartilage, 11, 102–103
Medial pterygoid, 2–3
  innervation, 71
Median palatine suture, 2, 102
Median raphe, 38
Meissner corpuscles, 207–208
Melanin, 237
Melanocytes, oral epithelium, 237
Meningeal nerve, 71

Mental artery, 67
Mental canal, 2–3, 69
Mental foramen, 2–3, 68–69
Mental nerve, 69–70
Mental protuberance, 2–3
Mentalis, 38
Menthol, free nerve endings stimulation, 55
Merkel cells, 207
  oral epithelium, 237
Merocrine glands, 79
Mesencephalic nucleus, 72, 209
Mesial, definition, 19t
Metabotropic glutamate receptors, 54–55
Metalloproteinases, 146
MG1 mucins, 81
MG2 mucins, 81
Microvilli, taste buds, 54
Middle superior alveolar artery, 68
Middle superior alveolar nerve, 70–71
Mineral crystal formation, 136
  crystal growth, 136
  nucleation, 136
Mineralization, 135
  bone, 136–137
  cementum, 137–138
  dentine, 140–141, 162–163
    biochemical aspects, 166–167
    interglobular, 166
    mantle, 166–167
    matrix vesicles, 166
    root, 136
  enamel, 137, 145, 147
  heterogenous nucleation, 136
  matrix vesicle-mediated, 135–136
  osteoid, 223
  predentine, 164, 166
  revision summary chart, 274f
  self-assessment
    answers, 140–141
    questions, 139
Minor salivary glands, 79, 239–240
  contribution to whole-mouth saliva, 82
  histology, 85
Mitral cells, 56
Molariform teeth, 18
Molars, 18, 22–24
  angulation/inclination, 24
  deciduous
    mandibular first, 23
    mandibular second, 24
    maxillary first, 23
    maxillary second, 23
    resorption/shedding, 118–119
    roots, 24
  dental notation, 18
  development (odontogenesis), 115
  innervation
    mandibular, 69
    maxillary, 70
  maxillary/mandibular differences,
    22–23
  permanent
    mandibular first, 23
    mandibular second, 23
    mandibular third, 23

Molars (*Continued*)
    maxillary first, 22
    maxillary second, 22
    maxillary third, 22
    third, eruption rates, 119
  revision summary chart, 257f
  root canals, 24
Monosynaptic reflexes, 42
Motor aphasia, 59
Mucins, 93
  salivary, 81–82
    functions, 81
Mucoceles, 92
Mucoperiosteum, 238
Mucous cells, 85
Muscle spindles, 11, 42, 209
Muscles of mastication, 36–38, 41
  chewing cycle, 41
  classification, 41
  innervation, 36, 71
  symmetrical/asymmetrical jaw move-
    ments, 49, 49t
Musculus uvulae, 39
Mutan, 96
Mylohyoid groove, 2–3
Mylohyoid line, 38
Mylohyoid muscle, 2–3, 38, 41, 80
  blood supply, 38
  innervation, 38, 71
Mylohyoid nerve, 48, 38, 71
Myoepithelial cells, 84

N-methyl-D-aspartic acid (NMDA) recep-
  tors, 54–55
Nasal aperture, 2
Nasal cavity, 71
  development, 101–102
  influence on speech
    resonance, 58
Nasal pits, 101
Nasal placode, 101
Nasal processes, 101
Nasal septum, 103–104
  primary, 102
  secondary, 102
Nasmyth's membrane, 94, 147
Nasolabial grooves, 1
Nasolacrimal duct, 101
Naso-optic furrows, 101
Nasopalatine artery, 68
Nasopalatine nerve, 1–2, 70–71
Nasopalatine veins, 68
Nasopharynx, influence on speech reso-
  nance, 58
Nausea-related salivation, 83
Neonatal lines, 19, 143–145,
  164, 168
Nerve growth factor, 171
Neural crest-derived cells, 113–114, 116,
  165
  dental papilla, 168
  melanocytes, 237
  odontoblasts, 169
Neuraminidase, 95
Neuropeptide Y, 171
Neuropeptides, pulp, 171

Nociception, 171
  neurones
    cell bodies, 172
    non-specific, 172
    periodontal ligament fibres,
      206, 210
    second-order, 172
    specific, 172
  neurotransmitters, 172
  revision summary charts, 281f
Nociceptors, 171
  algogenic activation, 171
  mechanical, 171
  polymodal, 171
  temporomandibular joint, 11
  thermal, 171
Non-amelogenin proteins, 137, 146
  enamel, 143
Noradrenaline, 172
Nucleation, 136
  enamel mineralization, 147
  heterogenous, 136–137
Nucleus of the tractus solitarius, 55
Nucleus ventralis posteromedialis, 209

Occipital artery, 37–38
Occipital somites, 104
Occlusal plane curvatures, 24
Occlusal surfaces, 19t, 40
Occlusion, 18b, 40–41
  permanent teeth, 24
  revision summary chart, 258f
  self-assessment
    answers, 33
    questions, 27–32
Octacalcium phosphate, 96, 142
Odontoblast process, 163, 165–166
Odontoblast-like cells, 164, 168
Odontoblasts, 115–117, 135–136, 144–145,
  165, 167
  cell junctions, 169–170
  dental pulp, 169–170
    development, 168
  differentiation, 165–167, 170
  growth factor responses, 170
  matrix vesicles, 166
  organic matrix secretion, 166
Odontoclasts, 118, 196
Odontogenesis See Teeth, development
Odorant membrane receptors, 56
Odorant receptor genes, 56
Odour
  classification, 56
  sensitivity thresholds, 56
Oesophageal sphincters, in swallowing,
  42–43
Oesophageal-salivary reflex, 83
Oesophagus, in swallowing, 42–43
Olfaction, 51b, 55, 66
  influence on behaviour, 57
  odorant membrane receptors, 56
  odour classification, 56
  odour sensitivity thresholds, 56
  self-assessment
    answers, 63–66
    questions, 60–62

Olfactory bulb, 55–56
Olfactory cortex, 56
Olfactory epithelium, 55–56
  odorant membrane receptors, 56
Olfactory nerve, 55–56
Olfactory pathway, 56–57
Olfactory receptors, 55–56, 66
Olfactory tubercle, 56
Olfactory-salivary reflex, 83
Ophthalmic artery, 67
Ophthalmic nerve, 69
Optic placode, 101
Oral cavity
  anatomy, 1–9
  development, 101–102
  innervation of musculature, 69, 71, 71t
  revision summary chart, 251f
  self-assessment
    answers, 7–9
    questions, 4–6
Oral epithelium, 235–237
  basal layer, 236
  gingiva, 238
  granular layer, 236
  keratinized layer, 236
  lining epithelium, 236–237
  masticatory mucosa See Oral mucosa,
    masticatory
  non-keratinocytes, 237, 247–248
  prickle cell layer, 236
  turnover time, 237
Oral mucosa, 235–249
  classification, 235–236
  epithelium, 235–237
  functions, 235
  lamina propria, 235, 237
  layers, 235
  lining, 236–237, 239–240
  masticatory, 235–236, 238–239
  mechanoreceptors, 207–208
  regional variation, 237–240
  revision summary chart, 287f
  self-assessment
    answers, 245–249
    questions, 241–244
  sensory innervation, 69–70
  specialized, 236
  submucosa, 235
  thermal sensitivity, 57
Oral nociceptor-salivary reflexes, 83
Oral seal
  anterior, 40–41
  posterior, 40–41
Oral vestibule, 1
Orbicularis oris, 38, 41
Orbital nerve, 71
Orbital plate, 2
Orbitofrontal cortex, 55–56
Orofacial musculature, 36, 36b
  facial expression, 38
  floor of mouth, 38
  muscles of mastication, 36–38
  revision summary chart, 259f
  self-assessment
    answers, 47–50
    questions, 44–46

Orofacial musculature (Continued)
  soft palate, 39
  tongue See Tongue
Oronasal cavity, 102
Oronasal membranes, 101
Oropharyngeal isthmus See Pillars of the
  fauces
Oropharyngeal membrane, 101
Oropharynx
  influence on speech resonance, 58
  swallowing, 42–43
Osmosis, 239
Ossification
  mandible, 103–104
  maxilla, 103–104
  woven versus lamellar bone, 104
Osteoblasts, 103–104, 135–137,
  221, 223
  bone remodelling, 224
  formation, 225
  periodontal ligament, 205–206
Osteocalcin, 136–137, 221, 223
Osteoclasts, 114, 223–224
  bone remodelling, 224
  formation, 224–225
  periodontal ligament, 205–206
Osteocytes, 104, 223
Osteodentine, 164
Osteoid, 136–137, 222–223
  matrix vesicles, 223
  mineralization, 223
Osteoid seam, 103–104
Osteon (Haversian system), 222
Osteonectin, 136, 162, 167, 195, 221
Osteopontin, 117, 136–137, 162, 167,
  195–196, 221
Osteoprogenitor cells, 225
Osteoprotegerin, 224–225
Otic ganglion, 70–71, 80
Overbite, 25
Overjet, 25
Oxytalan, 203–204

Pacinian corpuscles, 207–208
Pain, 171–173
  definition, 171
  dental, 172–173
  fast, 171
  gate control theory, 172
  neurophysiology, 171–172
  radiation, 172
  referred, 172
  slow, 171
Palatal, definition, 19t
Palatal gingiva
  blood supply, 68
  lymphatic drainage, 68
Palatal glands, 79, 85
Palatal shelves, 102
  elevation, 102, 111–112
  fusion, 102
    midline epithelial seam, 102
Palate
  anatomy, 1–2
  blood supply, 68
  development, 102

Palate (Continued)
  innervation
    muscles, 71t
    sensory, 70–71
  lymphatic drainage, 68
  masticatory apparatus, 40
  oral mucosa, 238
  venous drainage, 68
  See also Hard palate; Soft palate
Palatine aponeurosis, 39
Palatine bone, 2, 37
Palatine process, 2, 103
Palatine raphe, 1–2
Palatine rugae, 1–2
Palatine sutures, 102
Palatine tonsil, 1–2, 69
Palatoglossal fold, 1–2, 52
Palatoglossal glands, 79, 85
Palatoglossus, 1–2, 39, 52–53
Palatopharyngeal arch, 39
Palatopharyngeal fold, 1–2
Palatopharyngeus, 1–2, 39
Papillae
  circumvallate, 51–54, 85, 240
  filiform, 52, 240
  foliate, 52–54, 240
  fungiform, 52–54, 207, 240
  lingual taste buds, 53–54
Paracellular transport, 81
Parathyroid hormone-related protein, 114
Parotid capsule, 79
Parotid duct, 1, 79
  histology, 83
    collecting ducts, 84
    intercalated duct, 84
    striated duct, 84
Parotid gland, 79
  contribution to whole-mouth saliva, 82
  gross anatomy, 79–80
  histology, 84
    myoepithelial cells, 84
    serous cells, 84
  innervation, 80
    secretomotor, 70
  salivary proteins/glycoproteins, 80
Pars caudalis, 72
Pars interpolaris, 72
Pars oralis, 72
Passavant's muscle, 39
Passavant's ridge, 39
Peg-shaped lateral incisor, 20
Pellicle, 81, 94
  bacterial interactions, 95
Peppermint, free nerve endings stimulation, 55
Periamygdaloid cortex, 56
Periaqueductal grey, 172
Perikymata grooves, 143, 145
Perikymata ridges, 143
Periodontal disease, plaque microbial flora, 95
Periodontal ligament, 169, 194, 203, 222
  blood supply, 206
  cells, 205–206
  collagen, 203–204
    turnover rate, 204

Periodontal ligament (Continued)
  development, 116, 210
  epithelial rests, 116
  fetal-like characteristics of connective tissue, 210
  fibres, 203–204
    attachment to root dentine, 117
    principal, 204
  functions, 203
  mechanoreception, 207–210
    central pathways, 209–210
  mechanoreceptors, 207–208
    revision summary chart, 285f
  nerve fibres, 206–207
    autonomic, 206
    sensory, 206
  nociceptors, 206, 210
  non-collagenous matrix (ground substance), 204–205
  oxytalan, 204
  remodelling, 205
  revision summary charts, 283f, 285f
  self-assessment
    answers, 216
    questions, 212–215
  tissue fluid pressure, 204–205
  tooth eruptive mechanism, 120
    role of fibroblasts, 120–121
  tooth mobility studies, 210–211
    experimental, 210–211
    physiological, 210
  tooth support mechanism, 210–211
    adaptive response to mechanical loading, 205
    ultrastructural features, 211t
Periodontal pockets, 97
Periodontium
  blood supply
    mandibular, 67
    maxillary, 67–68
    role in tooth eruption, 121
  venous drainage, 68
Peristalsis, 43
Periventricular grey, 172
Permanent (secondary) dentition, 18
  alignment/occlusion, revision summary chart, 258f
  canines, 21
  chronology of development, 120t
  deciduous dentition comparisons, 19
  dental formulae, 18
  incisors, 19–20
  molars, 22–23
  premolars, 21–22
Peroxidase, 80–81
Peroxisomes, 206
PG1 proteoglycan, 204
pH, oral cavity, 80
Pharyngeal (branchial) arches
  first, 101–102, 104
  fourth, 104
  second, 104
  third, 104
Pharyngeal lymph nodes, 68
Pharyngeal nerve, 71
Pharyngeal plexus, 39, 53, 68

Pharyngeal pouch, first, tooth development, 115
Pharynx, taste buds, 53–54
Philtrum, 1
Phonation, 58
Phonemes, 58
Pillars of the fauces (oropharyngeal isthmus), 1–2, 42, 51–52, 69
  sensory innervation, 70
Piperine, 55
Piriform cortex, 56
Plaque, dental, 94–96
  bacteria
    attachment, 95
    host interactions, 95
  formation mechanisms, 95
  matrix, 95–96
    during diet, 95–96
  microflora composition, 94–95
  mineralization, 96–97
    oral hygiene product inhibition, 97
  polysaccharides
    extracellular, 95–96, 100
    intracellular, 96
  soluble dextrans, 96
Plasma cells, 237
Plexus of Raschkow, 171
Plosive consonant sounds, 59
Polymorphonuclear leukocytes, 237
Polyphosphates, 97
Polysynaptic reflexes, 42
Postcentral gyrus, 209
Posterior auricular artery, 37–38
Posterior nasal spine, 2, 39
Posterior superior alveolar artery, 67–68
Posterior superior alveolar canal, 70
Posterior superior alveolar nerve, 70–71
  anaesthesic block, 70
  dental branch, 70
Posterior superior nasal nerve, 71
Postsynaptic inhibition, 172
Pre-ameloblasts, 144–145
Predentine, 164, 166
  mineralization, 164, 166
  proteoglycans, 166
Premaxilla, 103
Premolars, 18, 21–22
  angulation/inclination, 24
  dental notation, 18
  eruption rates, 119
  innervation, 69–70
  mandibular
    first, 22
    second, 22
  maxillary
    first, 21
    second, 21–22
  revision summary chart, 256f
Presynaptic inhibition, 172
Prickle cell layer (stratum spinosum), 236
Primary dentition See Deciduous dentition
Primary enamel cuticle, 94, 147
Primary epithelial band, 113
Procollagen, 162
Profilaggrin, 236
Proline-rich peptides, 81

Proprioceptors, temporomandibular joint, 11
Prostaglandins, 224
Protease inhibitors, 239
Proteinases, enamel matrix, 146–147
Proteins, salivary, 80–81
Proteodermatan sulphate, 204
Proteoglycans, 11
  bone matrix, 221
  cementum, 118, 195
  dental pulp, 169
  dentine, 162, 166, 180
    mineralization, 136
  osteoid, 136–137, 222
  periodontal ligament, 204, 211
Proteokinetic secretion, 82
Psychic salivary reflexes, 83
Pterygoid fovea, 10, 37
Pterygoid venous plexus, 68, 77
Pterygoids, 37
  blood supply, 37
  innervation, 37
  lateral, 36–37, 41
  medial, 36–37, 41
    accessory, 37
Pterygomandibular raphe, 1, 11, 38
Pterygomaxillary fissure, 70
Pterygopalatine fossa, 67–68, 70–71
Pterygopalatine ganglion, 70–71
PU-1, 225
Pulp, 169
  age-related changes, 173, 193
  blood supply, 170
  cell-free zone, 168
  cell-rich zone, 168
  cells, 169–170
  composition, 169–170
  deciduous/permanent dentition comparison, 19
  development, 168
    innervation, 168
    vascularization, 168
  interstitial tissue fluid pressure, 170
  lymphatic vessels, 170
  morphology, 24
  nerve supply, 170–171
  neuropeptides, 171
  organization, 169–170
  revision summary charts, 280f
  self-assessment
    answers, 189–193
    questions, 186
Pulp chamber, 24, 169
  deciduous dentition, 24
Pulp horns (cornua), 24
  deciduous dentition, 24
Pulp stones, 173
Pyridinoline, 162, 166
Pyrophosphatase, 136
Pyrophosphate, 97

Ramus of mandible, 2–3, 79
  development, 103
RANK/RANKL, 224–225
Ranulas, 92
Raphe nucleus, 172

Reduced enamel epithelium, 94, 118, 147
Referred pain, 172
Remineralization, 80–81
Resonance, 58
Resorbing organ of Tomes, 118
Resorption lacunae See Howship's lacunae
Resorption/shedding of deciduous tooth, 118–119
Respiratory epithelium, maxillary air sinus lining, 2
Resting lines, 224
Rests of Malassez, 206
Reticular formation, 55, 72
Reticulin, 203–204
Retromandibular vein, 68, 79–80
Reversal lines, 224
Revision summary charts, 250
Ridge, 19t
Risorius, 38
Root, 19t
  deciduous/permanent dentition comparison, 19
  dentine mineralization, 136
  dentinogenesis, 167
  development, 103–104, 116, 210
    revision summary chart, 272f
    self-assessment answers, 130–134
    self-assessment questions, 122–129
  predentine, 116–117
Root canals, 24, 169
  deciduous/permanent dentition comparison, 19
Ruffini type endings, 11, 207–208

Saliva, 39–40, 79
  antimicrobial activity, 80–81
  biochemistry, 80, 267f
  composition, 80–81
  electrolytes, 80–82, 96
    modification, 84
  formation, 81–82, 93
    autonomic nervous system regulation, 81–82, 84
    bicarbonate secretion, 82
    primary stage, 81
    protein secretion, 82
    reflex activity, 82–83
    second stage, 81–82
  functions, 79–80
  glycoproteins, 80–81, 93
    bacterial protein interactions, 95
    plaque matrix, 95
  growth factors, 81
  mucins, 81–82
  physiology, 80, 268f
  proteins, 80–81
  reflex secretion
    gustatory-salivary reflex, 82–83
    masticatory-salivary reflex, 83
    oesophageal-salivary reflex, 83
    olfactory-salivary reflex, 83
    oral nociceptor-salivary reflexes, 83
    psychic reflexes, 83
    visual reflexes, 83

Saliva (Continued)
  self-assessment
    answers, 89–93
    questions, 86–88
  taste-related functions, 54
  whole-mouth, 82
    flow rates, 82
Salivary ducts
  histology, 83–84
  modification of acinar cell secretions, 81–82
Salivary enzymes, 80
Salivary gland tumours, 92
Salivary glands, 79
  age-related changes, 85, 92
  biochemistry, 80
  classification, 79
  connective tissue, 84
  gross anatomy, 79–80
  histology, 83–85
  innervation, 69
    secretomotor, 70–71
  masticatory apparatus, 40
  parenchyma, 83
  physiology, 80
  regeneration capacity, 92–93
  revision summary charts, 265f–266f
  self-assessment
    answers, 89–93
    questions, 86–88
  stroma, 83–84
Salty taste, 54–55
  reflex salivary secretion, 82–83
Secondary dentition See Permanent dentition
Self-assessment
  alveolar bone, 226–234
  cementum, 197–202
  craniofacial complex development, 105–112
  dental pulp, 172, 186
  dentine development, 181–182
  dentine structure/composition, 174–180
  enamel
    formation, 155–160
    investing organic layers, 98–100
    structure, 148–154
  gingival crevicular fluid, 241–249
  innervation, 73–78
  lymphatic drainage, 73–78
  mastication, 44–50
  mineralization mechanisms, 139–141
  occlusion, 27–35
  olfaction, 60–66
  oral mucosa, 241–249
  orofacial musculature, 44–50
  periodontal ligament, 212–216
  root development, 122–134
  saliva/salivary glands, 86–88
  speech, 60–66
  swallowing, 44–50
  taste, 60–66
  thermoreception, 60–66
  tongue, 60–66
  tooth
    development, 122–134
    morphology, 27–35
  vasculature, 73–78

Sensory nerve fibres
  gustatory neurones, 55
  periodontal ligament, 206
  terminals in dentine, 163
Serine proteinases, 146
Serotonin, 54, 172
Serous cells, 84
Serous demilunes, 85
Serous glands of von Ebner, 85, 240
Sharpey fibres, 104, 195, 204, 211, 221–224
Sialic acid, 95
Sialoliths, 92
Sialomicroliths, 92
Sinuses, influence on speech resonance, 58
Soft palate, 1–2, 9t
  lymphatic drainage, 68
  muscles, 39
    blood supply, 39
    nerve supply, 39
  role in speech production, 58
  sensory innervation, 70
  taste buds, 53–54, 240
  venous drainage, 68
Soluble dextrans, 96
Somatosensory cortex, mechanoreceptor
    pathways, 209
Sounds classification, 58–59
Sour taste, 54–55
  reflex salivary secretion, 82–83
Specialized oral mucosa, 236, 240
Speech, 51, 51b, 58, 80
  articulation, 58
  cortical centres, 59
  pathways, 59
  phonation, 58
  resonance, 58
  self-assessment, 60–66
  sounds classification, 58–59
Speech chain, 58
Sphenoid bone, 37, 71, 102–103
Sphenomalleolar ligament, 102–103
Sphenomandibular ligament, 11, 102–103
Spheno-occipital synchondrosis, 104
Spinal trigeminal nuclei, 209
Spongy bone See Cancellous bone
Staphne's cavity (cyst), 92
Statherin, 81
Stellate reticulum, 114, 144–145
Stem cells
  bone, 223
  dental pulp, 169
  osteoblast formation, 225
  osteoclast formation, 225
Stomodeum, 101–102
Stratum corneum (keratinized layer), 236
Stratum germinativum (stratum basale), 236
Stratum granulosum (granular layer), 236
Stratum intermedium, 114–115, 144–145
Stratum spinosum (prickle cell layer), 236
Streptococcus mutans, 81, 96
Striated duct, 83–85
Styloglossus, 52
Stylohyoid, 37–38
Stylomandibular ligament, 2–3, 11
Sublingual duct, 80
  histology, 85

Sublingual fold, 2, 80
Sublingual fossa, 80
Sublingual gland, 2, 79
  contribution to whole-mouth saliva, 82
  gross anatomy, 80
  histology, 85
  innervation, 80
    secretomotor, 70–71
  salivary proteins/glycoproteins, 80
Sublingual papilla, 2, 80
Submandibular duct, 2, 80
  histology, 85
Submandibular ganglion, 80
Submandibular gland, 79
  contribution to whole-mouth saliva,
    82
  gross anatomy, 80
  histology, 79–80
    mucous cells, 85
  innervation, 80
    secretomotor, 70–71
  salivary proteins/glycoproteins, 80
Submandibular lymph nodes, 53, 68–69
Submandibular parasympathetic ganglion,
    70–71
Submental lymph nodes, 53, 68–69
Submerged teeth, 119
Submucosa
  floor of mouth, 240
  hard palate, 238
  lining mucosa, 239
  lips, 239–240
Subnucleus caudalis, 172, 209
  nociceptive neurones, 172
Subnucleus interpolaris, 57–58, 209
Subnucleus oralis, 209
Subodontoblastic capillary plexus, 170
Substance P, 171–172, 210
Sulcus See Gingival crevice
Sulcus terminalis, 51–52, 240
Superficial temporal artery, 11, 37, 67
Superior alveolar artery, 206
Superior alveolar nerves, 70
Superior labial artery, 68
Superior labial vein, 68
Superior laryngeal nerve, 104
Superior salivatory nucleus, 70–71
Supporting cusps, 25
Supraorbital vein, 68
Supratrochlear vein, 68
Suspensory ligament, 210
Swallowing, 36b, 39–40, 42, 51, 80, 207
  control, 43, 50
  reflexes, 43
  revision summary chart, 261f
  self-assessment
    answers, 47–50
    questions, 44–46
  stages, 42–43
    oesophageal, 42–43
    oral, 42–43
    pharyngeal, 42–43
Swallowing centre, 43
Sweet taste, 54–55
  reflex salivary secretion, 82–83
Syndecan, 169

Synovial fluid, 11
Synovial membrane, 11–12

Taste, 51, 51b, 53, 65–66
  basic qualities, 54–55
    reflex salivary secretion, 82–83
  innervation, 104
    afferent gustatory neurones, 55
    chorda tympani nerve, 53–54
    glossopharyngeal nerve, 53
  self-assessment
    answers, 63–66
    questions, 60–62
  transduction mechanisms, 54–55
Taste buds, 52–54, 65–66, 236, 240
  epithelial stem cells (basal cells), 54
  innervation, 53–54
  intragemmal cells, 54
  receptor cells, 54
    reflex saliva secretion (gustatory-
      salivary reflex), 82–83
  transduction mechanisms, 54–55, 83
Taste pore, 54
Teeth See Tooth
Temporal bone
  mandibular (glenoid) fossa, 10
  styloid process, 52
Temporal fossa, 36–37
Temporalis, 2–3, 36–37, 41
  blood supply, 37
  innervation, 37, 71
Temporomandibular joint, 2–3, 10, 49
  articular surfaces, 11–12
  blood supply, 11
  gross anatomy, 10
  histology, 11–12
  innervation, 11, 72
  intra-articular disc (meniscus), 37,
    10–12, 16–17
  joint capsule, 10–11
  ligaments, 11
    accessory, 11
  masticatory apparatus, 40–41
  movements, 10
    symmetrical/asymmetrical, 49t
  revision summary chart, 253f
  self-assessment
    answers, 15–17
    questions, 13–14
  synovial membrane, 11–12
Temporomandibular joint disorders,
    16, 37
Temporomandibular (lateral) ligament, 11
Tenascin, 118, 169, 195–196, 222
  periodontal ligament, 205
Tensor tympani, innervation, 71
Tensor veli palatini, 39
  innervation, 71
Thalamus, 55–58, 72, 172, 209
Thermoreception, 51b, 57, 66
  afferent pathway, 55, 57–58
  self-assessment
    answers, 63–66
    questions, 60–62
Thermoreceptors, 57
  cold/warm types, 57

Thyroid cartilage, 39
Thyroid gland, 51–52
    development, 104
Tissue inhibitors of metalloproteinases
    (TIMPs), 205
Tomes process, 143, 145–146
Tongue, 51–66, 2, 236
    blood supply, 53, 68
    development, 102, 104
    dorsal surface, 51–52
        palatal, 240
        pharyngeal, 240
        specialized gustatory mucosa, 240
    innervation, 65, 71t, 104
        sensory, 53, 71, 104
    lymphatic drainage, 53, 68–69
        central vessels, 68–69
        marginal vessels, 68–69
    masticatory apparatus, 40
        pull-back process, 40
        squeeze-back process, 40–41
    mechanoreceptors, 207
    muscles, 52–53, 65
        extrinsic, 52–53
        intrinsic, 52
        nerve supply, 71t, 104
    palatal part, 51–52
    pharyngeal part, 51–52
    revision summary chart, 262f
    self-assessment
        answers, 63–66
        questions, 60–62
    speech articulation, 58–59
    taste buds, 53–54, 240
    thermal sensitivity, 57
    thermoreceptors, 55
    venous drainage, 68
    ventral surface, 51
        lining mucosa, 240
Tongue maps (basic taste-sensitive areas), 55
Tongue-tie, 51
Tonsils, 69
    lingual, 240
    palatine, 1–2
Tooth
    blood supply
        mandibular, 67
        maxillary, 67–68
    development (odontogenesis)
        amelogenesis, 144
        bioactive signalling molecules,
            115–116
        chronology, 119–120, 119t
        early, 113–114
        histogenesis, 115
        initiation, 115–116
        morphogenesis, 115
        presumptive incisor and molar
            regions, 115
        revision summary chart, 271f
        roots, 116
        self-assessment answers, 130–134
        self-assessment questions, 122–129

Tooth (Continued)
    innervation, 69–70, 69t
        mandibular, 71
        maxillary, 71
    lymphatic drainage, 68
    masticatory function, 40
    morphology, 18, 18b
        self-assessment answers, 34
        self-assessment questions, 27–32
        terminology, 19t
    remineralization, 80
    sockets, 222
    submerged, 119
    venous drainage, 68
Tooth eruption, 104, 118, 134, 147, 210
    active, 119
    alveolar bone remodelling, 210
    chronology, 119–120
        deciduous dentition, 119t
        permanent dentition, 120t
    dentogingival junction development, 118
    mechanism, 120–121
        role of periodontal ligament fibro-
            blasts, 120–121
        role of periodontal vasculature, 121
    passive, 119
    rates, 119
    revision summary chart, 273f
Tooth germs, 104, 113–114, 144
    bell stage, 114, 144, 165–166, 168
        early, 114–115
        late, 115
        layers, 144
    bud stage, 114
    cap stage, 114–115, 168
    epithelial-mesenchymal interactions, 115
    mandibular, 102–103
    tooth type specification, 115
Tooth support mechanism
    periodontal ligament, 210–211
    revision summary charts, 284f
Trabeculae, 222
Transcellular transport, 81
Transduction mechanisms, taste, 54–55, 83
Transforming growth factor beta-1, 114,
    162, 167, 170, 224
Transverse palatine suture, 102, 2
Trigeminal ganglion, 170–172, 209
Trigeminal nerve, 69, 71–72
    central connections, 72
    common chemical sense, 55
    nucleus of spinal tract, 72, 172
        pars caudalis, 72
        pars interpolaris, 72
        pars oralis, 72
    ophthalmic division, 69
    See also Mandibular nerve; Maxillary
        nerve
Trigeminal nucleus, 57–58
    motor, 41
    neurones responding to mechanical
        stimulation, 209
Trigeminothalamic tract, 57–58, 72, 172

Tropocollagen, 162, 166, 204
Tubal tonsils, 69
Tubercle, 19t
Tubercle of Carabelli, 22–23
Tuberculum impar, 104
Tubuloacinar glands, 79
Tufted cells, 56
Tuftelin, 137, 143, 146
Tympanic plate, 10

Umami taste, 54–55
    reflex salivary secretion, 82–83
Uvula, 1–2, 39
    sensory innervation, 70

Vagus nerve, 43, 53–54
Valleculae, 40–41
Vascular endothelial growth factor, 162,
    167
Vasoactive intestinal polypeptide, 54, 171,
    210
Vein accompanying the hypoglossal nerve,
    53
Venous drainage, 68
    self-assessment
        answers, 75–78
        questions, 73–74
Vermilion of lip, 1, 236, 239–240
Versican, 118, 136–137, 166, 169, 222
Vestibular fornix, 1
Vestibular lamina, 113
Viscoelastic properties, periodontal liga-
    ment, 210
Visual salivary reflexes, 83
Vocal folds, 58
    swallowing, 43
Volkmann's canals, 222
Von Ebner lines, 164, 168
Vowel sounds, 58

Waldeyer's tonsillar ring, 69, 240
Warm receptors, 57
Warmth sensitivity, 57
Waterbrash phenomenon, 83
Wernicke's aphasia, 59
Wernicke's area, 59
Whitlockite, 96
Wind-up, 172
Woven bone, 104, 222

Xerostomia in older people, 85, 91–92

Zinc salts, 97
Zygomatic arch, 36–37
Zygomatic nerve, 71
Zygomatic process, 2, 10, 36, 103
Zygomaticus major, 38
Zygomaticus minor, 38

Printed in the United States
By Bookmasters